Creative
Teaching Strategies
for the Nurse Educator

3rd Edition

Creative Teaching Strategies for the Nurse Educator

3rd Edition

Judith W. Herrman, RN, PhD, ANEF, FAAN
Consultant, Nurse Tim, Inc.
Professor Emerita/Adjunct Professor
University of Delaware
Newark, Delaware

F.A. DAVIS
Philadelphia

F. A. Davis Company
1915 Arch Street
Philadelphia, PA 19103
www.fadavis.com

Printed in the United States of America

Last digit indicates print number: 10 9 8 7 6 5 4 3 2 1

Publisher: Susan R. Rhyner
Manager of Project and eProject Management: Catherine Carroll
Content Project Manager: Amanda Minutola
Design & Illustration Manager: Carolyn O'Brien

As new scientific information becomes available through basic and clinical research, recommended treatments and drug therapies undergo changes. The author(s) and publisher have done everything possible to make this book accurate, up to date, and in accord with accepted standards at the time of publication. The author(s), editors, and publisher are not responsible for errors or omissions or for consequences from application of the book, and make no warranty, expressed or implied, in regard to the contents of the book. Any practice described in this book should be applied by the reader in accordance with professional standards of care used in regard to the unique circumstances that may apply in each situation. The reader is advised always to check product information (package inserts) for changes and new information regarding dose and contraindications before administering any drug. Caution is especially urged when using new or infrequently ordered drugs.

Library of Congress Cataloging-in-Publication Data

Names: Herrman, Judith W., author.
Title: Creative teaching strategies for the nurse educator / Judith W.
   Herrman.
Description: 3rd edition. | Philadelphia : F.A. Davis Company, [2020] |
   Includes bibliographical references and index.
Identifiers: LCCN 2019019758 (print) | LCCN 2019021778 (ebook) | ISBN
   9781719640305 (ebook) | ISBN 9780803694057 (pbk.)
Subjects: | MESH: Education, Nursing--methods | Teaching
Classification: LCC RT71 (ebook) | LCC RT71 (print) | NLM WY 18 | DDC
   610.73076--dc23
LC record available at https://lccn.loc.gov/2019019758

ACKNOWLEDGMENTS

This third edition finds me at a turning point of my life as a nurse and nurse educator. As I retire—or what I call "rewire"—from the role of full-time instructor (I still teach part-time) to one of consulting around the country, I find that I am truly grateful for the nurses, nurse educators, and nurse administrators who graciously share their insights, creativity, energy, and passion for our craft. I thank them for their ideas, strategies, and enthusiasm as we launch this third edition. I extend my sincere thanks to all at F. A. Davis for their ongoing support and guidance.

Finally, "the wind beneath my wings" is my wonderful family: my husband of many years, my mom who continues to be my guide to the English language, our three sons and their wives, and our seven grandchildren as they continue to inspire, enlighten, and enliven my life. Their devotion provides me the time, space, and imagination to continue to consider creativity as a critical element of nursing education.

— *Judith W. Herrman, RN, PhD, ANEF, FAAN*

CONTENTS

1 The Art of Innovation, 1

"The art of teaching is the art of assisting discovery." —Mark Van Doran

What Is an Innovation?, 1

A Focus on Clinical Judgment and the "Classroom Is Clinical", 2

How Do Innovative Strategies Enhance Learning?, 3

Enjoyment and Inspiration, 3

No Lecture Bashing Here, 4

What Are the Barriers to Innovative Teaching?, 5

Never Enough Time, 5

Out on a Limb, 6

Culture Versus Creativity, 6

What Kind of Instructor Are You?, 7

Assess Your Teaching Style, 7

Identify Your Strengths, 7

The Students' View, 8

How Can You Use This Book?, 9

2 Who Are New Learners?, 13

"Learning is a treasure that will follow its owner everywhere." —Chinese Proverb

Know Your Students, 13

Are Today's Learners Different?, 14

When Were They Young?, 15

Incivility or Just Different?, 19

Would You Enjoy Your Class?, 21

3 Making Nursing Stick: How We Learn, 23

"Smooth seas do not make skillful sailors."—African Proverb

The Brain and Learning, 23

Sensory Learning, 24

Hemisphere Dominance, 25

Making Nursing Stick, 25

4 Getting Started With Icebreakers, 31

"In the first minutes, you set the stage . . . you orchestrate how they talk to each other."—Michele Deck

Ideas, 32

Shapes Define Your Personality, 32

Get in Line, 33

Introduce Each Other, 34

"Why Are You in Nursing?" and Other Mysteries, 36

Let's Discuss, 37

Self-Test: How Creative Are You?, 39

Using Toys, Prizes, and Props, 41

Starting With Games, Puzzles, and Brain Teasers, 45

Common and Different, 46

Using Greeting Cards, Cartoons, and Pictures, 48

Why Are You Here?, 49

Critical Thinking Exercises (CTEs), 51

Dress-Up or Skits, 53

Tell 'Em Once, Tell 'Em Twice, Tell 'Em Again!, 55

Set the Stage, 56

Setting Priorities, 58

Past Experiences With . . ., 60

Be Prepared, 60

My Biggest Challenge, 62

Discussion Starters, 63

5 Strategies for Large Classes, 65

"The mediocre teacher tells. The good teacher explains. The superior teacher demonstrates. The great teacher inspires."—William Arthur Ward

Ideas, 66

Short Clips, 66

Read a Story, 68

Use the Star, 70

Case Studies: Quickie, 71

Preclass Case Studies, 73

Interspersed Case Studies, 74

Continuing Case Studies, 75

Unfolding Case Studies, 78

Reverse Case Studies, 79

Use the Book, 81

Worksheets, 82

All Things Being Equal, 86

When You Think of This, Think of That, 88

Current Events, 89

Bring in the Reinforcements and In-Class Applications, 91

Speak UP, 95

Quotation Pauses, 96

Group Thought, 97

Using Mnemonics, 103

Keep 'Em Awake Quizzes, Quickie Quizzes, Quizzes That Count, 104
Feedback Lecture, 108

6 Strategies for Small Classes, 111

"Implementing creative teaching strategies that will change a classroom from a four-walled room with educational hopes into an environment that is infused with excitement, curiosity, and genuine student learning."—Joseph S. C. Simplicio

Ideas, 112

Six Hats Exercise, 112
In-Basket Exercise, 114
The Right Thing to Do, 117
Gaming, 121
Imagine and Remember When, 125
Twosies, 128
What's the Point? or What's the Big Deal?, 130
Jigsaw, 132
Clinical Decision-Making Exercises, 134
Reality Check, 141
Muddiest Part, 143
In-Class Test Questions, 144
Email Exercises, 148
Group Tests, 153
Web Assignments, 157
Student-Led Seminars, 159
Self-Learning Mini-Modules, 161
Online Discussion Groups, 162
Learning Contracts, 164
Condensed Portfolios, 166

7 Strategies for Clinical Instruction and Orientation, 171

"I take one minute a few times a day to look at my goals and see what I want to learn . . . . I can teach myself what I want to learn more easily by taking one minute to catch myself doing something right. . . . We are at our best when we teach ourselves what we need to learn."—S. Johnson and C. Johnson

Ideas, 172

Scavenger Hunts, 172
Pass the Problem, 175
Cooperative Strategies, 177
Clinical Quick Writes, 180
One-Minute Care Plan, 182
Ah-Ha Journal, 185
Creative Lab Skills, 188

Equipment Conference, 191
Active Reading Conference, 193
Grand Rounds, 195
V-8 Conference, 196
Documentation Case Study, 198
Clinical Questioning, 202
Use the Book in Clinical, 204
Field Trips, 206
Learning From Each Other: Peer Teaching and Peer Team Leadership, 209
Clinical Puzzle, 211
One-Minute Class, 212
Film Clips in Clinical, 213
Let's Be Real in Clinical, 218

8 Strategies for Discussion Groups, 221

"Shared perspectives, shared knowledge, and shared experiences are the key foundational building blocks of creativity."—Joseph S. C. Simplicio

Ideas, 222

In-Class Debate, 222
Teaching Trios, 224
Same Information, 228
Think-Pair-Share, 231
Admit Ticket, 235
Write to Learn, 237
Group Concept Mapping, 240
War Stories and Clinical Anecdotes, 243
Nuts and Bolts, 245
Teaching Tools, 248
Day in the Life of a Client With . . ., 250
Invented Dialogues, 252
Guided Discussion Groups, 255
Out of the Hat, 258
Legal Cheat Sheets, 259
Mock Trials, 260
Learning Carts, 262
Pass the Stick, 264
Put It All Together, 265
FYI—Classroom Questioning, 267

9 Strategies for Teaching Research, 273

"Education is not the filling of a pail, but the lighting of a fire." —William Butler Yeats
"The highest result of education is tolerance."—Helen Keller

Ideas, 274

Market Research—Cookies, Candy, and the Research Process, 274

How Do You Pick Your Shampoo?, 275

Issues in Measurement, 277

Reliability and Validity Darts, 278

Mock Studies, 280

Group Research Critique, 281

Clinical Application of Findings to Case Studies, 282

Research Moments in Every Class, 284

Research Corners—Electronic or Bulletin Board, 285

Film Clips in Nursing Research, 286

Clinical Area Questioning—Research at Work, 287

Paper Towel Ideas, 288

Faculty Research Sharing, 289

Poster Sessions, 289

Research Concept Maps, 290

Campus or Unit Research and Nurse Interviews, 291

In the Know, 293

Bring on the Evidence, 294

Author Guidelines, 296

10 Creative Teaching Strategies to Enhance Clinical Decision Making and Test Taking, 299

"A good teacher can inspire hope, ignite the imagination, and instill the love of learning."—Brad Henry

Strategies to Build Test-Taking Skills, 300

Ideas, 300

Assess Your Own Learning Style, 300

Assessing the Learner, 301

Write Your Own Test Questions, 301

Alternate-Item Practice, 302

Take-Home Quiz on NCSBN Website, 303

Progressive Quizzes, 306

Strategies for The NCLEX® RN and PN Examinations, 307

Management of Care (RN)/Coordinator of Care (PN), 308

Ideas, 308

Case Management Case Studies, 308

Incident Report Exercise, 310

Delegation Exercise, 311

Nurse Practice Act Write to Learn, 312

"Call Bell" Examination Questions, 312

Safety and Infection Control, 314

Ideas, 315

What Not to Do or Find the Error, 315

Health Promotion and Maintenance, 317

Ideas, 317

Basics of Maternity Case Study, 317

End-of-Life Case Studies—Documents to Help, 318

Psychosocial Integrity, 321

Ideas, 321

Psychosocial Case Studies, 321

Reduction of Risk Potential, 324

Ideas, 324

Perioperative Care Case Study, 324

Pharmacology and Parenterals, 326

Ideas, 326

Pharmacology Field Trip, 326

Pharmacology Critical Thinking Exercises, 327

Basic Care and Comfort, 328

Ideas, 329

Pain Continuing Case Study, 329

Physiological Integrity, 329

Ideas, 330

Two Truths and a Lie, 330

What's the Big Deal and How Is It Treated?, 330

NCLEX® Integrated Processes, 331

Ideas to Reinforce QSEN Principles, 333

Patient- and Family-Centered Care, 334

Teamwork and Collaboration, 334

Safety, 335

Quality Improvement (QI), 336

Evidence-Based Practices, 337

Informatics, 338

Conclusion: A Charge to Nurse Educators, 339

11 Creative Evaluation Strategies, 341

"Everything that can be counted does not necessarily count; and everything that counts cannot necessarily be counted."—Albert Einstein

Basics of Evaluation, 342

Formative Evaluation, 342

Summative Evaluation, 342

Assessing Our Students, 343

Classroom Assessment, 343

Ideas, 343

It Starts With the Syllabus, 343

A Word About Examinations, 344

Clinical Assessment, 346

Ideas, 346

Preclinical Case Studies, 346

A Word About Assigning and Grading Written Work, 348

A Word About Clinical Evaluation Tools, 348

End-of-Program Assessment, 350

Ideas, 350

Clinical Preceptorships or Clinical Capstones, 350

Student Self-Assessment, 351

Ideas, 351

Reflective Journaling, 351

Conclusion: Newer Trends In Student Assessment, 352

12 Creative Strategies for Concept-Based Curricula, 355

"Concept-based teaching [demonstrates] the difference between memorizing facts related to the American Revolution and developing and sharing ideas related to the concepts of freedom and independence as a result of studying the Revolution."—H. L Erikson

Ideas, 358

Concepts, 358

Exemplars, 360

Compare and Contrast, 363

Reflection, 365

Clinical Application, 368

Conclusion, 371

13 Creative Strategies for the Flipped Classroom, 373

"Every one of us is both a student and a teacher."—S. Johnson and C. Johnson

Outcomes, 376

Ideas, 379

Preclass Strategies, 379

Class Strategies, 381

After Class Strategies, 386

Conclusion, 389

14 Creative Strategies for Technology and Online and Distance Education, 391

"Teaching Digital Natives proposes that educators focus on verbs (essential skills) and nouns (tools to learn skills). Teachers own the verbs; students own the nouns."—Marc Prensky

Ideas, 394

    Engaging Students in e-Learning to Prepare for Class, 394

    Technology and e-Learning in the Classroom, 396

    Technology and e-Learning in Online and Distance Education, 400

    Technology and e-Learning in the Clinical Area, 404

Conclusion, 408

15 Conclusion, 411

"Teaching was the hardest work I have ever done, and it remains the hardest work I have done to date."—Ann Richards

"My joy in learning is partly that it enables me to teach."—Seneca

General Hints for Using Creative Strategies, 411

    Start Slowly, 411

    More Ideas for Groups, 412

    Set the Rules, 412

    Develop Your Style, 412

Make Learning Fun, 413

Advantages and Disadvantages of Creative Strategies, 413

Finding the "Teaching Fuel", 414

Guidelines for PowerPoint, 414

Evaluate Your Strategies, 416

Some Words about Motivation, 417

Strategy Locator, 419

Index, 425

Chapter 1

The Art of Innovation

WHAT IS AN INNOVATION?

To examine creative teaching strategies clearly, we must define innovation and its relationship to teaching. Innovation in teaching methods is the use of new, different strategies to engage learners. One characteristic of human nature is the desire for novelty—the need for new and different stimuli to attract our attention and thus make something deserving of our learning energy. This is where innovation—the use of nontraditional methods in learning settings—comes in. In essence, an innovation is any educational strategy that is not usually performed by the instructor or that has not been witnessed previously by a class.

"The art of teaching is the art of assisting discovery."—Mark Van Doran

Previously, the literature about nursing students' engagement in learning and the effectiveness of creative, innovative teaching strategies was limited. Research affirming the enhancement of nursing and other students' learning by engaging them in active learning strategies and fostering "deep thinking" is growing.[1,2,3] Chapter 3 will discuss how we learn and how to enhance learning based on current knowledge about the learning process.

Nowhere does the definition of innovation mention the extent or degree of creativity. Therefore, the innovation doesn't have to be major; any deviation, large or small, from custom is considered an innovation. Anything you haven't done before or don't usually do can fall within this category. It's important to remember that any strategy new to the students is considered an innovation, even if it isn't new to you. In addition, the innovation lies not only in the teaching strategy but also in the method that the individual nurse educator uses to present content in the learning environment.

New methods can and should be used to enhance learning for nurses and to educate nursing students. Innovative strategies provide a foundation from which to design classroom activities, assignments, approaches to content, new ways to teach previously taught material, and evaluation methods. New nurse educators may find these creative methods helpful in developing their own teaching style. Instructors who have taught for several years or who have taught the same material several times may appreciate the need for novel, creative, and objective-driven strategies.

A FOCUS ON CLINICAL JUDGMENT AND THE "CLASSROOM IS CLINICAL"

In an effort to enhance public safety and the safety of nursing practice, the National Council of State Boards of Nursing (NCSBN) launched a long-term project focused on ensuring the effective measurement of clinical judgment. NCSBN defines clinical judgment as the outcome of critical thinking and clinical decision making.[4] The model developed to portray the deliberate, rationale process indicates key tasks of clinical judgment, including:

Although this model has fundamental similarities to the nursing process, the clinical judgment model illustrates variables that provide an operable foundation for nursing practice to generate innovative test items that replicate reality in healthcare.

In concert with the work by the NCSBN, considerable attention has been devoted to reconceptualizing the classroom as a component of clinical.[5] Students often see classroom and simulation or laboratory settings as separate from clinical learning. This dichotomous framing of classes as different from the "real world" slows student learning and often may hinder the development of practice-oriented clinical judgment. Bringing concepts of clinical into the classroom and laboratory creates a seamless educational experience and reinforces the realities of nursing practice. Innovative teaching strategies revealed in this book provide methods to bring clinical into your classroom and simulation lab.

HOW DO INNOVATIVE STRATEGIES ENHANCE LEARNING?

Enjoyment and Inspiration

Many nurse educators teach the way they were taught. For some of us, that's a recent experience; for others, it is more remote history. We remember the learning experiences we found most powerful. We retain information that was delivered in a unique, innovative, and enjoyable way. Perhaps most important, we chose to teach because we believe that these positive and negative learning experiences, information gathered throughout our practice, and a desire to "pass it on" are key in the teaching-learning process.

Differences in learning styles warrant new and different ways to interact with students and promote learning. Many nurse educators practice their craft year after year. There's a saying, "Anyone can face a crisis—it's the day-to-day living that wears you out." Teaching on a one-time basis to a crowd of excited learners may require a different level of creativity and innovation than a routine teaching session or a class that teaches less popular material. Creative teaching strategies really earn their merit in the routine situations. Innovations slipped into current teaching methods can provide a diversion and reinforce material that might otherwise be forgotten.

Not only are today's learners different from those of previous generations—so are their expectations of the learning experience. Today's students are consumers with high standards for instructors, sometimes presenting a challenge to even the most accomplished and seasoned instructors. By increasing the level of enjoyment in learning, creative teaching strategies can inspire students to attend class, prepare for class, and maintain vigilance during the session.

No Lecture Bashing Here

I wrote *Creative Teaching Strategies for the Nurse Educator* from a belief that the time-honored method of teaching—the lecture—is effective, efficient, and meets the needs of most learners. Oermann[6] states that lecturing is time efficient, especially with larger classes, and that most nurse educators are comfortable with this technique. According to Oermann, however, lecture is more effective when it is interlaced with active learning experiences that ensure retention and the ability to retrieve information on a long-term basis.[6]

The lecture as a teaching method has come under a lot of fire lately. Many consider it passive, traditionalist, and less in tune with the needs of current learners. Others contend that nursing education literature has taken to "lecture bashing." This book does not lecture-bash. Instead it recommends interspersing creative strategies with tried-and-true lecture methods as a way to enhance active learning. Often educators are charged with assuming new teaching methods that "throw the baby out with the bath water." Instructors are told of great disservices imposed by traditional ways of teaching and are urged to make huge changes in their methods. The nurse educator of today probably doesn't have time to overhaul teaching methods or to update previously taught materials to a radically new method of instruction.

The strategies discussed in this book are presented as short, purposeful innovations meant to complement and reinforce lecture material. Attention spans have changed, students are more stressed, and teaching now uses a variety of media. We must consider innovative methods that break into traditional content yet still allow us to cover material and meet class objectives. In essence, the lecture method presents information effectively; creative strategies provide diversions that reinforce key material or areas of emphasis. These strategies are grounded in the belief that students are more likely to remember content presented in an atmosphere of creative learning and fun.

You can use innovative teaching methods to highlight key points of a class. This method helps to focus the content, allowing students to sort out information and establish priorities. Setting priorities is a challenge in nursing education and practice alike. Using an innovative strategy to highlight selected content helps students to hone in on vital information. These strategies, when applied to priority class objectives, can assist instructors in focusing the exams and evaluation methods. This emphasis on priority information ensures that instructors *and* students recognize and think about the priority information.

Another challenge of nursing school teaching may be summarized in the following statement: "We keep adding content to nursing education and don't take anything out—we just talk faster." This sentence reflects our need to differentiate the "need to know" from the "nice to know" and the "nuts to know." A creative teaching strategy can put the "need to know" label where it needs to go. Review your class objectives and consider the most important parts of your lesson and the "muddiest points." These "muddiest points" are defined as concepts that are unclear or are exceptionally difficult to comprehend even after a teaching session.[7] Creative teaching strategies may be used to assess for "muddiest points" and may provide the means for educators to address and clarify difficult concepts.

WHAT ARE THE BARRIERS TO INNOVATIVE TEACHING?

Now that we've discussed reasons to introduce creative teaching strategies, it is time to address some of the barriers that instructors encounter when attempting to weave creative strategies throughout their material. Barriers to innovative teaching may be time, instructor self-confidence, and resistance in the work environment. These are described in more detail. Others, including adherence to tradition, past educational experiences, the physical setup of the classroom, and personal teaching and communication skills, may also be considered as potential barriers.

Never Enough Time

Years of teaching and presenting this material to nurse educators has distilled the barriers to a few categories. The most formidable perceived barrier is time. It takes time to prepare a strategy: the instructor has to relate it to class material, assemble equipment, and practice a smooth transition so that the strategy will fit naturally into the class. In addition, class time may be limited, and creative strategies leave less time for traditional methods.

Nursing educators feel the need to cover content. We all think, "If I don't say it, they won't learn it, and it will be my fault." Instead, we should be thinking of ways to use valuable classroom time to clarify concepts, reinforce more difficult elements, and synthesize other learning methods. Such methods may include assignments, readings, and hands-on experiences. By changing our mindset about the goals of the classroom, we can better incorporate creative strategies despite limited time.

I say "perceived barrier" because these strategies don't take as much time as you might think. You need time to think of, plan, and prepare each strategy, but once it's developed, it can be adapted for several class contexts. In Chapter 15, we discuss sources of material for developing a toolbox of adaptable creative strategies. We may also borrow strategies from other successful nurse educators and share effective methods with fellow instructors.

Out on a Limb

Another, more subtle barrier is self-confidence. Creative teaching strategies include an element of risk. Instructors may need to step out of their usual role or perhaps convey a different image than usual. Some strategies may "crash and burn" because they do not meet the students' needs, do not work well with a particular group, or fail in some other way.

Don't worry—you can mold creative strategies to your specific teaching style and comfort level. You may need to stretch outside your usual classroom techniques, but you should never feel uncomfortable or awkward. A good rule is that if you feel uncomfortable, the students will, too, negating the value of the teaching strategy. You'll need to prepare in advance and be comfortable with your strategy; it should flow smoothly, fit well with the class objectives, and not interrupt learning.

So this is a key point: you, the instructor, must understand and feel comfortable with the material. You need clinical experience with the content, familiarity with your lecture material, and a clear idea of your learning objectives and teaching goals for the session. The first time you teach a topic, use only one or two creative strategies to make your points—holding back a little will ensure that you deliver the content. As you start covering the same material again and again or in greater depth, you can get more creative with your strategies and feel more confident that the information is getting across. It's especially important to remember that in today's teaching environment, instructors must frequently teach varied topics, may teach outside their own skills or specialty, and be given the opportunity to teach on a repetitive basis.

Culture Versus Creativity

The final barrier may be the teaching culture of the institution. A school or service agency with a traditional culture may not accept new or innovative strategies. The administration may adhere to certain teaching habits or may simply not see the value of creativity in teaching. Some view the change to creative teaching strategies as a "disruptive innovation." Thompson[8] shares the definition of disruptive innovation in terms of past references, including "permanent white water" and "creative destruction." Authors affirm that disruptive innovation is critical to solving critical issues in learning and healthcare.[9] Nursing instructors are finding the impetus to change teaching methods in the best interest of their students and student learning. Individual instructors may need to confront this issue and teach in the way they believe will best serve the students. Teaching cultures are clearly changing. By developing individual teaching styles, instructors can support institutions as they begin to embrace innovation.

Students may reject new methods, preferring passive listening and pre-printed spoon-fed information to active engagement in class preparation, participation, and rigorous studying. This is particularly difficult for new instructors or the lone instructor who implements active learning strategies in a unit more inclined to use traditional methods. As will be noted in Chapter 3, research on deep learning, retention, building a knowledge base, and retrieval (especially important for examinations and National Council Licensure Examination [NCLEX®]) substantiate the impetus for creative and active teaching and learning.

The number of barriers is almost unlimited, but let's focus instead on the reasons you can and should use innovations in your teaching.

WHAT KIND OF INSTRUCTOR ARE YOU?

Assess Your Teaching Style

An important foundation for creative teaching strategies is an honest and accurate assessment of personal teaching style, ability, and knowledge level. Instructors are often hired or delegated to teach because of their ability to speak in public. Although public speaking is an important skill, building a teaching environment that encourages learning requires much more. To make a significant impact, instructors must take a comprehensive, holistic approach. This is where self-assessment and creative teaching strategies enter the picture.

Sometimes self-assessment is as simple as asking yourself, "Why do I teach?" By analyzing your personal attraction to teaching while assessing your strengths and weaknesses, you can begin to explore personal teaching philosophies and styles. Self-assessment can overcome some of the previously mentioned challenges of infusing creativity into the classroom.

Identify Your Strengths

Some factors to assess are previous experiences with teaching, clinical experience with certain populations, and interpersonal skills. Instructors may take on the roles of sage, mentor, information juggler, expert, colleague, and entertainer—nursing instructors often feel like all these characters at different times. The following questions can help you to assess your teaching as well as to set personal goals:

- Are you comfortable enough with the material to deliver it in an understandable manner?
- Do you have enough expertise with the subject matter to provide a personal perspective? If not, can you glean the more subtle aspects from reading, talking with others, or capitalizing on the experience levels of class participants?
- Do you have the talent to create a learning environment in which students feel free to ask questions, clarify material, and consider alternatives?
- Can you use feedback and evaluative information to give students a clear picture of their progress in the class and to help them improve understanding and performance?
- Do you present a positive role model for the profession and for the need for lifelong learning?
- Do you foster cooperation among students, encourage active learning, and communicate high expectations?
- Do you respect divergent learning styles and adapt teaching to meet the needs of various learners in the group?
- Do you organize your presentations, class conduct, and class structure? Although some instructors are more organized than others, new students need structured methods, which give them a foundation on which to learn, organize their thoughts, and pattern concepts so that they make sense.
- Do you feel comfortable presenting material in various settings and with different-sized groups? Can you adapt your teaching methods and styles in these circumstances to provide the greatest benefits for the class?
- Do you have the energy to teach with enthusiasm?

The Students' View

It's also important to consider what each class expects from the instructors. Students indicate that they want their instructors to:

- Be caring and promote personal growth.
- Include creativity and a variety of strategies in their teaching.
- Be willing to learn as well as teach, demonstrate approachability and availability, and foster an interactive environment.

- Maintain instructor-student boundaries.
- Demonstrate respect for others and personal qualities deserving of respect.
- Provide feedback to their students.

These statements provide an acceptable consensus on what students perceive as the qualities needed for instructor success. By assessing how we teach, considering the expectations of our learners, and determining the characteristics of our learners (to be discussed in Chapters 2 and 3), educators may ensure meaningful integration of creative teaching strategies to meet the needs of students effectively.

HOW CAN YOU USE THIS BOOK?

The ultimate goal of *this book* is to increase learning and retention by making teaching more enjoyable and effective. For many of us who teach nursing students or nurses, our goals are to enhance clinical judgment, encourage teamwork, foster a sense of lifelong learning, facilitate problem solving, and stimulate active learning. We hope that meeting our goals increases the number of intelligent, skilled, and high-quality nurses in the workforce.

Whether you use an isolated creative strategy in your teaching repertoire or decide to create a more substantial revision in your teaching style, this book is here to help you. Here are a few suggestions to assist you in using it:

- Use your own creativity and teaching needs to mold the teaching strategies. Your own style and content may dictate adaptation. For example, you may need to change a strategy to fit the room setup. Or, as you "read" your class, you may sense that a strategy as planned will not work with this group. Adapt each strategy as you find necessary.
- Strategies in specific chapters may be transferred to other teaching venues easily. For instance, a strategy discussed in the clinical teaching chapter may be revised for use in a large or small classroom. The strategies in this text were chosen on the basis of their previous success. It's up to you to determine their usefulness elsewhere and modify them as needed.
- To avoid "creativity fatigue," make sure you use creative teaching strategies appropriately and in small doses. Suddenly incorporating 20 strategies in an hour-long class will not only exhaust and frustrate the class, thereby hampering learning, but will also steer

you away from your objectives. Instead, use one or two strategies per class to emphasize key points, provide transition, or break up difficult material.

- Remember that these strategies are designed to be interspersed with your customary teaching styles and methods. They are not intended to replace current methods or to demand a total overhaul of your teaching.

- Staff development educators probably need no reminder that nurses are tired and overworked. Creative strategies that are fun and contribute to a collaborative learning atmosphere will help the students pay attention and remember the material. Generational differences may be even more pronounced in the workplace than in academic settings, increasing your need to attend to a variety of learning styles and customs (see Chapter 2).

   Nurses who work long hours feel pulled from their client-care priorities and demand incentives to pay attention to new concepts. In addition, nurses may perceive educational days in the practice setting as time off. Innovative teaching strategies may help center nurses on class priorities and provide an incentive for learning and application to practice.

- I invented many strategies as the need arose during active teaching of nurses in academic and practice sessions. I experienced other strategies as a student in nursing continuing education classes and derived still others from fellow nurse educators. The importance of sharing for the common good, while giving credit to developers of strategies if they are known, is key to the enhancement of nursing education.

- Most important, have fun with this book. Pick it up and put it down whenever you want to. You may choose to read it cover to cover or peruse it like a reference book to find what you need. If you can create an environment that promotes sharing, mutual respect, and active learning—an atmosphere that establishes rapport with each student—you will have a positive impact on the learning experience of your class.

Enjoy!

References

1. Oermann MH. Evidence-based teaching in nursing: What's new and what's missing. Baltimore, MD: University of Maryland Institute for Nurse Educators' Conference, 2018.

2. Breytenbach C, Ha-Baolyi WT, and Jordan PJ. An integrative literature review of evidence-based teaching strategies for nurse educators. Nursing Education Perspectives, 38(4): 193–197, 2017.

3. Popkess AM and McDaniel A. Are nursing students engaged in learning? A secondary analysis of data. Nursing Education Perspectives, 32(2): 89–94, 2011.

4. National Council of State Boards of Nursing. Measuring the right things: NCSBN's Next Generation NCLEX® endeavors to be beyond the leading edge. In Focus, Winter, 2018.

5. Cole LG, Graves A, and Turner S. Transforming the nursing classroom into a clinical setting. Nursing Education Perspectives, 39(1): 46–47, 2018.

6. Oermann MH. Using active learning in lecture: Best of "both worlds." International Journal of Nursing Education Scholarship 1(1): 1–9, 2004.

7. Aycock M, Sikes ML, and Stevens G. Physician assistant student perceptions of "muddiest point" classroom assessment technique implementation. Journal of Physician Assistant Education, 29(2): 115–117, 2018.

8. Thompson CJ. Disruptive innovation in graduate nursing education. Clinical Nurse Specialist, 30(4): 241, 2016.

9. Stey A, Kanzaria H, and Brock R. How disruptive innovation by business and technology firms could improve population health. Journal of the American Medical Association, 320(10): 973–974, 2018.

Chapter 2

Who Are New Learners?

> *"Learning is a treasure that will follow its owner everywhere."*
> —Chinese Proverb

Traditional methods of teaching are not always effective with today's nursing students or novice nurses. Nursing educators must assess and potentially change the way they teach. Student populations have become more diverse, and public expectations and healthcare demands have changed. Learning about our students may have a great impact on our ability to build effective, meaningful, and innovative strategies.

KNOW YOUR STUDENTS

In a learning situation, responsibility lies on both sides. Both learners and educators must devote some effort to building a learning relationship. Two of the educator's responsibilities are to assess the students and to develop strategies aimed at their individual and collective needs.

Several methods may be used to describe today's learners and their specific learning needs. First, as with any cohort, we must remember that they are a heterogeneous lot, reflecting different ages, cultural backgrounds, contexts, beliefs, and learning styles. Today's nursing students and novice nurses may be more diverse than ever before. In fact, their heterogeneity may create the greatest need for innovative teaching strategies. A participative lecture interspersed with creative strategies, rather than a straight lecture format, may satisfy a greater number of learning styles and needs.

13

Our learners represent the increasing diversity of our world, and our teaching benefits from reflecting on the unique needs of today's learners. This diversity may be characterized by the culture and background of each individual learner. When we think of culture, we often think of race or ethnicity. Additional factors, such as region or locale, religion or spirituality, gender or gender identification, sexual orientation, community/family characteristics or values, learned norms, and age or generation may also be considered. Our discussion will focus on age as it applies to specific learning characteristics of each generation, although I encourage you to reflect on the additional factors listed previously as they inform your teaching.

Are Today's Learners Different?

One characteristic of many present-day learners is the need to have fun, in essence, to be entertained while learning. This is not to say that creative teaching strategies should "dumb down" the lesson or make it less meaningful. However, generations that have been entertained with rapid-fire stimulation may need increased impetus to pay attention to class content, especially if it's delivered in a dry manner. These types of learners benefit from strategies to enhance retention and enjoyment in the classroom.

Conversely, many of today's learners catch on to concepts more quickly than previous generations did, increasing the likelihood that they may lose interest in boring or repetitive material. It is not enough to provide keen insights and experiences to augment material. Today's learners expect the material to be enjoyable and perhaps intriguing.

Other students in the class many learn at a more traditional pace, adding to the challenge for teachers. In fact, as discussed in Chapter 1, students often refute the value of creative teaching strategies, seeming to prefer passive "spoon feeding." Students from different cultures and backgrounds respond to creative strategies in various ways, which may be especially true for students with many conflicting priorities. Those with families, who work extended hours, or who have complex lives often consider class time their sole or most critical dedication to their studies. Instructors often expect material provided in class merely to provide the foundation for further study of material. Creative strategies may provide mechanisms for individual study and provide tangible assignments to ensure that students attend to their own learning responsibilities (see Chapter 3).

Although creative strategies don't guarantee fascination, they may provide diversion and enjoyable breaks in the rhythm of class. Marketers tell us that the television viewer's attention span is approximately 6 minutes or less. This statistic is reflected in the current interval between commercials during television shows, potential for instant accessing of information on the internet, and propensity for scrolling smartphones to find information. Therefore, methods paced to the prevailing attention span of the class may be the most effective in reinforcing material and keeping students attentive.

When Were They Young?

Chester notes that, in identifying and determining teaching applications for generational differences in learners, "The question is not, 'How old are you?', but, 'When were you young?'"[1] Asking students to remember whether their experiences in grade school were dominated by a blackboard or a computer screen may offer insights into their current learning needs. Students who are used to the computer, smartphones, and newer technologies learn at a more rapid pace. This indoctrination causes learners to demand interesting, relevant content. I must also note here that all students learn best, regardless of age, when the content is relevant to their experiences and contexts.

Some recent studies have focused on generational thinking and the impact of generational differences on education, interests, and performance in the workplace. Several newly available resources delineate generations according to common learning characteristics.[2-7] Although you may find several versions of the generational categories, I've summarized them to be useful as we investigate teaching strategies.

Veterans

Traditionalists, Silents, or Veterans, born between 1922 and 1945, are very rarely in our current classrooms, and few instructors represent this cohort. Despite this, and to provide context, Veterans tend to be attentive, respectful, and passive learners. They respond to more traditional lecture methods and are usually motivated to learn and work. Veterans build on previous knowledge, respect wisdom in others, and learn best when respected for their current levels of competence and experience.

This group tends to find creative strategies the most unpleasant. They want to stay in their comfort zone, the lecture format, and their ideals of traditional teacher-student roles. They also may resist group work. In contrast, they tend to follow orders or directives in the classroom. This tendency may result in their cooperation, albeit reluctant, with creative strategies.

As noted, few of our learners are Veterans. In contrast, many of our passive, teacher-focused teaching practices reflect the needs of these few learners or are the relics of tradition. As we explore other age groups, contemplate how the characteristics of each should inform more progressive and learner-focused strategies.

Baby Boomers

Baby Boomers, born between 1946 and 1964—now both a few students and the parents of students—have come to realize their role as a large generation of consumers. They make up a majority of the nursing workforce, nursing faculty, and those in nursing leadership roles. Because of this, Baby Boomer characteristics are often thought of as the "norm," with little respect or tolerance for the diversity of learning or priorities. Nurse leaders encourage Baby Boomers to be more inclusive and have more respectful mindsets in order to embrace new ways of knowing and learning.[7]

Both demanding and accepting, this group may or may not endorse technology, but Baby Boomers have high standards for teaching. Boomers frequently place the responsibility for learning on the quality of the teaching. They tend also to devote considerable effort to learning if they perceive the information to be valid, relevant, and ultimately useful in their future lives or work.

The Baby Boomers learn from experience. They want to be respected for their current levels of experience and learn best with experiential teaching strategies. This group expects some level of sacrifice to be associated with learning. They may oppose other students who may not accept or who may resent personal sacrifice to be part of the learning experience. In contrast, this group of students, as a rule, seeks monetary reward for work and sees level of pay directly commensurate with the quality and the complexity of the task completed.

Generation X

Those born between 1965 and 1980, sometimes known as Generation Xers or Gen Xer's, respond well to creativity in learning and teaching methods. This group finds that the innovations and complexity associated with technology and health are intriguing and represent challenges rather than obstacles. They enjoy learning, but learning needs to be enjoyable. Gen Xer's may not remember life without a television, and they were adolescents during the onset of the computer age.

Individuals in Generation X see education as a necessary step toward another goal, and they work toward achieving a balance between work and play. It is frequently this desire for life balance that elicits conflict with other age groups, where learners may expect that learning and school should work around their personal lives. Other age cohorts may believe instead that those personal elements take a lower priority to nursing or other school obligations. Generation X students may see life balance as a way to attain and maintain health, while Baby Boomers may wonder, "Do they really want to be a nurse?" The potential clash in differing priorities may be apparent here and warrants discussion, negotiation, and a focus on objectives and expectations. Gen X students may see each training and job and/or position as a piece in their career-long skill building, and they may or may not see agency longevity as a priority. However, education is perceived as a means to attaining more fulfilling and rewarding positions in their career trajectory. They seek out feedback but resent being controlled, micromanaged, or stifled in creating new and innovative means to reach goals. Freedom is critical in their educational and professional goals.

Millennials

Millennials, Generation Y, or Generation Why? represent a large proportion of nursing students and nurses just entering the workforce; they often require intensive educational interventions and comprehensive workplace orientations. This group learns at a rapid pace, is comfortable with innovation, and expects learning to have a creative side. Millennials are also referred to as digital natives, and they learn and live at one with technology. They see technology as a tool for learning; compare this to previous generations, who often view technology as a challenge and are often called digital immigrants. One concern for secondary educators about this age group is the diversity of educational backgrounds and the broad range of preparation for the demands of higher education.

This cohort generally embraces group work because of indoctrination in group methods throughout their education. Like others, however, this age group may shy away from group work when the output receives a grade. The implications of group grading in a competitive academic environment often lead students to prefer to work on their own. Instructors often need to reinforce the teamwork that is so vital in the healthcare working environment and create specific rubrics that ensure fair grading practices. This group also benefits from interprofessional education in order to function in the transdisciplinary workforce; they need to understand the roles and responsibilities of other professionals and nonprofessionals in healthcare environments. The insulation of nursing students from roles such as calling healthcare providers, conducting admissions or discharges, or interfacing with the electronic health record may create problems as individuals enter the workforce, indicating fertile ground for innovative education.

Millennials are also known to advocate for their own learning needs and to be vocal about curricula, assignments, and requirements. Although this may be disturbing to other age groups, it is important to consider the question, "Did we get what we asked for?" The subservient, nonassertive nurses and nursing students of the past have been replaced by assertive, outspoken, and personally focused learners who demand quality experiences and who often require some coaching about the learning process and the need for grit in their personal responsibilities and roles in the educational process. On the other hand, this generation is extremely altruistic, dedicated to service, and focused on societal and global issues once their personal basic needs are met. This group, as a cohort, is less money-oriented, less materialistic, and less focused on financial rewards. They also function in the paradigm of high expectations for teaching and are less inclined to dedicate a high level of personal effort without a clear understanding of how it relates to success. With this generation, discussion of active learning, personal effort, and the role of the learner has the most impact.

Millennials may also seek and expect lots of feedback, want positive affirmations, and solicit constructive criticism as means for improvement. This may be in contrast to the Baby Boomers and Gen Xer's' perceptions that "no news is good news." Again, communication and discussion of expectations is critical to ensure that you meet everyone's learning and evaluation needs.

Although an older resource, I encourage readers to seek out "The One Minute Teacher."[8] This component of the *One Minute* series reinforces the need to "teach students to teach themselves" and to set up environments so that "learners have the tools to teach themselves."

Generation Z

Depending on your academic or practice setting, individuals who are in Generation Z may make up a large percentage of your students and will soon join the workforce. This category, also called the Centennials or iGen, includes those born between 2000 and 2016. This is now the largest group of the world's population, having surpassed Baby Boomers as the largest demographic group. Members of Generation Z have never been "disconnected" and generally depend on smartphones for all aspects of their personal, academic, and professional lives. These individuals have been described as digital natives on steroids.

iGen individuals are extremely social, although texting and social media may dominate their modes of communication. This may clash with members of other generations who value the role of interpersonal communication in nursing practice and in the need for age-related interventions to ensure safe and caring nursing practice. This may also warrant policies and education related to confidentiality and privacy. Members of Generation Z do not consult textbooks or research journals. They prefer the internet and learn from videos. Although this is characteristic of Generation Z, this reliance on search engines and video instruction has had an influence on all age groups. The need to assess the quality and validity of these resources is critical in nursing education and practice.

This group of learners is often called experts at multi-tasking, although current controversies exist related to the value of multi-tasking and the potential for superficial learning of many topics instead of deep learning of critical components of practice. Members of Generation Z are socially focused, and their global focus and precarious future infuses their worldview and perceptions of the role of education and personal improvement. Many see education as a way to pave the way to their personal role in the betterment of the world. This cohort may be reigniting the caring and humanistic role of nursing while being informed by a high-technology healthcare world. This age group has high expectations, is willing to work hard, and sees themselves as entrepreneurs in the workforce. They are dedicated and devoted to their causes and seek to better their world.

Incivility or Just Different?

During our discussion of the generations and their priorities and needs, one can quickly recognize the potential for conflict, altercation, and confusion. Communication, clear policies, and mutual respect may provide the foundation for dealing with these issues. To address issues with generations, readers are encouraged to focus on selected components, which are listed in Box 2–1.

Box 2–1.
Components of Generational Teaching

- Knowledge
- Caring
- Perspective and empathy
- Clear expectations
- Engagement

As instructors, our role is to teach learners to teach themselves, pass on the knowledge needed to function, and guide their exploration. Despite differences in learning, our role allows us to ensure that our students have accurate and useful knowledge about their practice. This may also include specialty- and agency-specific knowledge. A wise nurse educator once told me, "You can't critically think about things you don't know yet." Our students deserve current, evidence-based information, when available, to build their knowledge base so that they can develop critical thinking, decision-making, and clinical judgment skills.

It goes without saying that we, as instructors, should exude caring about our students. It has been said that, to develop caring nurses, we must provide caring instruction. Caring includes compassion, consistency, constructive criticism, and competence in interpersonal relations. This definition does not include making excuses, changing standards, or alleviating work. It does mean that we demonstrate caring behaviors to foster professionalism and competence in our craft.

In line with caring is our need to see the perspectives of our students and be empathic as we interact with them. Again, this does not mean that we should lessen expectations, change the rules, or set the bar lower. It does mean that we should understand the perspectives of students, explore their personal issues, and assist them in solving their own conflicts in order to be successful in our academic programs or in their employment. Empathy may be confused with solving the problems of another. In contrast, we need to remember what it was like to feel new, unsure, unaware, and scared, and we need to provide the support and skills to succeed. We must examine our own biases and use perspective and empathy to ensure professionalism in our teaching environments.

Consistency in rules, policies, and guidelines may also assist in addressing generational discord. Clear deadlines and other policies may alleviate confusion, arbitrariness, and feelings of injustice. As learners take on the characteristics of consumers, there is a natural tendency to see themselves as advocates for their rights and personal needs. Although this is an admirable quality, it is paramount to ensure that standards are adhered to for fairness to the group and to ensure high-quality education and competent practitioners.

It is often said that a great way to ensure civility in the classroom is to be a great teacher. Assessing and meeting the learning needs of your students, respecting each student as an individual, and fostering civility in the classroom is largely the product of a skilled classroom manager. Keeping students' attention, adhering to preset policies, and teaching with a love for nursing and a desire to share this love with others contribute a great deal in creating an atmosphere of learning and growth. Using creative teaching strategies, gearing teaching methods to foster student success, and relating to students as you would want to be treated may go a long way in attaining healthy learning communities. Mentoring the next generation of nurses and embracing diversity in learners are critical components of nursing education and practice.

Would You Enjoy Your Class?

How we assess our learners can be distilled to a common concept: respect for the learner. The educator who responds to the needs of students, assesses groups for learning needs and styles, and demonstrates a sincere attitude of caring and a desire to teach will have the greatest success with innovative teaching strategies. You can ask yourself this question to assess your own teaching: "If you had you for a teacher, would you enjoy coming to class?"[1]

References

1. Chester E. Generations. Accessed on December 18, 2018 from https://ericchester.com.
2. Hopkins M and Merilatt J. Bridging the generation gap. ModRN, 56–60, Fall 2006.
3. Shatto B and Erwin K. Teaching millennials and generation Z: Bridging the generational divide. Creative Nursing, 23(1): 24–28, 2017.
4. Pardue KT and Morgan P. Millennials considered: A new generation, new approaches, and implications for nursing education. Nursing Education Perspectives, 29(20): 74–79, 2008.
5. Johnson SA and Romanello ML. Generational diversity: Teaching and learning approaches. Nurse Educator, 30(5): 212–216, 2005.
6. Robinson J, Scollan-Koliopoulos M, and Kamienski M. Generational differences and learning styles preferences in nurses from a large metropolitan medical center. Journal of Nurses in Staff Development, 28 (4): 166–172, 2012.
7. Alexander GR. Building capacity: President's message. Nursing Education Perspectives, 39(4): 199, 2018.
8. Johnson S. The one minute teacher. Willow Morrow Company, 1986.

Chapter 3

Making Nursing Stick: How We Learn

THE BRAIN AND LEARNING

"Smooth seas do not make skillful sailors."—African Proverb

The learning process is so important that I think it deserves its own chapter in this edition of *Creative Teaching Strategies for the Nurse Educator*. Although controversial related to age-old theories about physiology versus social learning, the link between neuroscience and learning lends credence to many of our thoughts on active learning and means to foster learning in the classroom.[1,2] For our purposes, when we talk about the classroom, we refer to the larger learning environment, including the clinic, simulations, the community, the home, or anywhere students interact with information.

Newer research about learning identifies the role of the neurons in being energized by other neurons and transmitting information to subsequent cells for encoding, consolidation, organization, storage, and future retrieval. The brain is described as having neuroplasticity, or the capacity for learning and growth. One of the principles we often refer to in the context of learning is the need for repetition. Termed mental aerobics, repeating phrases or words, interacting with material a few times in different ways, and engaging in learning about material repeatedly are thought to exceed the action potential threshold of a neuron, thus allowing the cell to be energized and to pass the impulse to the next neuron.[3] Although difficult to quantify, engaging in material two to four times has been shown to achieve this action potential threshold in order to form new neuronal connections, pass messages to subsequent parts of the brain for responses, and send messages for organization of memories in the hippocampus and for storage throughout the neocortex of the brain for future retrieval.[1,4] These memories are stored during sleep, reinforcing the need for adequate rest to support learning.[4]

As will be discussed later in this chapter, mindless repetition or chanting is not enough. Learners must interact with information and exert effort for information to be learned. Although mnemonics provide tools for memorizing, deep thinking about information, making connections, and placing information in context are required to incorporate memories into mental models, build new neuronal connections (essentially rewiring the brain), and engage in conscious rumination about concepts.[4] As new information is learned, we force new connections and networks between neurons in our brains. We are challenged to practice, use repetition, and engage in conscious thought in learning.[3,5]

Sensory Learning

Also important are the categories of learning styles: visual, auditory, and kinesthetic.[6] Do your students learn predominantly by sight, hearing, or feeling and touching? Different learning styles warrant different teaching strategies. In the general population, 80 percent of learners are thought to be visual; 10 percent, auditory; and 10 percent, kinesthetic.

Many contend that nurses have a greater propensity toward kinesthetic learning, or learning by feel, demonstration, or manipulation. This idea is no surprise to teachers of psychomotor skills, in which demonstrating, touching, practicing, and proving competency are the most effective ways to achieve mastery. Learners who can identify their style may also discover the study methods that enhance their learning.

Although sensory dominance may assist students in developing study habits, newer research indicates that multisensory learning experiences are actually best for most learners. Engaging strategies that predominantly engage one sense may be effective for some learners, but using a variety of strategies may lead to critical mass. Newer studies indicate that innovative strategies that allow for the greatest sensory stimulation may be the most effective.[3] Several of these strategies engage more than one sense, allowing divergent learners to assimilate information on their own personal level. For example, showing a film clip in class may appeal to both visual and auditory senses, whereas using bargain and novelty stores appropriate to content may stimulate both the kinesthetic and visual senses. In addition, experiences in which learners sustain an emotional response are more likely to be remembered. Students who are asked to remember a time in their lives when they experienced a loss and compare that to the emotional experience of their clients' lives may be able to remember concepts of loss, grief, and bereavement by connecting with personal experiences and thus empathize with their clients.

Hemisphere Dominance

Other authors have recommended analyzing brain dominance in the learner to evaluate learning styles. Left-brain-dominant people are analytical and detail-oriented; right-brain-dominant people are more global and creative in their learning styles. The need to adapt teaching styles to both left- and right-brain-dominant individuals is a key responsibility of teachers. The left-brain learner may be resistant to creative teaching strategies, seeing them as trivial. The right-brain learner may need to focus on objectives to ensure that the teaching strategy is valuable and goal directed rather than merely fun. Assessing your class for a predominant "brain side" may help you create effective, well-received class strategies. Remember, however, that each of us uses both brain hemispheres and that both are essential to learning.

MAKING NURSING STICK

It might be odd to recommend another book while readers are engaged with this one, but I will nonetheless. *Make It Stick*,[4] by Brown, Roediger, and McDaniel, was recommended to me by a colleague and continues to inform how I think of learning, creative teaching, and affecting nursing practice through education. I will synthesize what I consider the key points and apply it to nursing education, but I do think *Make It Stick* should be your next read. Other fields, such as clinical lab stories and podiatry, reinforce the value of these perceptions about student learning.[7,8]

Make It Stick emphasizes the importance of individual responsibility in learning, the mutual roles in the teaching-learning process, and the need to rethink some of our ideas about enhancing learning. The most salient point of learning is that, to be effective, the learner must have self-discipline and devote effort, perseverance, and time to the study process. Learning is stronger when the content matters, when it is relevant to our lives, and when hard work is exerted in the learning process. Learning that is "easy" is not usually retained, leading to our current issue in nursing education where students learn it, spit it out on a test, and then forget it. Unfortunately, human nature dictates that we like to study what we like and what we are good at, often avoiding concepts that are difficult for us to grasp or topics in which we are less interested. We like to take the easy route, the path of least resistance. Researchers contend that we are often very poor judges of what we learn and do not learn. We think we know something when we actually may have just a superficial understanding of the concept. Brown et al.[4] discussed the "curse of knowledge," where we tend to underestimate how long it takes to learn something, and poor performers tend to overestimate their level of knowledge (they don't know what they don't know). Massed practice, which includes reading and rereading the text, going over notes, and intensive study (cramming), are effective for familiarity and immediate recall, but these practices are largely ineffective in long-term retention for later retrieval. Therein lies one difficulty with teaching nursing: students often resist innovative teaching strategies such as flipped classrooms, preparatory work, classroom exercises, or standardized testing. In actuality, these methods, and others, subscribe to new research findings about learning.

Several basic principles noted by Brown and colleagues[4] may assist you in more clearly applying learning principles in your classrooms, clinicals, and labs. See Box 3–1 for more information.

Box 3–1.
Making Nursing Stick: Concepts

- Effort
  - Deep learning
  - Persistence, perseverance, self-discipline
- Retrieval practice
  - Spaced practice
  - Quizzing and testing
  - Compare and contrast
  - Interleaving
- Elaboration
  - Reflection
  - Layering
- Calibration
  - Frequent testing
  - Self-quizzing
- Mindsets
  - Growth
  - Fixed

Source: Adapted from Brown PC, Roediger HL, and McDaniel MA: Make it stick. Cambridge, MA: Belknap Press of Harvard University, 2014.

No one wants to work harder to learn, and as educators, we don't want to make learning more challenging for our students. However, effortful strategies are what enhance learning information and concepts that can be applied in nursing practice. The generation effect, wherein we are receptive to new learning experiences and put work into learning, is found to solidify memories. Strategies that enhance effort include trying to solve a problem before looking it up or being told the answer, working through case studies and other exercises individually or in groups prior to class discussion, and methods that generate deeper thinking and require effort. These strategies are more effective than passive listening, taking notes, and being distracted in class. Including PowerPoint slides with incomplete information, information out of order, or the briefest of outlines ensures that students devote increased effort to learning. Personal experience taught me that, although my intentions were in the right place, students often complained about my slides. Reinforcing the principles of active interaction with the information and effortful learning alleviated, or at least reduced, some of my students' resistance.

Other components of effort include perseverance, self-discipline, and motivation to study. Difficult information that is revisited frequently is remembered and applied to nursing contexts and mental models. Nursing instructors may foster effortful learning by encouraging students to think for themselves and reason through questions. Both in clinical settings and in the classroom, instructors may say, "Why don't you look it up?" "What do you think?" and "What is the highest priority in this situation?"

The concepts of retrieval practice may also be applied to nursing education. First, spacing out practice has been noted to be more effective than squeezing learning into single, long time periods. In this case, revisiting information, whether via spaced-out quizzing and testing, putting away a topic and restudying it later, or delaying the review of an exam a week or two after the exam, allows the learner to recall information, strengthen memories, and reconsolidate learning. Providing feedback and the correct answers is critical, but delaying feedback and allowing students to remember content after a delayed period of time actually increases student learning. Unsuccessful attempts increase learning the correct response and encourage processing.

Spacing out learning interrupts forgetting and strengthens memories. Spaced-out retrieval practice has been noted to increase student retention in programs and increase student attendance while reducing participant test anxiety.[4] Students involved in self-testing, low-stakes quizzing, and other methods of self-assessment often space out their learning naturally, based on time and other constraints. This allows for time delay and the effort associated with effective studying. Counseling students to revisit information, study a little bit each day, review difficult information, and to space out studying ensures more effortful and productive studying.

A current teaching practice is to ask students to compare and contrast newly learned with previously learned information. A common application of this is comparing clients previously cared for in clinical situations with current clients. How does infection look the same and different in clients? How does the care of an 18-month-old infant differ from a 4-year-old child? What manifestations of increased intracranial pressure does one see in adults versus children? How does aging affect the ability to metabolize medications and thereby change the nursing care of adults and older adults? How does one provide deescalation strategies with a client with schizophrenia, and how is that the same and/or different when a client is in the manic phase of bipolar disorder? All of these questions prompt students to build on knowledge and scaffold information to enhance learning.

Interleaving is a concept discussed by Brown et al.[4] that fosters effortful retrieval. By discussing information out of context, out of order, and interspersed with other information, the learner must exert extra energy to sort out, organize, and retain information. Learning feels slow to the learner, but the increased effort, through variation and increasing complexity, ensures that the learner engages in deep thinking and is more apt to retain information. Interleaving may also increase conceptual knowledge, discrimination skills, and the ability to compare and contrast. Students can be told to move from one topic to another to interleave their studying. Instructors may bring up previously learned topics and compare and contrast, encouraging their students to consider previously learned information. This may also assist in learning new information, building on previous concepts, and stretching or adding to memories. Memories come alive, ready to be added to and used to layer mental models. One benefit of concept-based curricula is the inherent interleaving of material and concepts and the building of mental models that is a product of the learning of concepts. Many believe this addresses content saturation by focusing on processing rather than on information overload.

Elaboration refers to the need for learners to express what they have learned in their own words and to connect new information with previously learned information. By making an emotional connection with material, putting the new information into a larger context, layering information, and creating mental models of how different pieces of information are interrelated, learners make memories for future application. Layering knowledge by retrieving information from earlier experiences, connecting with new ones, and rehearsing in different ways reinforces learned information. Reflection on what was learned, rephrasing information, teaching others information or explaining content to others, peer interaction, rehearsing content from a new vantage point, contemplating the true meaning of a concept, or visualizing information from different perspectives may assist students to elaborate. The use of journaling, ah-ha journals, quick writes, write to learn, self-assessments, case studies, and debriefing of simulation learning all may assist in elaboration.

Calibration refers to gauging areas of strength and weakness and studying accordingly. As stated, people tend to study what they like and what they are good at, consciously or subconsciously avoiding areas that are less fun or make them feel inadequate. Newer research indicates that calibration, through frequent testing and quizzing, provides a barometer of success for learners. Self-testing, in-class quizzing, Quizlets, group study with quizzing, standardized testing, collaborative testing, group testing, and self-assessment allow for calibration. These activities may be student- or faculty-led. Both announced and unannounced quizzes allow for student calibration. Performance in simulations with self-assessment and debriefing may also enhance calibration efforts.

The concept of mindsets may further inform our ability to foster success in nursing students.[4] As noted by Williams,[9] variables such as motivation, perseverance, effort, and the ability to stick with the rigors of academics shape learners' ability to learn and to become competent. These variables may be categorized as mindsets. The growth mindset indicates that individuals have ample quantities of these qualities for success, enabling them to meet the challenges of academics. Growth mindset learners can increase their learning based on their focus on personal choice and their desire to meet their learning goals.

In contrast, individuals with fixed mindsets focus on "proving" intelligence to others rather than on "improving" their personal abilities.[9] Fixed mindset learners may resort to memorizing; learning for the next test; and immediate, short-term success rather than deep learning or learning for future application.[9] Those with fixed mindsets may not seek to remediate or improve previous performance, fear failure, and may quit quickly rather than invest in long-term efforts. Fixed mindset learners perceive themselves as helpless when they are unable to meet their performance goals.

Learners with a growth mindset embrace the precepts of effortful and effective learning, and they employ methods such as studying material that is unfamiliar or difficult, interleaving, retrieval practice, and calibration. Those with fixed mindsets adhere to traditional cramming, learning for the moment, and focusing on information they know and are good at rather than seeking out learning experiences that challenge them and may prove difficult. As noted by Williams, a growth mindset may be fostered through awareness, assessment, and support and by sharing the potential successes associated with hard work, stamina, and devotion to learning and future goals.[7] Brown et al.[4] emphasize that educators should provide positive feedback and rewards based on effort dedicated to a project rather than praising innate intelligence to foster learning.

Critical in these new views of learning is the need to pass this information on to our learners. We need to teach students how learning works, teach them how to study, and create effortful learning exercises in the classroom. We need to use frequent testing and quizzing to assist students in calibrating their own level of knowledge, studying areas in which they are weak, and becoming aware of their strengths. This entire process needs to be very transparent rather than keeping any details a secret from learners. As one can imagine, students may resist these concepts because they may be uncomfortable with ambiguity and want expedient and expedited ways of learning. In contrast, creative classroom, clinical, lab, preparation, homework, and study exercises may assist nurses and nursing students to learn more deeply and to make nursing concepts stick. Ultimately this translates to improved clinical judgment, higher NCLEX® pass rates, improved program completion rates, and enhanced patient care and clinical outcomes.

References

1. Ruiter DJ, Marlieke TRV, and Fernandez G. How to achieve synergy between medical education and cognitive neuroscience? An exercise on prior knowledge in understanding. Advances in Health Science Education 17: 225–240, 2012.
2. DeBruin ABH. The potential of neuroscience for health sciences: Toward convergence of evidence and resisting seductive allure. Advances in Health Science Education 21: 983–990, 2016.
3. Wingeier B. What processes are taking part in our brains when we learn new things? Quora, www.forbes.com/sites/quora, 2018.
4. Brown PC, Roediger HL, and McDaniel MA. Make it stick. Belknap Press of Harvard University, 2014.
5. Stevens AP. Learning rewires the brain. Science News, www.sciencenewsforstudents.org, 2018.
6. Wilmes B, Harrington L, Kohler-Evans P, and Sumpter D. Coming to our senses: Incorporating brain research findings into classroom instruction. Education 128 (4): 659–666, 2007.
7. Oja J, Wright S, and Cummins K. Make it stick: Methods for improving student learning. Clinical Laboratory Science 29 (2): 102, 2016.
8. Shapiro J. Learning to learn. Podiatry Management, 69–70, January 2018.
9. Williams CA. Mindsets may matter in nursing education. Nursing Education Perspectives 39 (6): 373–374, 2018.

Chapter 4

Getting Started With Icebreakers

"In the first minutes, you set the stage . . . you orchestrate how they talk to each other."—Michele Deck

Challenges

- Classes in which the students don't know each other may take on an impersonal quality.
- If you don't know the students, they may be more difficult to teach because of the lack of a sense of community and mutual learning.
- If the students don't know you, the class may lack the level of trust required to allow creative teaching strategies to flourish.
- As the instructor, you have the responsibility to set the stage for learning—it's efficient to simply jump in, but you may miss a great opportunity for team building and creating an active learning environment.
- Creative teaching strategies may surprise some learners and therefore may be met with resistance. Breaking the ice at the beginning of class may allow for more comfort with subsequent strategies.
- Participants may enter a class with disparate expectations and motivations for learning.
- Participants may be reluctant to talk within a class. Icebreakers, pairing exercises, and group work provide students with a voice in the learning environment.
- Whether a class is a one-time event or an ongoing experience, students may be less comfortable in a formal learning environment. Effective, entertaining icebreakers may warm them up.
- You may need to be able to anticipate the dynamic of your class to determine their responsiveness to interactive or more personal types of icebreakers.

Using introductions and icebreakers helps set the tone for the class and provides a forum for the creative teaching focus. With these techniques, you can get the class on the right wavelength for innovative teaching and learning methods. These strategies also give you an opportunity to quickly assess the students; you can discover their levels of motivation, backgrounds, objectives for the class, and openness to innovative teaching strategies. Icebreakers may initiate conversation, allowing for future participation and group discussion. Most important, they provide a means for you to build rapport with the class and to ensure that both you and the students are comfortable and ready for learning.

IDEAS

Shapes Define Your Personality

General Description. This strategy displays shapes on an overhead projector, in PowerPoint format, or as regular slides. Participants choose a shape on the basis of selected criteria, and then discussion ensues.

Preparation and Equipment. You'll need a blackboard or PowerPoint setup and writing implements. You may draw the pictures in front of the class or bring them already prepared.

Example of the Strategy at Work. To break the ice, participants are asked to determine which shape matches their nursing style, personality, learning style, or any other personal characteristic (Fig. 4–1). As an additional icebreaker, encourage class members not to pick shapes that resemble their body types. The instructor then explains the psychogeometric interpretations of each shape. Psychogeometric theory, according to Dellinger,[1] states that the following shape choices appear to correlate with certain personality types.

- Squares: Organized, structured, rigid, task-oriented, concrete, no ideas—all "do"
- Circles: People lovers—caring, nurturing, harmonious
- Rectangles: In transition—confused, don't know what to choose
- Triangles: Leaders—make decisions, work well with squares, take charge, delegate, may be ruthless in their leadership styles and management methods
- "Squiggly" line: Creative, relaxed, idea people—little work, few results

Participants should be given the choice about whether or not to divulge their shape in class. The instructor should "read" the class to determine whether this disclosure would encourage group dynamics.

ICEBREAKER EXAMPLE:

Which shape best describes you as a nurse?

Team building . . .

Fig. 4–1. Which shape best describes you as a nurse?

Ideas for Use

- This strategy provides unique insights into the group and into individual personalities, and how each individual relates and contributes to group functioning.
- Simply by knowing the group better, students may become more comfortable and be more ready to participate.
- **Shapes Define Your Personality** may provoke some self-exploration into priorities, thoughts, and abilities.
- This strategy makes a good team-building exercise. After students select their shapes, the class can discuss how the shapes may be used to diagnose group strengths and weaknesses. A group of triangles—all leaders—may have a difficult time reaching consensus. A group of squiggly lines might never produce results, but the group members would be very creative.
- As discussion continues, members can appreciate the valuable role each shape brings to the group process. They can begin to understand that a diversity of talents and ideas is needed to optimize group functioning.
- This strategy is great for building a collegial spirit in a clinical or orientation group.

Get in Line

General Description. This strategy is great for the first day of class or for a one-day class. It's especially useful for classes in which students will be asked to participate actively or to work in groups, or when students appear rooted in their seats and not engaged in the learning process. The strategy is limited to a group of approximately 10 to 20, although larger groups may be divided.

In this exercise, students line up according to age, birth month, number of years in a position or with an agency, or alphabetically by first or last name. The fun in this exercise is that the students are forbidden to talk or write. They must use nonverbal communication, such as lip synching, hand gestures, and facial expressions, to determine the correct order.

Preparation and Equipment. No preparation or equipment is required. The efficacy of this exercise may be limited by the size of the room.

Example of the Strategy at Work. I have used this exercise at the beginning of the semester to get students out of their seats, active, and acquainted with each other. Quiet or nonparticipative students may become more comfortable after having this opportunity to interact with others. Faculty often notice that students who are up and moving are more responsive to new information and creative strategies, further reinforcing the value of active movement in class.

Ideas for Use

- If the class is large enough to divide into several groups, each group may try to finish the task first, adding the element of competition.
- This strategy exemplifies the value of nonverbal communication, the frustration of being unable to talk, and the difficulties of being unable to understand the dominant language spoken in a particular setting.
- The group finishing first may be offered a prize.
- Classes may be asked to develop their own ideas for the order of the line.

Introduce Each Other

General Description. This strategy is just what the title states: the class members pair up, talk for a designated period, and then are asked to **Introduce Each Other** to the class at large. Pairs may be given a discussion topic, such as "What is your name?," "Why are you taking this class?," "What type of nursing do you do (want to do)?," "What's the most significant aspect of your life?," and "What was the most significant event in your life?"

Preparation and Equipment. No equipment or preparation is required. This strategy is most feasible with groups of about 20.

Example of the Strategy at Work. This initiative is most successful if all groups have the chance to **Introduce Each Other,** so you must allow adequate time. The most valuable time to use this exercise is at the beginning of a class session, when group comfort is being established. You can ask the class to **Introduce Each Other** to their neighbors or ask them to get up and move to another part of the room.

Ideas for Use

- The strategy may be limited to an introduction within each pair of students. This version omits the need for students to **Introduce Each Other** to the larger group. It is valuable in larger classes or when the available time is restricted. Some classes prefer this version of the strategy because it's less intrusive.
- Introductions may assist in breaking up cliques or forging new relationships within a class. You can set a ground rule requiring participants to pair up with someone they don't know.
- Use this strategy to combat the after-lunch "sleepies" or with a characteristically nonparticipative class.
- Introduction questions may be tailored to meet specific needs, which can be determined by the objectives of the class. For example, you can ask a class of nurse educators to discuss educational challenges, the most creative strategies used, or the most embarrassing teaching moment. Any of these subjects will inspire discussion. As you use this strategy, you may stumble on questions that are both fun and relevant to your teaching topics.
- A great way to use **Introduce Each Other** is to have students pair up. They stand face-to-face and observe each other for several seconds. Each person then turns around and makes three changes in his or her appearance: removing glasses, changing jewelry or hairstyle, moving clothing around, or altering position in some way. The pair then turns back around, and each tries to identify the changes in the other. This tactic reinforces the observation skills needed in nursing and assessment.
- The **Introduce Each Other** exercise can also stimulate creativity: the pairs of students can repeat it to see how many changes they and their partners can undergo. The pairs then **Introduce Each Other** and discuss the changes. Not only does the strategy focus on assessment and creative problem solving, it gets students up and moving. This version is fun and works well in large classes.

A Brush With Fame

My colleague Michele Deck uses an innovative icebreaker to work with groups of various sizes and compositions. She calls it **A Brush With Fame.**

In this strategy, students pair up and share their experiences of meeting a famous person. Deck has found that this exercise provides just the right balance between personal information and privacy. To illustrate the need for privacy in healthcare, she emphasizes the need to keep professional **Brushes With Fame** confidential, although they can be shared freely in personal life. She tells the amusing story of a class participant who won over the class by going on a double date with a famous rock star. Pairs can share their **Brushes With Fame** and develop a rapport with the whole class by selecting one **Brush With Fame** that's particularly special.

"Why Are You in Nursing?" and Other Mysteries

General Description. As in the previous strategy, class members form groups of two or three and explore a question posed by the instructor. Pairs or trios may or may not be asked to report the results to the group. Questions may be general or may be specific to the class content or objectives. This strategy can facilitate active listening and active learning and can loosen up the class.

Preparation and Equipment. You can print the questions and directions for the activity on a PowerPoint or regular slide, or you may simply ask the question or questions out loud.

Example of the Strategy at Work. I've found that this strategy works best when students are given a focused amount of time (5 minutes) and are asked to list a specific number of items. In the exercise shown in Box 4–1 (which was done at the beginning of a pharmacology course), students are asked to come up with five reasons why nurses need to know pharmacology. Then the group shares their ideas. Rather than accept a list of reasons from the instructor, students become more invested in the topic by contributing their own ideas and discussions.

Box 4–1.
Why Do Nurses Need to Learn Pharmacology?

Why must nurses learn about medications: their actions, their uses, and their nursing implications?
- Think about the question.
- Talk about it with your neighbor.
- What five reasons did you list?
- Share your thoughts with the class.

Ideas for Use

- Consider this strategy any time you plan to teach a list of ideas.
- New nursing students or new graduates may be asked, "Why are you in nursing?," "Why did you pick this agency?," and "Why is it important for nurses to know about _____?"
- For continuing education, you'll need to ask, "Why is it important that nurses know Advanced Cardiac Life Support (ACLS)?," "Why is it important for nurses to know the legal aspects of nursing practice?," or any other question that relates to the class objectives.
- **"Why Are You in Nursing?" and Other Mysteries** can be used at the end of a class to review key concepts, do a mini-evaluation of learning, or set the stage for questions. Students are asked, "How do you think the information in this class will enhance your nursing practice?" and discussion follows.
- This strategy may be done in pairs or trios.
- **"Why Are You in Nursing?" and Other Mysteries** can set the stage for further participation in class, whether the students answer your questions about difficult material or formulate their own questions.
- You can ask the same questions to the entire class without dividing them into small groups. Be aware that only certain people tend to participate in class. Those who don't generally participate are allowed to remain passive during this version of the exercise. The questions do set the stage, however, for later questions that may be put to the class. At that time, you should encourage the quiet students to speak up.

Let's Discuss

General Description. To set students at ease, you may want to begin class with an informal, conversational tone. This will entice learners to listen more attentively. Facial expressions may cue the instructor to the timing of this and other strategies.

Let's Discuss develops rapport among the students by building collegiality. In this method, the instructor stimulates discussion by saying, **"Let's Discuss** your past experiences with _____," **"Let's Discuss** this material: _____," or, **"Let's Discuss** the meaning of _____ in nursing practice." This method tells your students that you appreciate their knowledge levels and their experience. It also allows students to understand that not all experiences are positive, and it may introduce some ways of dealing with negative encounters.

Preparation and Equipment. No preparation or equipment is required for this strategy.

Example of the Strategy at Work. This method has been used many times with a variety of topics. By simply posing a question, you urge students to share their experiences. You might begin an infant resuscitation class with **"Let's Discuss** your previous experiences with neonatal resuscitation." This strategy guides a preliminary discussion of the issue, clarifies what the class knows, and identifies any misconceptions. Other topics have included **"Let's Discuss** your previous experience with diabetes," **"Let's Discuss** your previous experiences with nurses," **"Let's Discuss** your previous experiences with cross-training," **"Let's Discuss** how you were able to learn about a new procedure or piece of equipment," and **"Let's Discuss** your previous experiences with cancer."

A cautionary note: **Let's Discuss** requires students to participate. Your role is to judge the success of the strategy by determining whether you can get students to talk. Part of the value of this strategy is to highlight complex concepts that students don't find particularly interesting or relevant to what they think they should be learning. For example, in a community nursing course, the topic was the value of community assessment. Several community assessment charts and criteria were scanned into PowerPoint and shown to the class. Conversation began with **"Let's Discuss** where you grew up." Students described their neighborhoods and compared them with those they might work in during clinical rotations. In this situation, community assessment was made real through a discussion about communities in which the class had lived, worked, and socialized.

Ideas for Use

- **Let's Discuss** is useful for new or controversial topics.
- Using PowerPoint allows you to scan in portions of text or questions to spur classroom discussion.
- **Let's Discuss** sets the stage for classroom participation so that other group or active learning strategies may be used.
- This strategy may be used following another icebreaker to continue to build group process.
- I've used this strategy to summarize a section of study before going on to other topics. **Let's Discuss** opens the discussion to questions, comments, and free interchange about the topic or material.
- **Let's Discuss** may be used as a segue to other topics, for review after breaks, or to reinforce key points. You can use it in the middle of a class when you sense the need for a break or when you see confusion on the part of the students.
- **Let's Discuss** may be the perfect strategy to use when you sense students puzzling over a **Muddiest Part** or **Muddiest Point.**

- This strategy changes the mood of a class from lecture to discussion. Simply saying **"Let's Discuss . . ."** gives the students license to participate.
- In academic settings, this strategy reinforces test materials, parts of the text to be reviewed, and areas that may be confusing. It helps students realize that they aren't the only ones having difficulty with a tough section.
- In nonacademic settings, **Let's Discuss** allows participants to share their experiences while learning from the experiences of others.

Self-Test: How Creative Are You?

General Description. This strategy is most effective when students arrive at different times—for example, when some are unavoidably late and the rest of the class has already arrived, or when there is a prolonged or staggered registration period. **Self-Test** also helps when the instructor is not quite ready. In this method, a quiz is distributed to the class. The quiz usually doesn't relate to the topic; it's meant to get creative juices flowing. I first encountered **Self-Test** at a scout leader orientation, where it was used to break the ice and demonstrate the flexible and inquisitive mind needed to work with young boys.

Preparation and Equipment. You can copy the quiz out of this text (see below), or you can scan it into PowerPoint. I have found, however, that students take it more seriously when they are working from their own copy.

Example of the Strategy at Work. Here is the quiz; the answers follow.

Creativity Quiz

1. A friend gives you two U.S. coins that equal 55 cents. One of them is not a nickel. What is the other coin?
2. How many species did Moses take on the Ark?
3. Some months have 30 days, some 31. How many have 28?
4. How much dirt is contained in a hole 2 ft by 2 ft by 1 ft?
5. A farmer had 17 sheep. All but nine died. How many does he have left?
6. Each country has its own Independence Day. Do they have the fourth of July in England?
7. Is it legal in California for a man to marry his widow's sister?
8. How far can a dog run into the forest?

9. Two women are playing chess. They played five games and each won an equal number of games. There were no ties. How can this be?

10. An archaeologist found two coins inscribed "46 BC." How old are they now?

11. How many Fs are in this sentence: Fine infants' and children's shoes are the result of decades of scientific research combined with years of experience.

12. A patient has been injured in an automobile accident in which the patient's father was killed. The doctor refuses to operate because the patient is the doctor's son. How can this be?

ANSWERS

1. *A nickel.*
2. *Moses wasn't on the Ark; Noah was.*
3. *All 12 months have 28 days.*
4. *None, it's a hole.*
5. *Nine.*
6. *There is a fourth of July in every country.*
7. *No, he's dead.*
8. *Halfway, then he's running out of the forest.*
9. *They are not playing each other.*
10. *They are bogus, nothing is dated "BC."*
11. *Six lower- and uppercase or one uppercase F.*
12. *The doctor is the mother.*

Ideas for Use

- **Self-Test** can be used any time your goal is not only to break the ice but also to stimulate creativity, inquisitiveness, and team spirit. It has been used in many teaching venues to open a discussion about creativity. Creativity is presented as a habit to be learned and cultivated rather than as an innate or inherited trait.

- To hone test-taking skills, students may take this quiz and then discuss the need to read questions carefully. Invariably, some don't catch Moses versus Noah or some of the other subtle but generally easy questions.

- Froman and Owen[2] used a similar quiz in teaching about innovative methods to teach research. Although an old reference, this resource provides several highly effective icebreakers and exercises to teach research and evidence-based practice (see Chapter 9).

Their quiz, entitled "Logico-perceptual Thinking—A Test for Intelligence," was used as an assessment of validity. The authors administered several creativity questions and then discussed whether the results should be used to determine performance evaluations, pay raises, and other rewards. Subsequent discussions focused on the valid use of the quiz results in those situations, and on the valid use of tools to measure parameters outside their intended scope. The same quiz has been used to stimulate interest in research.

- You can do **Self-Test** in pairs or trios as a way to build team spirit for future exercises.

- When flexibility is discussed, this quiz helps to drive home points such as "You need to be able to think differently." It's valuable in classes about conflict resolution, problem solving, or nursing decision making.

- A colleague* used the strategy to get the group started in a publishing workshop. She presented publishing as a process that requires flexibility and creativity, and asked the class to reframe the task and think about it a little differently. She then gave the following quiz, which the class worked on in pairs or trios. As a result, the students got to know one another and learned to regard publishing as a less formidable task.

1. How do you get a giraffe in the refrigerator?
   You open the door, put the giraffe inside, and close the door.
2. How do you get an elephant in the refrigerator?
   You open the door, take out the giraffe, put in the elephant, and close the door.
3. The Lion King has a party. All the animals come except one. Which animal doesn't go to the Lion King's party?
   The elephant—he's in the refrigerator.
4. A river is known to be full of crocodiles. You need to get to the other side. How do you get across?
   You wade or swim—all the crocodiles are at the Lion King's party.

*This exercise was originally conceived by Dr. Lucille Gambardella, RN.

Using Toys, Prizes, and Props

General Description. This strategy is based on the premise that we learn with toys across our life span. Any physical object that creates a memory can assist with learning. These physical objects can include props, visual cues, prizes, and objects that must be manipulated.

Preparation and Equipment. This strategy takes more preplanning than preparation. If you use props, toys, and/or prizes, they should have a relevant connection to the material. Ensure that the objects provide a visual cue for the class that will be remembered later. If you plan to distribute prizes or props to the entire class, select items that don't cost much, and make sure that you have enough for the entire class. If you use props, make sure they're large enough to be seen by the whole class.

Example of the Strategy at Work. **Using Toys, Prizes, and Props** has many uses. While teaching a class on stress management, I distributed Chinese finger traps from a discount toy store. Each student placed the index finger of each hand into one end of the trap. Then I asked the students to get their fingers out on their own. The students learned that the harder they pulled, the greater the tension on their fingers and the tighter the trap became. If they relaxed and allowed the trap to loosen, it slipped easily off their fingers. Many lessons may be taken from this exercise: the harder we try to deal with stress, the more stress we experience. The more we relax, the easier it is to deal with life's conflicts, and so forth.

Ideas for Use

- Use a sneaker to describe the learning process. In this exercise, students learn to tie their shoes all over again. First, they are given a written description of how to tie a shoe and asked to forget that they know how to do it. They must use only the written guidelines. Then they are shown step-by-step pictures of shoe tying and asked to complete the job. Next, they are given a demonstration of shoe tying.

  Finally, the students learn the children's method: "Make one loop—that's the tree. Make another loop—that's the bunny. The bunny runs around the tree. Now he jumps in a hole under the tree. Now he comes out the other side and quickly runs away." We then discuss how slip-on shoes and Velcro fastenings have removed the challenges sneakers used to present and have created new ones.

  All of these examples provide visual cues about the learning process. They also provide nurses, nursing students, and clients with specific strategies for teaching and learning psychomotor skills.

- I've used a toolbox to teach decision making in nursing. Each tool represents a step in the process. In one demonstration, a hammer stood for psychomotor skills, the pliers for critical thinking, the screwdriver for a knowledge base, and the wrench for organizational skills. We then discussed the vital function of each "tool" and the negative effect on nursing care if a single tool is missing.

You can also show students how the nurse uses each tool to arrive at a decision. Different tools represent assessment, diagnosis and analysis, planning, implementation, and evaluation. Again, each tool, representing each step of the nursing process, is important, but no single tool is more important than the others. For some jobs, tools must be used in a specific order.

- A Koosh Ball may be used to demonstrate how necessity breeds creativity. This toy was invented by a grandfather who enjoyed playing with his grandchildren. His wife frequently scolded them all about playing ball in the house for fear something would be broken. The grandfather's response was to create a ball out of rubber bands. The ball became the Koosh Ball. Not only is it safe for in-house play, but its inventor made millions of dollars. I've used the same story to illustrate concepts such as creative problem solving and personal achievement. I also use it to introduce a subject that may require an open mind, such as a change in agency policy, a difficult topic, or a problem warranting creative solutions or a shift in thinking.

- Give out "learning favors," much like party favors, to help students remember both the class content and the association with the favor when they look at it. Fortune cookies, magic tricks, and other novelties may be aligned with class objectives and encourage later recollection of the material.

- Use a flashlight to describe the nursing process. Let's say that you turn on the flashlight and it doesn't work. At that point you make assessments. You determine whether there are batteries in the flashlight, the bulb is intact, the batteries are in correctly, and the switch is working. You then analyze all the data to develop a diagnosis of the problem. On the basis of your data, you determine that the batteries are dead and you plan to get a new set. You decide that dead batteries are the priority diagnosis and set about intervening, in this case replacing the batteries.

  In the evaluation phase, you discover that the light still doesn't work. You revise the care plan, using the cyclical nature of nursing decision making, and discover that you may have inserted the batteries incorrectly. You plan, then intervene by reinserting the batteries. In your evaluation, when the light shines, you determine that the nursing diagnosis was correct and the problem is resolved.

- Bring a funnel to class. Use the funnel to describe the information coming into a nurse's consciousness. The nurse must churn through all of this information to meet client needs, establish priorities, develop organizational skills, or learn a new specialty.

- Bring stretchy body parts found in the toy aisles of stores to reinforce assessment skills. Students are asked to describe the object using technical assessment terms and to discuss methods of physical examination relative to the type of body part. For example, a finger can be used to assess capillary refill, a foot can be used to assess pedal pulses, or an eye for the red reflex and condition of the cornea and color of the sclera.

- Combine several teaching strategies by using **Starting With Games, Puzzles, and Brain Teasers** in class and providing prizes. Inexpensive trinkets, food products, nursing-related company giveaways, and tokens may be used. One summer, my children spent lots of good times "winning" boardwalk prizes for my students' fall games. Discount stores, toy stores, and magic stores can supply ideas for **Using Toys, Prizes, and Props.** Some mail-order companies gear their products specifically toward this type of market, in which large volumes of inexpensive items may be purchased.

- I've used a blender in class to demonstrate the analytical part of the nursing process, in which all sorts of data must be mixed together to create a homogenized product, the nursing diagnosis. The blender can also denote the brain's role in neurological functioning, the need to mix different types of people in groups, and many other topics. This example illustrates the use of common household items to provide a visual cue.

- Show healthcare equipment and let the students pass it around the room. This visual cue helps students to learn and understand difficult new equipment.

- Candy, gum, sugar-free products, and healthy snacks may be used. Food is always a welcome diversion.

- In teaching about conflict management and assertiveness, one colleague brings an assorted collection of stuffed and plastic sharks to class. She describes each to the class, emphasizing the characteristics and methods of dealing with well-dressed sharks, sharks in sheep's clothing, big sharks, little sharks, sharks with no teeth, and human-eating sharks. She passes out the sharks to the class and asks participants how they would react to and manage such a shark in their personal work environment.

- Bubbles are a common birthday party and wedding favor and may be purchased inexpensively at party stores. You need to connect the bubbles with class objectives: enhanced ventilation, celebration of a newly learned skill, or a creative teaching method. Then have the students blow the bubbles to provide a memory cue. You can also ask students to come up with their own associations—as long as the bubbles stay linked to course objectives or content.

- You can use bells and whistles to "reel in" the class after spirited group activities. You also can distribute them as visual cues; for example, whistles are effective in replicating breathing exercises. The bell or whistle may also be an auditory cue that you are moving to the next topic or section.
- A colleague* brings a "Hot Potato" to class. This marketed toy is passed around until a buzzer goes off. The instructor poses a question and whoever has the potato when it buzzes needs to answer it. This strategy really wakes up the class!

*Karin Sherrill is the owner and user of this strategy.

Starting With Games, Puzzles, and Brain Teasers

General Description. When students come to class, they see a puzzle, game, or brain teaser on the overhead or PowerPoint screen (see Boxes 4–2 and 4–3). This strategy is especially valuable for large classes, when lots of discussion and participation may become unwieldy. It provides an activity for early arrivals or students who don't know one another. Instructors can also pass out puzzles or games to get student thinking started.

Preparation and Equipment. You just need to find the brain teasers and have them available for the class, whether in audiovisual form or on paper.

Example of the Strategy at Work. Boxes 4–2 and 4–3 show only two of many possible brain teasers.

Box 4–2.
Brain Teaser

To Start You Thinking

1. A client is to receive 500 mg of ampicillin. It is diluted in 75 mL of normal saline solution and is to run for 45 minutes. The drop factor is 15 gtt/mL. What is the rate of the IV?
   (Answer: 25 gtt/min)
2. A client is to receive 0.5 mg of naloxone, available in a 400-mcg/mL solution. What is the dose?
   (Answer: 1.25 mL)
3. A client is to receive 500 mg of phenytoin, available in a 75-mg/mL solution. How many milliliters should she or he receive?
   (Answer: 6.6 mL)

Box 4–3.
Brain Teaser

To Keep You Thinking

A client is to receive lidocaine at a rate of 2 mg/min. A 250-mL bottle of D_5W contains 1 gm of lidocaine. The IV set is labeled "Microdrip." At what rate should the nurse set the IV?

$1000 \div 250 = 4$ mg/mL
2 mg $\div 4 \times 1 = 0.5$ mg/min

Answer: 60 × 0.5 = 30 gtt/min

Ideas for Use

- Obviously, the examples shown in the boxes have been used for pharmacology calculations. They can be used, however, for any material that has complex concepts or a **Muddiest Part.**
- Email the questions or brain teasers to the students. Ask them to bring the answers to the next class. You can also ask the students to answer you orally. Give prizes in front of the class to the ones who answer correctly. You can combine this strategy with **Admit Ticket.**
- Send the **Brain Teasers** in the confirmation letter or in the registration materials. Use them to stimulate interest in a topic and discuss the answers in class as an icebreaker.
- Post the **Brain Teaser** to the class or to the organization's Web page. Provide prizes for those who enter the class with the right answer.
- Post answers to the class website or on a common class bulletin board.
- Include a **Brain Teaser** used in class as an extra credit option on an examination. This rewards class attendance, punctuality, and memory for the answer.
- If you include really difficult **Brain Teasers,** current class topics may not seem so formidable.
- Critical thinking texts provide puzzles and **Brain Teasers** relevant to nursing that may be adapted for any class content.

Common and Different

General Description. This may be one of my favorite icebreakers. It's valuable for students who don't know each other. Students are asked to form pairs or trios. Remind them not to select people they already know. They talk within their groups for a short time, perhaps 5 minutes. In that time, they must think of four similarities and four characteristics unique to each group member. Invariably, gender, occupation, marital status, and parenting experience are mentioned.

Thinking of eight characteristics requires students to delve somewhat into each other's lives. The most rewarding aspect of this method is that the students who do this exercise together become bonded for the duration of the class. Thus, collegiality increases among students who have not previously worked together. Be aware that some students won't participate in this (or any other) icebreaker. This one is less threatening, however, and appears to engage students more intensely than other strategies.

Preparation and Equipment. One of the greatest assets of this strategy is how much reward it produces with little effort. The only preparation you need is memory; just remember to introduce the strategy at the beginning of class. You can also prepare a screen with instructions that stimulate action and cut down on your need to give directions.

Example of the Strategy at Work. Box 4–4 shows one version of the slide I use for this exercise.

Ideas for Use

- Use **Common and Different** for nursing clinical groups or orientation groups. It's effective in creating team spirit, especially when small numbers of participants know each other and others may feel left out.
- This exercise may be done in pairs, trios, or larger groups.
- You can alter the number—it doesn't have to be four—to fit the class time frame and objectives.
- **Common and Different** may be used to open meetings. Even people who have worked together may discover some interesting new facts when they reach out to discover each other's common points and differences.

Box 4–4.
Common and Different

- Talk to your neighbor on the left.
- Find four things you have in common.
- Find four differences between you.

What's harder—finding common ground or finding differences? Now you know each other!

- You can stimulate discussion after the exercise by asking the group, "Which was harder, finding commonalities or finding differences?" The answers may provide insight into the group process and composition.
- **Common and Different** may also generate discussion about differences and similarities, transferring to cultural, professional, ethical, or controversial topics.
- A variation of this strategy from the literature uses confirming communication to set the stage for intensive care simulations and standardized patients.[3] Students and standardized patients engage in personal discussions before and after the simulation and examine commonalities and differences in their perceptions of the experience. Students found that these communications reinforced their roles and explored the empathic elements of caring for clients in critical-care situations.

Using Greeting Cards, Cartoons, and Pictures

General Description. This approach has been readily embraced by nurse educators. If you use it, you must be always on the lookout for greeting cards, cartoons, pictures, appropriate jokes or stories, and other material to open the class with a smile. The Internet has opened up a whole new world of email jokes, interesting pictures, and other material. You can also search through calendars, newspapers, and magazines. The material should be amusing, relevant to the class content, and culturally and politically correct for general classroom use.

Preparation and Equipment. Materials may be scanned into PowerPoint files. This strategy requires you to consider the fair use of copyrighted materials. Although attorneys provide varying opinions in their counsel on fair use, most stipulate that such materials can be used for educational purposes if you follow certain guidelines. You may not sell admission to a class solely on the basis of another's creative work, and you may not sell a copy of any written document that contains copyrighted material unless you have written permission. This means that PowerPoint slides or handouts should not include copies of such material or scans of cards, photos, or cartoons. Credit should always be given when it's appropriate.

Example of the Strategy at Work. I have used this strategy as an opening tactic. When students see slides with comics, pictures, or jokes on the screen, they feel welcomed and a friendly tone is set for the class. Here is one I have used, and it was met with lots of laughter:

> A frog goes into a bank and approaches the teller. He can see from her nameplate that her name is Patricia Whack. "Miss Whack, I'd

like to get a $30,000 loan to take a holiday." Patty looks at the frog in disbelief and asks his name. The frog says his name is Kermit Jagger; his dad is Mick Jagger; and that it's okay, he knows the bank manager. Patty explains that he will need to secure the loan with some collateral. The frog says, "Sure, I have this," and produces a tiny porcelain elephant, about an inch tall, bright pink, and perfectly formed. Very confused, Patty explains that she'll have to consult with the bank manager and disappears into a back office.

She finds the manager and says, "There's a frog called Kermit Jagger out there who claims to know you and wants to borrow $30,000, and he wants to use this as collateral." She holds up the tiny pink elephant. "I mean, what in the world is this?" The bank manager looks back at her and says, "It's a knickknack, Patty Whack. Give the frog a loan. His old man's a Rolling Stone!"

Ideas for Use

- You can show greeting cards, cartoons, and pictures in the middle of lecture content to break up sections of material or as a transition to the next topic.

- Personal photos may be used with some content. Photos of others should always have a record of consent to use them for educational purposes.

- Again, the use of these materials requires the utmost in educator discretion. The strategy is effective in stimulating interest, but it should not insult students or make them uncomfortable. You must use care with jokes and cartoons that use colorful language or innuendo, and you must keep in mind the purpose of the strategy. Discretion must also be exercised with fair use parameters.

- Frequent use of pictures from clip art, the Web, and scanning provides visual cues for learners. When creating handouts for class, make sure that you delete all pictures. This is important for legal reasons and also to decrease the time it takes to download handouts from the Web.

Why Are You Here?

General Description. This strategy explains itself, you simply ask, **"Why Are You Here?"** before the start of a class session. You're trying to determine the students' goals for the class and examine their internal versus their external motivations for participating. You then can use this information with the class.

Box 4–5.
Why Are You Here?

- My boss told me to come.
- What choice did I have?
- A good nurse needs to know this.
- I'm trying to get to the next step in my career.

This strategy sets clear boundaries, ensuring that expectations are in line with planned teaching topics or content. You may be able to gear class objectives toward student needs or provide creative teaching strategies for less-motivated students. By determining the motivation level, you can employ creative teaching strategies to enhance internal motivation.

Preparation and Equipment. No preparation is involved. All you have to do is remind yourself to ask the question at the beginning of class.

Example of the Strategy at Work. I frequently use this strategy to open a semester or class. I show the sentence **Why Are You Here?** and solicit group responses (see Box 4–5). The answers are sometimes amusing—for example, "Because my manager told me to come," "Because I have to," or "It's required." We then discuss what people want to learn from the class, how they want to be different at the end of it, or why they need the class to improve their current or future job performance. Some students have a sincere desire to attend the class and will answer, "Because nurses need to know this," or "I need to know this to go on in my career."

By collecting student responses, I am more able to assess the needs and abilities of the group. I then introduce class topics, class objectives, or both. This information allows all of us to determine whether the class will meet the students' needs and gives me the opportunity to change gears or clarify class objectives. It also reinforces what the class will include after a discussion of **Why Are You Here?**

Ideas for Use

- Use a flip chart to write down student responses. Go back to the flip chart at the end of class to determine whether most of the topics were addressed. You may want to briefly address topics that were missed.
- Some classes—for example, "the mandatories"—suffer from low levels of student motivation. **Why Are You Here?** gives you an opportunity to spur interest by using creative strategies, instilling

motivation through stories and exercises, and discussing the reasons these courses are required.

- This strategy is effective in opening up classroom dialogue and getting students primed for later class participation.
- You can answer the question yourself, disclosing your love of teaching, your belief in the importance of the material, and your personal motivation to provide high-quality instruction.

Critical Thinking Exercises (CTEs)

General Description. **Critical Thinking Exercises** are a great way to get the thinking juices flowing. Used early in the class, they encourage participation and ground the students in the class content. You can base them on class material or include them in the syllabus or in preparatory reading. This method encourages students to learn something about the topic before class, peruse the readings, and think about content before the class begins.

One frustration that students and novice nurses often encounter is the difficulty of setting priorities and "thinking like a nurse." Use of CTEs that pinpoint these priorities allows participants to determine what is integral to a problem. **Critical Thinking Exercises** in every class allow students to routinely practice internalizing and applying new concepts.

Use of **Critical Thinking Exercises** allows students to:

- Recall information.
- Get in the critical thinking habit.
- Spend pre-class time thinking about content.
- Put a new twist on known concepts.
- Reflect on content after class.

Students can also assess their own learning before the rude awakening of an examination.

Preparation and Equipment. **Critical Thinking Exercises** can be introduced spontaneously or planned in advance. Questions such as "What role does the nurse have in caring for this client?," "What is the highest priority for the nurse and client?," and "How would the nurse cope with this situation?" allow students to see the "realness" of content and begin problem solving.

Example of the Strategy at Work. For each nursing class, I provide four to six CTEs (see Box 4–6). I make sure that these exercises, whether used to introduce or reinforce a topic, are well represented in the class objectives and on the evaluation material. I also make sure that my CTEs relate to test questions for academic classes. For continuing education classes,

Box 4–6.
Critical Thinking Exercises

- A client receives a new diagnosis of diabetes mellitus (DM). The client doesn't need much insulin at this point. Why not?
- A client tells you her blood glucose levels are always within normal limits. She also tells you she only takes her insulin every other day to save money. What can you do to determine her past blood glucose values?
- Why are some organs more prone than others to hyperglycemic changes?
- What societal trends have influenced the increase in DM in the United States? What is the role of nursing in this issue?

CTEs presented at the beginning of class help the students gain interest and give them a preview of the topics to be discussed.

Ideas for Use

- You may want to use this strategy at both the beginning and the end of class so you can evaluate learning and provide closure.
- I use the term **Critical Thinking Exercises (CTEs).** You may want to come up with another term, such as *Medical–Surgical Thinking Exercises,* to add interest and individuality for specific courses.
- These exercises may be adapted for email use. You can make them sound friendly by calling them **Email Exercises.** These exercises may be uploaded into your learning management system (LMS) and submitted and graded via the assignment or other appropriate function in the LMS.
- **Critical Thinking Exercises** encourage class attendance, especially when the topics lead to test questions. They also provide students with ready cues to use as study guides.
- Sometimes questions posed as **Critical Thinking Exercises** may be more user friendly than objectives, which students may find formidable.
- For continuing education programs, include **Critical Thinking Exercises** in class brochures, registration letters, or class advertisements and brochures. Well-articulated CTEs entice students.
- In an academic setting, you may want to design **Critical Thinking Exercises** after examination questions, base

examination questions on CTEs, or both. Either way, examination questions and CTEs should reflect key concepts and learning priorities.

- These representative examples may be used as **Critical Thinking Exercises** and to provide the foundation for examination questions:
  - You make a medication error as a nursing student. Who is accountable?
  - Why does helping a client sit up ease respirations?
  - How do the signs of end organ perfusion differ in hypovolemic shock and in septic shock?
  - How can you assess the mental status changes in a client with hepatic encephalopathy?
  - What are the classic signs of hypoglycemia? Compare them with the classic signs of hyperglycemia.
  - A client is in congestive heart failure. What medications or classes of medications would you anticipate to be part of her or his care?
  - How do you assess pain in a nonverbal client?

Dress-Up or Skits

General Description. At the beginning of class, the instructor dresses up or organizes a skit to provide relevant content or to introduce the class. These costumes or skits may be simple or elaborate and are focused on class objectives.

Preparation and Equipment. This strategy takes a lot of self-esteem and some preparation. Keep class objectives in mind so the costumes or props enhance learning and retention. You can find dress-up materials by shopping in costume and thrift stores and by raiding the closets of your friends and family.

Example of the Strategy at Work. I have steered toward the simpler aspects of this strategy. I've worn some unlikely articles to help a class loosen up and focus on topics: a clown nose for a discussion of how humor is addressed in nursing theories, a boardwalk T-shirt with an antistress message for a class on nursing and stress, and a jester's hat to introduce nursing communication principles.

One group of students designed a class fund-raiser with a sweatshirt showing "nursing diagnoses" (Fig. 4–2). I wore the sweatshirt to class and showed it as a slide to introduce the class to nursing diagnosis and analysis. Beginning nursing students have trouble embracing this rather dry concept, but the sweatshirt made it seem real and useful to their

READ MY SHIRT:

Alteration in Mental Status
Related to Nursing School AEB...

Weight Gain × 30 LBS.

Increased dementia

Alternating constipation
with diarrhea

Sleep deprivation,
2h q night x 10 weeks

Social isolation

Junk food dependency

Instructor phobia

Stooped posture
(heavy book syndrome)

Empty pocket syndrome

Problem?   Etiology?
Identifying characteristics?

Fig. 4–2.   Read my shirt: Alteration in mental status related to nursing school.

nursing careers. The strategy worked especially well because more senior students in the program had designed the shirt.

Ideas for Use

- A colleague arrived in class dressed in camouflage to represent the immune function of the T-cells and their responses to immunosuppression. This same faculty member used a superhero theme for the graduation address, wearing a belt, helmet, and other insignia borrowed from her preschool son to depict a "Supernurse."

- A well-known nursing speaker has been known to arrive at classes dressed as Mother Goose, a good fairy, and a nurse from ages past. Dressing up as part of the class theme truly does break the ice; it also enhances retention of the material.

- Amusing hats, perioperative garb, historical costumes, scrubs, old uniforms, or any other odd clothing relaxes participants and helps you to teach serious material whimsically.

- Again, **Dress-Up or Skits** can be as elaborate or as simple as you choose. The idea is to provide a visual reminder of the material—an image that novice nurses, students, or even experienced nurses can summon up to remind them of a topic.

- In addition to costumes and props, a script or skit helps with retention. Students can simulate a client interview or assessment, conduct a dialogue with a nurse from the past, respond to a mock resuscitation code, or act out the symptoms of a condi-tion. I had two students videotape their skit of a client suffering from gastroesophageal reflux disease, demonstrating the signs, symptoms, and lifestyle issues that exacerbate the condition. We showed this video before class to reinforce the material for the session. Skits may be part of class assignments, extra credit, or performed on a volunteer basis, depending on the size of the class, the rapport among the students, and the time available. Your simulation lab personnel may help with props and moulage.

Tell 'Em Once, Tell 'Em Twice, Tell 'Em Again!

General Description. Each class session should begin with an introduction and end with a summary. This teaching strategy is a great icebreaker. Repetition, a valuable teaching tool, allows students to organize their thoughts in a structured format and to hear the key priorities of the class again and again.
Preparation and Equipment. No special equipment is required. You should prepare a succinct, articulate introduction and summary to keep the students as focused as possible.
Example of the Strategy at Work. For each class I teach, I first introduce and later summarize the talk. When using PowerPoint, I create a screen for both the introduction and the summary (see Boxes 4–7 and 4–8).

Ideas for Use

- Use this method to begin and end every class. This gives your classes a level of predictability and closure.
- Many students live by the "get it, spit it, forget it" method of studying. Providing repetition of material improves long-term retention.

Box 4–7.
Drug Action: Introduction

- Why nurses need pharmacology
- Three phases of drug action
- Four pharmacokinetic processes
- Terms used in pharmacology
- Prototype medications
- Nursing implications of herbal therapy
- The nursing process
- Client teaching

> ### Box 4–8.
> ### Drug Action: Summary
>
> - Determinants that affect drug therapy
> - Nursing assessment and analysis
> - Client teaching

- Be warned that when students see the summary screen, they start packing up and leaving. I've started to put testing information, important learning hints, and other announcements on the last screen to discourage this behavior (I call these the "Secrets of the Universe").
- Repetition is a sound principle of adult learning. **Tell 'Em Once, Tell 'Em Twice, Tell 'Em Again!** uses that principle as a framework for every class. It allows you to ensure that all content is being covered and that each area is reinforced.
- A colleague ends class with the question "What's your takeaway?" Students share their thoughts on paper, type it into their notes, or discuss them in pairs or with the entire class. This provides a reinforcement much like **Tell 'Em Again!**

Set the Stage

General Description. In the first few minutes of a class, whether in an academic or a clinical setting, the instructor primes the students for learning. **Set the Stage** is an icebreaking strategy that establishes the ground rules, introduces the class, and sets the tone. This also is a great time for housekeeping details, setting important dates, and making necessary announcements. One colleague lamented that a student entered class with the question "Are you going to say anything important today?" **Set the Stage** ensures that something important will be covered in class!

In **Set the Stage,** the instructor may read poems or short stories, play music, discuss class policies, or introduce speakers. Many speakers prefer to introduce themselves; some let others introduce them. My personal preference is to avoid the common litany of educational and employment histories and ask speakers to decide what they'd like the class to know about them.

Preparation and Equipment. The equipment depends on the type of stage-setting method used. If you're reading a piece, you just need to bring it to class. If you're playing music, you need to prepare the music via the computer. An audio cable or speakers may be needed with PowerPoint.

Example of the Strategy at Work. I use one of my favorite stage-setting examples in a continuing education and academic class on adolescent health. At the beginning of this class, I read the following quotation to illustrate the characteristics of adolescent thinking:

> You work with children with diabetes. You notice Caitlin is hospitalized—again! Caitlin is a 14-year-old with type 1 diabetes. This is her third admission in the last year—it is always the same. Caitlin gets busy with school and activities. She forgets to check her blood sugars. She doesn't know when her levels are high and when to check ketones. She forgets to calculate her carbohydrate-to-insulin ratio, doesn't correct her lows using her correction formula, and sometimes forgets her insulin altogether. She proceeds to be admitted with diabetic ketoacidosis. You sigh as you enter Caitlin's room. As you stand at her bedside you ask, "Caitlin, what were you thinking?" With wisdom far beyond her years or her recent behavior, Caitlin replies, "That's just it—I wasn't thinking!" This confirms what you have believed all along—teens think differently!

This quotation, based on teen thinking, depicts some of the realities of treating adolescent clients.

Ideas for Use

- Play a popular song to set the tone for the class. You might use "Haven't Got Time for the Pain" by Carly Simon for a class in pain management, songs about heat for fever management, "Hope You Dance" by Lee Ann Womack for launching into publishing, and "These Are the Good Old Days" by Carly Simon to open a talk on the history of nursing. Some connections aren't as clear as others. For example, "Hope You Dance" embraces an active involvement in life and love. A colleague used this song to invite class participants to collaborate in publishing and enjoy the experience of writing for publication. Look for tunes and play short excerpts to open the class. Song clips are especially effective in opening topics with an affective component. A word of caution: Preview any audio files to ensure they are appropriate for classroom listening.

- You can use a strategy called **Quiz About Me.** Tell the students several facts about yourself: years spent in nursing, your nursing specialty, your hobbies, or the way you spend your free time. Then turn around and ask them to tell the class the same facts about themselves. After a few students have shared their thoughts, ask, "How many people spend their time _____?" or

"How many people enjoy _____?," using the students' ideas to get to know the group. This strategy allows you and the class to get acquainted and puts you on a more human plane. It can take as little as three minutes.

- A colleague discusses using a "Stump the Professors" strategy to set the stage. Students are encouraged to come up with a fact or question to challenge the instructor. Keeping this strategy good-natured reinforces mutual respect and learning.

- **Set the Stage** is especially valuable in continuing education or staff development classes.

- Several ground rules in any class are important. In this day of smartphones, you need to send a clear message about turning them off or silencing them. Even in the vibrate mode, the phone can be a disruption. Also, policies about the use of phones can be articulated here.

- Latecomers may also disrupt a class. Some instructors follow the theater model, in which the door is locked after the class has started. That way, students can't come in later and disturb the class. Of course, sometimes we're so glad to see students come to class, we may overlook infractions of punctuality.

- It's important to make clear that you and any speakers who come to class need quiet so they can present the material. All instructors have experienced the hassle of undercurrent conversations, which are very distracting for teachers and students alike. Setting the stage for a professional class atmosphere can go a long way toward creating the proper learning environment. Policies for classroom management are critical in setting the stage.

- Stephens and colleagues[4] discuss the use of sports games as icebreakers for interprofessional simulations. The developers discussed how using the metaphor of a football game for instruction about rules, roles, and relationships also provided an effective mechanism for reflective learning.

Setting Priorities

General Description. Setting priorities is one of the foremost challenges of nursing and nursing education. The more students learn, the more often they encounter this challenge. This strategy allows students to draw on their own experience, helps them clarify values, and validates the importance of thoughtful priority setting.

Preparation and Equipment. To use this strategy most effectively, give each student three index cards. If index cards aren't available, ask each student to tear off three small pieces of paper. You may want to prepare a PowerPoint slide to introduce the exercises.

Example of the Strategy at Work. I use this icebreaker to introduce a class on the planning stage of the nursing process. Each student is given three index cards. The students list something that matters greatly to them, something they value highly, and something they believe is important—one item on each card. I have also asked them to list the three most important "things" in their world, reinforcing that it does not need to be a thing. It can be a person, entity, value, or anything they hold dear. I then ask the students to look at these three cards and arrange them in order of personal importance.

I ask the students to take their time to consider the criteria they use in priority ranking. Then comes the clincher: I ask them to rip up one card and throw it away. How does it feel to lose something they value so much?

The next step is to rip up another card. By now the whole class is groaning and suffering a sense of loss. We then discuss how it feels to lose things that we value. This topic leads us to the importance of setting priorities carefully and in turn how priorities depend on the individual. If there's time, students may share their real priorities, their reactions to loss, and the insight they gained from this exercise.

Ideas for Use

- **Setting Priorities,** like **Common and Different,** allows students to get to know each other.
- Students can share their thoughts with a partner, adding to the team-building quality of this exercise.
- This strategy demonstrates the difficulties of setting priorities in any situation that requires it.
- **Setting Priorities** demands a level of self-reflection and thought—students are asked to consider the impact of lifestyle or situational changes.
- To set client priorities, list three or four client needs and have the students write them on cards. Then, as previously described, have students rip up cards and essentially develop a list of priorities among the concepts. This is a great way to introduce priority setting to novice students and nurses.
- In giving up what they treasure most, students may better understand the sacrifices imposed by aging, poverty, injury, or illness. This strategy can be used to reinforce choices made by those living in poverty, how it feels to lose things and abilities as we age, and so on.
- For some students, this exercise provides a chance to practice both priority setting and the need to deal with loss.

Past Experiences With . . .

General Description. Some of the common reasons that nurses enter the field are some past experience with healthcare, illness, or trauma; and acquaintance with nurses. Individual experiences can be valuable if shared among the students. This strategy simply calls for a brief discussion of the students' past experiences with any aspect of the class content.

Preparation and Equipment. No equipment is necessary. You just need to plan which topics to address and when to ask the questions during those classes.

Example of the Strategy at Work. **Past Experiences With . . .** works especially well with a group of 30 or fewer participants. I simply ask, "What have your past experiences with nursing been like?" or "What past experiences have you had with nursing?" Students often share very candid stories of both positive and negative experiences with nurses. These experiences, whether positive or negative, spark an interest in pursuing a nursing career.

Ideas for Use

- Seasoned nurses and continuing education students may be asked, "What past experiences have you had with nursing students?" as a way to generate discussion about the next generation of nurses.

- Personal experiences with illness, trauma, healthcare, and disability may provide a unique opportunity to share and learn. Although **Past Experiences With . . .** is introduced here as an icebreaker, students who know each other well may feel especially free to share intimate personal details.

- Sharing in a large classroom may be difficult. You can ask larger classes to reflect quietly on **Past Experiences With . . .** or to write down a short synopsis of their thoughts.

- Students in clinical groups may discuss hospital routines, nursing staff, and other subjects to generate discussion and share clinical experiences.

- For specific class material, it's effective to link the class topic with the students' past experiences. For example, if you're teaching a class on diabetes, you could ask, "What is your previous experience with diabetes?" or "When you hear the word *diabetes*, what do you think of?" This tactic introduces class material, provides a brief assessment of the class, and sets the stage for learning.

Be Prepared

General Description. Much as the Boy Scout phrase implies, students need to **Be Prepared** for class and learning. Often, though, they don't know how to prepare effectively for a class or learning session. Lack of preparation slows learning and frustrates the instructor and the class alike.

This strategy opens the class discussion with how students should **Be Prepared** for that particular session. You should share your hopes and expectations. The end of the class should include your suggestions about how the students should prepare for the next class. You'll use that closing strategy as the introduction to the next class.

Preparation and Equipment. An important element of **Be Prepared** is a critical analysis of what class preparation requires. Frequently we burden students with entire chapters and other long passages. Students may learn from experience that reading an entire assignment is a waste of time. Many students today may not do readings at all, and some may not even buy or rent the book. Others postpone the readings until after class so they can focus on information they've just heard. Meanwhile the instructor assumes that the group is prepared, only to be asked to spell some of the simpler words in the assignment.

Review the course content and objectives and consider what preparation is essential for classroom learning. Abbreviated sections of readings; charts, pictures, or boxes; and questions and exercises within chapters often highlight key points of the content.

Example of the Strategy at Work. Nothing is more discouraging for an instructor than a class in which students walk in and ask, "What are we talking about today?" Obviously, these students didn't complete the reading or think about class objectives. When this happens, I use **Be Prepared** to help students get ready for subsequent classes.

At the end of one class and the beginning of the next, I focus on three to four aspects of each chapter or exercise that assist in class preparation. For example, when presenting congestive heart failure (CHF) and medications, I ask students to review their pathophysiology notes about CHF. I remind them of the importance of the terms *preload, afterload,* and *contractility.* Then I tell them we'll be using these terms to describe the actions of selected medications. This technique sparks interest—now they understand the need to remember these words. I do this exercise a few minutes before class ends to keep the students from putting away their notebooks in the middle of my discussion.

Ideas for Use

- Textbooks are great resources for questions, terms to define, case studies, and chapter synopses.
- Sometimes just reading the chapter summary helps students get a glimmer of what the next class will cover. You should reinforce the importance of reading more deeply, but busy students may benefit from some shortcuts.

- Preparation is difficult to expect from busy nurses attending continuing or in-service education. Signs or email messages hinting at discussion topics may spark interest in attending a class. The mention of words or concepts learned in nursing school and perhaps forgotten can also generate interest. This also is true if the content represents a new skillset or job expectation.

- Articles or outlines for class preparation may be posted online, in the learning management system, or in public areas. Some schools and agencies have found the restrooms a great forum for educational materials! One academic setting calls this "Elimination Illumination." Another called it "Stall Street Journal."

- Gather some "Do you know?" questions under the **Be Prepared** heading. Post them on a sign or in an email. They'll stimulate questions, encourage thought, and increase the likelihood that your students will be prepared.

- Any material used to entice your students must be discussed in class and included in tests. This kind of follow-up is necessary to drive home the value of the strategy.

My Biggest Challenge

General Description. Students and practicing nurses may enter class in a passive mode, expecting the instructor to do all the work. **My Biggest Challenge** is a great way to "get the thinking machine" going and encourage participation in the active teaching strategies that follow. As in several other icebreakers, participants are asked to consider their biggest challenge—in life, nursing, school, or any other area. Tying this challenge to the class content reinforces that content and engages the students in active thinking about the material.

Preparation and Equipment. Little equipment is needed for this strategy. The only preparation is to plan when and how you'll ask, "What was your biggest challenge?" Your approach may vary depending on the size of the class.

Example of the Strategy at Work. I use this strategy to develop empathic skills about some of the challenges faced by healthcare clients and their families. It's especially effective in the class dealing with spinal cord injury. I start the class by saying, "Okay, class. First, before we address our topic for today, I want you to consider what is the biggest challenge you have encountered in your life." After several minutes of discussion about personal health and life challenges, I ask, "What challenges confront the client sustaining a spinal cord injury?" The class readily mentions paralysis, potential need for a ventilator, loss of bowel and bladder activity, sexuality issues, and many other challenges these clients face. Some may note depression and other psychosocial issues.

Continued discussion of spinal cord injury management may highlight technological advances, medical treatments, and prevention of complications. The importance of high-quality nursing care in confronting and surmounting these challenges reinforces the key role of the nurse in caring for a client with spinal cord injury.

This 5- to 10-minute introduction engages students in considering the personal experience of clients with spinal cord injury and the need to see the individual rather than the medical diagnosis. A brief comparison of personal challenges with those of clients who are ill or injured provides a meaningful perspective for beginning practitioners.

Ideas for Use

- This strategy attaches value to the students' experiences. Too often, students are never asked to share their own experience, level of knowledge, or perspective. **My Biggest Challenge** communicates respect for background and experience and allows everyone to participate actively in the group.
- This strategy works well at a conference after clinical rotations. The small group encourages sharing. Personal experiences may be compared and contrasted with those encountered in a clinical setting.
- Clinical groups often need some icebreaking if the participants don't know one another. **My Biggest Challenge** promotes discussion, focuses on personal abilities to meet challenges, and provides insight into the strengths and weaknesses of each group member.
- **My Biggest Challenge** is valuable for novice nursing students and anyone who doesn't understand the obstacles imposed by illness or injury. It gives learners a frame of reference for contact with clients who have different needs and perspectives.

Discussion Starters

General Description. As the title indicates, this strategy gets the ball rolling. It's really a catch-all for the different tactics instructors use to generate discussion.

Individual teachers often establish particular phrases to signal to students that it's time to start class. When students hear, "What are we discussing in class today?" "How many of you have cared for clients with _____ ?" or "What do your readings say about this topic?," they know it's time to learn. **Discussion Starters** engage the participants, begin the class, and alleviate any discomfort associated with the material.

Preparation and Equipment. Planning and rehearsing your statement is all you need to do.

Example of the Strategy at Work. In teaching a large class, I found my standard "Let's get started" doesn't always command attention as well as I'd like. I selected a statement to open every class: "Thanks for coming to class. Today we're going to talk about _____ ." Before long I noticed that the students saw this **Discussion Starter** as a signal for class. Much like the bell in grammar school, it ended personal conversation; suddenly the pencils were poised to write and laptops were ready. Some students glared at others who were still talking or entering the classroom late.

Ideas for Use

- Use **Discussion Starters** any time you need to get students' attention. It only takes one or two to disrupt an entire class, regardless of size. **Discussion Starters** provide an established signal that it's time to learn.

- In a continuing education program with several sessions, a **Discussion Starter** can tie material together or provide a segue between different parts of the class.

- **Discussion Starters** may be used in smaller classes in which you seek active participation. The statement lets the class know when they can share and when you would like to manage the discussion.

Now that you've broken the ice and set the stage for learning, you can sail into teaching with many creative strategies at your command.

References

1. Dellinger S. Psychogeometrics: Communicating Beyond Our Differences. Jade Ink, 1996.
2. Froman RD and Owen SV. Teaching reliability and validity: Fun with classroom application. Journal of Continuing Education in Nursing 22: 88–94, 1991.
3. Karlsen MW, Gabrielsen AK, Falch AL, and Stubberud DG. Intensive care nursing students' perceptions of simulation for learning confirming communication skills: A descriptive qualitative study. Intensive and Critical Care Nursing 42: 97–104, 2017.
4. Stephens J, Abbott-Brailey H, and Pearson P. "It's a funny old game." Football as an educational metaphor within induction to practice-based interprofessional learning. Journal of Interprofessional Care 21 (4): 375–385, 2007.

Chapter 5

Strategies for Large Classes

Challenges

- Large classes inevitably include students with diverse learning styles, expectations, and attention spans.
- Large classrooms may present space and noise issues that impede creative teaching strategies and group work.
- Room lighting and size may challenge the instructor's ability to relate to students and establish eye contact. Sometimes the instructor may even have trouble seeing all the students and may feel isolated from the class.
- Physical distance in the classroom may create a formal and impersonal learning environment, making it difficult to engage all the students.
- An instructor in a large class may find it difficult to recognize students, recall their names, and relate to them in general.
- Because large classes encourage anonymity, students may be unprepared, uninvolved, or inattentive.
- Conversely, students may find large classes frustrating because the instructor can't give personal attention or be aware of individual learning needs.
- Less assertive students may be reluctant to participate in large classes, leaving their questions unanswered and their contributions unshared.
- Students who don't know each other may be uncomfortable with, and therefore resistant to, creative teaching strategies.

"The mediocre teacher tells. The good teacher explains. The superior teacher demonstrates. The great teacher inspires."—William Arthur Ward

Although I've noted challenges, don't despair. With a little skill and effort, you can easily use engaging strategies. In addition, large classes necessitate the use of innovative strategies to help you increase your students' comfort, engage them in the material, and stimulate their interest. If you intersperse the traditional large lecture class with quick, uncomplicated strategies, you will reinforce concepts, grab your students' attention, and create a warm and inviting learning atmosphere. Today, people use YouTube to learn. Gone are the days of checking a book, or even Google, to learn a new skill or task. We watch YouTube videos about how to ice a cake, catch a fish, paint a room, or do our hair. As instructors, we also need to use YouTube videos, along with other forms of media. We need to view them first before we use them in class, however, to ensure that they are valid and appropriate.

IDEAS

Short Clips

General Description. Showing short film clips in the middle of class is an attention-grabbing way to emphasize a point and break up material. Most students today watch television and frequent movie theaters, so this strategy capitalizes on their frame of reference. **Short Clips** may come from commercials, television serials about healthcare, or popular movies. Clips may portray positive or negative images of nursing and healthcare related to class topics, or they may depict patient responses to crisis or illness.

This method promotes thinking and direct application of information. For **Short Clips** to have the greatest effect, you should focus on class objectives and develop "thinking questions" or exercises to provide focus. See Herrman, "Using Film Clips to Enhance Nursing Education,"[1] for more details.

Preparation and Equipment. You can use various methods to present **Short Clips.** Cueing of DVDs allows you to play the clip in class, provided a DVD player is available. DVD software lets you bookmark selected clips and play them on a laptop or desktop computer. The newest version of PowerPoint lets you add cueing signals to presentations to trigger the appearance of specified scenes. Other software packages let you copy short clips onto a CD. Fair use may be interpreted to allow the making of limited, short clips for use during class, to meet learning objectives. This method requires a significant amount of technological knowledge. Check your agency resources for support in this area.[1] For YouTube videos, you need to have access to the internet. You can cue the video and toggle between PowerPoint and YouTube, or copy and paste the URL into the slide to be clicked on during the class.

Example of the Strategy at Work. I frequently use this strategy to teach both in the classroom and in staff development settings. Popular movies provide fertile ground for discussion of health and illness issues, current societal conflicts, and day-to-day living.

Examples of video clips from popular movies that I have used include *Pearl Harbor, Patch Adams, A Beautiful Mind, Save the Last Dance, Remember the Titans, The Notebook, Young Frankenstein,* and others. I've used *John Q* to discuss access to healthcare and the use of medical jargon. *How the Grinch Stole Christmas* demonstrates the stages of change as the Grinch is transformed into a caring soul. I have used scenes from *A Beautiful Mind* to carry through the entire nursing process discussion, providing examples of assessment, analysis, planning, implementation, and evaluation. *Patch Adams* can demonstrate what not to do in nursing grand rounds, the value of humor in wellness, and the use of group therapy in the care of clients with mental health issues.

Prepare thinking questions in advance, show them to the students before you show the clip, and discuss them afterward. Appropriate questions include "What are the nursing implications of this clip?," "How should a nurse respond in this situation?," and "How does this clip relate to the subject matter of today's class?"

Ideas for Use

- Tired learners, both students and working nurses, may appreciate the use of film clips to enhance the discussion topic and provide entertainment.
- **Short Clips** may deal with emotions and the affective realm better than lecture or other methods.
- You can use **Short Clips** in each class or in just one. You can show several clips from one video in a single session and discuss related topics as the story unfolds.
- Make sure that you reinforce points of discussion, or thinking questions, so that students see the film clips as a learning method, not just time off from class. Show a slide with the questions prior to the clip and then discuss the questions after the clip. This ensures that the students relate the clip to class objectives and content.
- **Clinical Decision-Making Exercises** and **Critical Thinking Exercises,** discussed in other chapters, may be combined with this strategy.

- Movie clips can stimulate engaging conversations because videos and television are such a comfortable method of communication for today's learners.
- Some video clips depict clinical signs and symptoms that are difficult to demonstrate in the classroom. *A Beautiful Mind* contains a scene showing seizure activity; *Awakenings* demonstrates extrapyramidal, parkinsonian symptoms; and *Patch Adams* shows catatonic behavior.

Read a Story

General Description. This commonly used strategy allows instructors to use some creativity by interjecting fiction, poetry, and other literature into class content. Information from popular books, business texts, social media, the internet, parenting books, personal nursing stories, comics, newspaper columns, and children's literature provides great teaching aids and adds relevance to potentially dry content. Business success guides may offer inspirational and encouraging messages. Children's books may provide poignant stories about life conflicts, illness, death, or personal experiences from the eyes of a child—often very compelling for adult learners.

Preparation and Equipment. Stay alert, especially if you go into a bookstore or pass a newsstand. Poignant stories trending on social media may be integrated into class content. Resources providing interesting quotations or passages may appear at surprising moments.

Example of the Strategy at Work. The story in Box 5–1, given to me by a colleague, helps me when I discuss poverty and global health issues. I hope that you can also use it.

For another example of this strategy, I read from an 1885 nursing textbook that I found at an antique show. I have read many excerpts about

---

Box 5–1.
A Village of 100

Imagine the world reduced to 100 people. Fifty-one would be female. Seventy would be nonwhite. Eighty would live in substandard housing. Seventy would be unable to read. Fifty would suffer from malnutrition. One would be near death, and one would have just been born. One would graduate from college, and no one would have a computer. Fifty percent of the world's wealth would be in the hands of six people—all living in the United States.

nursing in that era, and my students and I have discussed the significant advancements made since that time. Here is a selection I especially like when discussing nursing research:

> Try to find out why things are done, to be familiar with the underlying principles as well as details of practice. Learn to nurse by reason rather than by rule, for no rule can be laid down to which exceptions will not arise. Do not fancy that after you have been through a training-school you will know all there is to know about nursing; in fact, you will only have been taught how to learn, how to appreciate and profit by experience which you will get. Every new case will teach you something new.[2]

Ideas for Use

- Don't rely exclusively on books. Newspaper articles, columns, social media, the internet, and editorials also provide great material.
- Nursing journals have begun to publish works reflecting the art of nursing. Poetry, haiku, and short stories may carry powerful messages.
- Readers are encouraged to search the internet for interesting stories or anecdotes to emphasize class content. One option is to search Sir Winston Churchill, Sir Alexander Fleming, and penicillin. There is a great story that, though often refuted, I have used in my pharmacology class to introduce antibiotics.
- The coloring book *I Might Be a Nurse*[3] is a great resource for early nursing students.
- Children's books such as *The Fall of Freddy the Leaf*[4] and *Bob and Jack: A Boy and His Yak*[5] provide insights into children's concepts of aging and death. *The Three Little Pigs From the Wolf's Point of View*[6] shows how viewing problems from various perspectives can illuminate the real meaning of an issue.
- Old copies of *Cherry Ames* books and other novels about nurses may provide historical images of nursing.
- Two Golden Books, *Nurse Nancy*[7] and *Doctor Dan*,[8] can assist students in delineating professional roles and provide a historical view of nursing and medicine.
- Other, newer books offer myriad opportunities to integrate childhood literature into class sessions. *The One and Only Ivan*[9] and the *Wonky Donkey*[10] have been used to reinforce topics like loyalty, diversity, and humor.

Use the Star

General Description. Students have a difficult time determining priorities and identifying key study materials. Novice nursing students frequently highlight every word in the chapter and can't distinguish vital information from the rest. In a similar way, students struggle with delineating priority concepts in a PowerPoint presentation.

In this easy strategy, stars are used to distinguish the most important material from the rest. Asking students to **Use the Star** will give them useful visual and auditory prompts. You can use stars in PowerPoint presentations or traditional handouts, or you can simply ask the class to "put a star next to this." Stars highlight important material to be used later as study tools.

Preparation and Equipment. No preparation is required. Stars may be added either before or during class.

Example of the Strategy at Work. This strategy can be used spontaneously. During class preparation, I've added PowerPoint stars to areas that need emphasis. I realized this strategy was a success when a teaching assistant told the class, "Pay attention to the stars."

It's important to make sure that test questions coincide with starred material; if you don't follow this rule, students will learn not to trust the stars. This doesn't mean you need to "teach to the test," however; **Use the Star** keeps the focus on key points and helps the students identify potential material for test questions (see Fig. 5–1).

ETHICAL PRINCIPLES

- Beneficence
- Nonmaleficence
- Autonomy
- Paternalism
- Justice
- Allocation of resources
- Informed consent
- Accountability
- Confidentiality
- Self-determination
- Fidelity
- Veracity

Fig. 5–1. **Use stars to illustrate important points in class.**

Ideas for Use

- **Use the Star** is a great way for faculty to ensure that tests represent key factors in class content. Often tests are constructed before the first class meeting, making it difficult to ensure that vital facts are tested. By basing your test questions on starred material, you can stick to the important facts, ensure test content validity, and avoid minutiae. You can also be sure that the students know what information matters the most.

- Ask your students what information deserves to be starred. Use frequent pauses as an opportunity to ask, "Okay, what facts covered in the last 20 minutes deserve a star?" Given this opening, students will revisit and repeat information while developing skills in priority setting.

- This strategy is important for new nurses or those new to a clinical specialty. Even nurses who have been practicing for a while may need to learn the priorities specific to an unfamiliar clinical area. Starred material provides a way for nurses at all levels to focus on new and vital information.

- **Use the Star** ensures that students are actively writing and attending to notes during class.

Case Studies: Quickie

General Description. The use of case studies in nursing education is well documented and has demonstrated effectiveness as a teaching tool.[11] Nurses and nursing students share and learn via clinical anecdotes, real-life experiences, and so-called war stories. Case studies teach reality-based information within a story developed according to specific class content and objectives.

The drama of a case study allows nurses and nursing students to embrace information on a human level. Because the case study is fictitious, the teacher can mold it to include relevant details and emphasize key information.

Case studies may take a while to write but can be used again and again. They can be brief or as extensive as class and preparation time allow. The next several strategies describe several uses of case studies in teaching. Case studies work well with large classes when other creative strategies prove unwieldy, but they may be used in any teaching venue. **Quickie Case Studies** are just that—a brief introduction to the client and the main clinical issue. **Quickie Case Studies** may be used to introduce topics, segue from one area to another, emphasize priorities, or show how concepts fit together.

Preparation and Equipment. This strategy takes more cognitive effort than anything else. Once the content and objectives are established and the lecture is written, you can write your **Quickie Case Study.** This can be read out loud, written onto a slide, or included in a handout.

Example of the Strategy at Work. I use **Quickie Case Studies** to differentiate type 1 and type 2 diabetes mellitus. The class can differentiate the diagnosis, characteristics, and management of the two types. This **Quickie Case Study** provides a transition in the discussion from type 1 to type 2 diabetes, highlighting several of the differences and nursing implications.

Quickie Case Study

Type 1 Diabetes Mellitus

A. C., a 6-year-old boy, is taken to the pediatrician by his mother. He says he feels "bad" and "tired all the time." His mother notes that he has been drinking and eating a lot and is "always going to the bathroom." She adds that he appears thinner and lacks his usual energy. She also comments that his breath smells sweet. A peripheral blood glucose level is 450 mg/dL. A. C. is referred to the endocrinology clinic.

Quickie Case Study

Type 2 Diabetes Mellitus

J. C. is a 58-year-old man with a history of hypertension and cerebrovascular accident. He is African American and is 40 lb overweight. His mother is being treated for type 2 diabetes mellitus. J. C. has been drinking and urinating more than usual but says that he feels well. He is on disability leave from work and lives a sedentary life. When asked about his diet, he replies, "I eat what I want to. I don't like to diet." Routine blood work reveals hyperglycemia, and he is referred to the endocrinology clinic.

Ideas for Use

- Use **Quickie Case Studies** to open or close a class session. They can also be used as transitions from one topic to another, ensuring that students are caught up with the changes in class subjects.
- Use case study content to provide a test review. **Quickie Case Studies** can provide the context for later test questions.

- One hazard of using case studies is the possibility that the students will overgeneralize. It's important to emphasize that the case study is an example of issues and characteristics. Novice students or nurses may assume that all clients with certain characteristics present the same issues. Make sure you include a preliminary statement that the case represents a prototype rather than a "standard client" with all the same issues.

- **Quickie Case Studies** are valuable when clinical pictures are closely aligned or when differences are subtle. Students can analyze the differences within a short, tight framework.

- Handouts may include the case study and appropriate study questions. You can combine **Quickie Case Studies** with **Email Exercises** or **Online Discussions.**

- Case study strategies may be coupled with **Group Thought, Think-Pair-Share,** and **Teaching Trios**.

Preclass Case Studies

General Description. **Preclass Case Studies** are especially valuable if some preliminary study is needed before class. Examples include technical information that may depend on background reading, preparation for class, or classes that need to cover more content than time allows. **Preclass Case Studies** also reinforce learning by requiring students to read, write and complete, and hear the material.

Preparation and Equipment. **Preclass Case Studies** need to be written in advance and should be fairly detailed. These case studies can then be posted on the internet, included in the class workbook, or distributed as a handout. Class time is set aside to discuss the case study and the accompanying questions.

Example of the Strategy at Work. I developed this strategy while teaching a class on pediatric gastrointestinal problems. The class contained far more content than I could cover in 2 hours.

I decided to develop a case study about cleft lip and palate. This study allowed an extensive discussion of the medical, surgical, nursing, and multidisciplinary approach to managing cleft lip and palate disorders. Students were instructed to read the case study before class and to underline key words associated with organic changes, assessments, and management and nursing considerations. Study questions, discussed in class, were based on the case study information.

Students who had prepared well understood the rather brief discussion that reflected the case study. Students who didn't prepare appeared lost, especially when I mentioned that the test questions on this content would be drawn directly from this case study. The next time I used a **Preclass Case Study** on another topic in that class, I found most of the students were prepared, and we completed the material quickly.

Ideas for Use

- Use **Preclass Case Studies** when you need to spend less time on a single topic.
- **Preclass Case Studies** help when preparation before class is vital to understanding material. Have students read the case study, answer key questions, and hand in the answers on admission to class (see **Admit Ticket**).
- **Preclass Case Studies** may be used in continuing education and staff development settings to ensure that all participants are on the same page. If you include a case study in registration materials, students can look over the case, do background reading, and consider answer options.
- Ensure that the topic of a **Preclass Case Study** is represented on a test or examination. Use the basic elements of the case study to develop multiple-choice items or quiz questions.
- Case studies done before class may be part of an **Email Exercise** or an **Online Discussion.**

Interspersed Case Studies

General Description. Like the previous case study formats, **Interspersed Case Studies** allow for a short pause in the lecture to discuss a case. These mini-cases are simply used to reinforce key points or to emphasize important content. They are based on single concepts and are directed toward starting thinking about one area of discussion. You can design them to clarify difficult concepts or to help students establish priorities among conflicting demands.

Preparation and Equipment. Write **Interspersed Case Studies** after the content and objectives are established and the lecture is written. You can read the case studies out loud, write them as a PowerPoint or any other type of slide, or include them in a handout.

Example of the Strategy at Work. I use **Interspersed Case Studies** to break up lecture content and to reinforce key information. In a class on stress management, I found that students often internalized class content as part of their own personal situations; they rarely considered the role of the nurse in helping clients to cope with stress. **Interspersed Case Studies** ask students to consider what sort of assistance they can offer a client. They're called on to identify the client's major stressors, the signs and symptoms of stress, and potential nursing interventions to use in stress assessment and management. Using **Interspersed Case Studies** helps students begin to assimilate their role as practitioner.

Interspersed Case Study

A Stressed Client

K. L. is a 36-year-old man. He is married and has four children, 1 to 5 years old. He smokes two packs of cigarettes per day, is 20 lb overweight, does not exercise, and admits to drinking five or six alcoholic drinks every day. He expresses frustration with his job, family situation, and life in general. He feels that stress is his most significant problem.

Ideas for Use

- Use **Interspersed Case Studies** any time you believe students are finding information difficult or confusing. Put the information on a personal level to help them understand complex concepts.
- Conclude a class with a brief **Interspersed Case Study** to reinforce information.
- To discuss the case study and related **Critical Thinking Exercises,** have students split into groups for **Think-Pair-Share, Teaching Trios,** or **Group Thought.**
- If using **Group Thought,** choose cases that differ slightly to help students understand the subtleties of different situations. Ask students to report back to the class with conclusions (see **Group Thought**).
- If you're using objective examinations, use **Interspersed Case Studies** in each class to emphasize test material. Help students see the entire spectrum of the nursing process by asking questions that represent each step. This strategy is important in preparation for the National Council Licensure Examination (NCLEX®).

Continuing Case Studies

General Description. **Continuing Case Studies** develop throughout the class as content is presented. I like to expand on the same case study throughout one class session because it allows my students to get to know the client; revisiting the study creates a holistic picture of the client and his or her nursing care. **Continuing Case Studies** provide a human element—the subject of the case study becomes an old friend to be revisited—and students can apply the information as it's discussed.

This strategy is especially valuable when single, complex topics are taught in one session. The case continues to develop as content becomes more complex, as the client's status changes, or as the information branches off into related topics. The **Continuing Case Study** is introduced at the beginning of class, discussed during class, and used to summarize issues at the end of the session. **Continuing Case Studies** are beneficial when the course of a complex condition is discussed, allowing students to witness the diagnosis, assessments, treatment, client response, and nursing implications.

Preparation and Equipment. Write **Continuing Case Studies** after the content and objectives are established and the lecture is written. Like **Interspersed Case Studies, Continuing Case Studies** can be read out loud, written onto any type of slide, or included in a handout. I like to decorate my slides with humorous drawings, which help students remember the material.

Example of the Strategy at Work. I have used **Continuing Case Studies** to teach concepts across the nursing process, such as pain assessment and management. In the first slide, I present the client.

Continuing Case Study

A Postsurgical Client

L. W. is 13 years old and has scoliosis. She had a posterior spinal fusion today. The surgery took 6 hours, and the incision is 18 in. long. She is on postoperative bedrest for 24 hours, has two IVs and a urinary catheter, and is receiving patient-controlled analgesia.

We then discuss pain assessment and the physiological, behavioral, and subjective criteria we use to measure pain. Then the client's assessment information is presented.

Continuing Case Study

Postsurgical Assessment
- Denies severe pain
- Pulse 130 bpm, respirations 36/min, blood pressure 118/88 mm Hg
- Restless, refuses to move, moans with turning and care
- Verbalizes pain at 7 on a scale of 1 to 10
- Refuses to breathe deeply or cough
- Reports pain at incision and graft sites
- Parents at bedside—very anxious

The lecture then turns to pain management. Pharmacological and nonpharmacological methods are discussed. I reinforce the lecture with a slide.

Continuing Case Study

Management
- Patient-controlled analgesia with continuous morphine
- Morphine bolus with care and position changes
- Distraction
- Dark, quiet room
- Warm cloth on forehead
- Client and parent education

Finally, I present the concept of evaluation as integral to pain assessment and management. In summary, we discuss the importance of evaluating and reevaluating pain from the client's perspective.

Continuing Case Study

Evaluation
- Verbalizes pain at 4 on a scale of 1 to 10
- Logrolls freely in bed; urinary catheter discontinued
- Using female urinal
- Breathing deeply and coughing
- Vital signs within normal limits
- Sipping liquids
- Interacting with parents
- Watching TV
- Expressing fears but excited about getting out of bed tomorrow

Ideas for Use

- **Continuing Case Studies** work well for single topics in which the content develops detail and complexity throughout the class. Extensive class time is often needed for topics such as shock, cardiac emergencies, the surgical process, and various aspects of cancer management.

- **Continuing Case Studies** may be used for examination review to reinforce material that may have been taught several weeks ago.
- This strategy is especially valuable in continuing education and staff development, in which experienced nurses learn best with real-life scenarios. Providing the case study with discussion points every 15 minutes or so appeals to listeners and accommodates the attention span of busy learners.
- Have students develop a **Continuing Case Study** as part of an **Email Exercise** or **Online Discussion.**

Unfolding Case Studies

General Description. This innovative strategy was developed and documented by Glendon and Ulrich.[12] Although an older book, it contains more than 50 case studies that are still relevant today. Each case divulges an increasing amount of detail during the course of the study. As the story unfolds, students are asked to consider the many facets of the client's care. The ability of these cases to enhance real-life application may be superior to more linear, unidimensional case studies.

The merit of these cases lies in the lifelike, dynamic nature of the stories, which weave in clinical status changes and the results of assessments and interventions. As each case develops, students must consider the increasingly complex details and use them to influence decisions. The students discuss the study as it grows more complex. Educators may use the published **Unfolding Case Studies,** which represent all nursing specialties, or create their own. Those included by Glendon and Ulrich represent all nursing specialties, various nursing settings, and different phases of clinical expertise.

Preparation and Equipment. As with other case studies, **Unfolding Case Studies** need to be developed as part of class preparation. After the class is organized, an **Unfolding Case Study** can be developed to include its various aspects.

Example of the Strategy at Work. I have used several of the cases developed by Glendon and Ulrich.[12] One unfolding case study addresses legal and ethical aspects of professionalism and highlights the need for patient confidentiality: Two student nurses are working in labor and delivery. Each has a client. One mother discusses her husband Jim and his steadfast nature. The other mother talks about her boyfriend Jim and their future marriage. A man named Jim comes to visit both, and the nursing students decide he is the same man and spread rumors all over the unit. The visiting Jim turns out to be both women's pastor, and the students learn the lesson of jumping to conclusions, the inability to "right" a previous wrong, and the hazards of breaching patient confidentiality.

Students love the drama associated with this case. They recognize the students in the study and compare it with their own professional roles in the clinical area. I use **Think-Pair-Share** with this case to have students discuss the legal and ethical implications of this issue.

Ideas for Use

- Develop your own **Unfolding Case Studies** to emphasize key points. Add more information to the case as it unfolds to challenge students further and to reinforce important issues.
- Ask students critical thinking questions through **Email Exercises** or **Online Discussions** to keep them thinking.
- Use the **Unfolding Case Studies** developed by Glendon and Ulrich[12] to enhance your personal teaching materials.
- Use the unfolding nature of these cases to demonstrate unexpected yet common changes in client status. Discuss the postoperative client who develops a wound infection, the client who develops congestive heart failure after a myocardial infarction, a client going through the stages of sickle cell crisis, a client who received a medication that does not produce the anticipated effect, or the laboring mother who experiences a placental abruption. By adding details as the case unfolds, you can introduce students to the dynamic nature of client care and the need for ongoing assessments and decision making.

Reverse Case Studies

General Description. Published by Beyer in 2010,[13] this type of case study is a collaborative, interactive, and active strategy developed for group work. Students receive a list of home medications or those the client is prescribed to receive while in the agency and a two- to three-sentence description of the current clinical situation or "picture" of a client. With only this information, students must develop a comprehensive case study or concept map as a result of group process.

Preparation and Equipment. Instructors can develop a slide or dictate aloud the home or agency medications and client scenario for issues, concepts, or disorders discussed in class. If the students are creating concept maps or brainstorming ideas, a flip chart or computer with concept map software is often helpful.

Example of the Strategy at Work. I use this strategy in both clinical and the classroom. When teaching about adult respiratory disease, I found that simply including bronchodilator inhalers, a steroid, and an antibiotic, and noting that the client was on oxygen, smoked cigarettes, and lived alone created a rich description of a client's life with emphysema and the challenges that would ensue in the management of this client's care. Students were asked to develop these areas and others as they documented using a concept map on a flip chart and then presented "their client" to others in the class.

Reverse Case Study

- Home or agency-prescribed medications
- Brief description of current course of events
- Previous Medical History (MH)
- Assessment data
- Nursing diagnosis
- Nursing interventions
- Labs/diagnostics
- Outcomes

Ideas for Use

- This is a great strategy for clinical groups. Although designed as a group activity, **Reverse Case Studies** are also great for individual assignments.
- **Reverse Case Studies** may also be used as postconferences for common problems on the unit. This is an effective way to introduce this common disorder in the first few days of a clinical rotation at a new agency.
- **Reverse Case Studies** can also be effective in orientation for novice nurses or nurses new to a specialty. They can learn about the most common disorders at an agency or on a unit and also foster a holistic picture of client care.
- You may alter the criteria noted above. For example, a mental health course may focus on previous traumas/stressors, coping mechanisms, and other variables. A pediatric nursing course may discuss developmental history, favorite toys, current developmental status, and others.
- In class, use of **Reverse Case Studies** may be group work following a unit, may be incorporated into a flipped classroom, or may supplement lecture material.
- A colleague discussed a strategy called **Build a Patient.** Much like **Reverse Case Studies**, this technique requires students to create a client by brainstorming characteristics, presenting signs and

symptoms, relevant health history components, and other traits. Students are asked to use creative knowledge to demonstrate their learning and reinforce key information. A class discussion follows to reinforce the potential for individual variations, potential complications, and key nursing interventions.

Use the Book

General Description. This strategy encourages both students and instructors to **Use the Book.** Nursing education and other textbooks often include resources that go unused because of time, lack of knowledge, or just habit. Today's students view textbooks as research resources rather than as tools to assist in daily class preparation. In addition, students frequently use class notes to study for a test; today's learners don't seem to read to supplement knowledge.

Use the Book encourages use of the ancillary resources included with books. Many texts offer critical thinking exercises, test questions, CD-ROMs, and scenarios; publishers encourage authors to develop these materials because they make textbooks more marketable. Probably the greatest benefit of this strategy is that students learn the hidden uses of their textbooks. They can go back and **Use the Book** to learn material and study for the tests.

Preparation and Equipment. The only preparation for this strategy is to peruse the text and view the available resources. Use exercises that enhance class content or align with class objectives. This strategy may use key textbook information—boxes, charts, tables, examples, and pictures—which is then reinforced in class. By citing page numbers, scanning pictures into the lecture slides, using publisher-developed audiovisuals, using exercises and case studies from assigned chapter readings, and asking students to use the resources in the book, you emphasize the value of the book and its features.

Example of the Strategy at Work. This strategy can enhance learning in two ways. The first method simply uses the resources available to reinforce content. For pharmacology, I've used the case studies at the back of the chapter, and others, to summarize the class content. The case studies were geared toward lesson content and asked poignant questions related to the material.

Another way to use this strategy is to scan in pages of the book and selected information and import it into a PowerPoint presentation to show students. I scanned in a box from the readings with the steps of case management. You may also ask the students to open their textbooks to a page with the list of these steps. Then develop a case study using the information. The slides help students **Use the Book** and apply it to a case study you've developed. Following is an example in which I applied the steps of case management to a class-related study.

The Case Management Process

You are a nurse caring for C. C., a 14-year-old boy who sustained a spinal cord injury in a motor vehicle accident. He has a tracheostomy, is dependent on a ventilator, and is wheelchair bound. Use the steps of the case management process to consider his needs.

Ideas for Use

- Most textbooks provide a wealth of material that you can use to reinforce your teaching. Test questions, case scenarios, critical thinking exercises, graphics and image files, supplemental case studies and exercises, and test banks may all be used to enhance classroom discussion.
- Instructors may ask students to identify **Muddiest Parts** and, via the learning management system (LMS), suggest small chunks of readings and hints to encourage students to exert their own effort to discover and address their misconceptions. This encourages students to take responsibility for their own learning.
- Students can use text resources in studying for tests and to clarify **Muddiest Parts.** Once they get comfortable with all the resources a book provides, students may become more eager to use it for class preparation and to do the assigned readings.
- Some students need the reinforcement of a postclass review. **Use the Book** gives them tangible exercises or review materials to look at after class. By reinforcing what they've learned in class, students can study in small, manageable chunks and avoid last-minute cramming before examinations.

Worksheets

General Description. Some of us recall **Worksheets** as important study tools, classroom activities, and teaching strategies from grammar school. These valuable tools take some time to prepare in advance, but you can use them in class again and again.

Preparation and Equipment. Class material must be prepared in advance so the **Worksheets** supplement the class content and increase the students' active participation in class. They also supplement student notes and PowerPoint handouts. Providing PDF files with type-in fields allows students to amend files during class.

Example of the Strategy at Work. Table 5–1 shows a worksheet I use for a discussion of pulmonary deficits with cystic fibrosis. I used this worksheet to clarify complex conditions such as the pulmonary deficits associated with cystic fibrosis. Other topics conducive to **Worksheets** include endocrine disorders, arterial blood gases, acid–base balance, and dysrhythmias. I try to leave off arrows indicating elevations or decreases in lab values or

Table 5–1. Management of Cystic Fibrosis: Pulmonary Changes

Pathophysiological Problems	Signs and Symptoms	Management and Nursing Implications
Short-Term Respiratory Changes		
_____ Mucus (viscosity, amount)	_____ Dyspnea	CPT, P&PD, CBD, percussor vests
_____ Dilatation	_____ Cough	Exercise
_____ Fibrosis	_____ Aeration (especially lower lobes)	Forced fluids
_____ Ciliary action	_____ Wheezes	Adequate nutrition
_____ Mucus stasis	_____ Fatigue (hypoxia)	Bronchodilators
_____ CO_2, O_2 exchange	_____ Respiratory rate	Antibiotics (inhaled) Tobramycin
_____ Leukocyte-rich sputum	_____ Symptoms of URI	O_2 (low-liter flow)
_____ Risk for infection	_____ Sx of pneumonia	Expectorants, flutter valves

Continued

Table 5–1.   Management of Cystic Fibrosis: Pulmonary Changes (cont'd)

Pathophysiological Problems	Signs and Symptoms	Management and Nursing Implications
Long-Term Respiratory Changes		
_____ Fibrosis	_____ Sx of atelectasis	Relaxing
_____ Organ function	_____ FEV1	Forced exhalation (huffing)
_____ Potential for pneumothorax	_____ FCV	Nebulizers
_____ Cor pulmonale, pulmonary hypertension	_____ Barrel chest	Dornase alfa
_____ Multidrug resistance	_____ Clubbing	Ibuprofen (to decrease inflammation)
	_____ Signs of respiratory distress	Home care: Timing, skills, equipment
	_____ Rhonchi	Surgical management: lung transplant

CBD = coughing and deep breathing; CPT = chest physical therapy;
P&PD = percussion and postural drainage; Sx = symptoms; URI = upper respiratory;
FEV₁ = forced expiratory volume; FVC = forced vital capacity

symptoms and to omit several words in each block of the **Worksheet.** When the students realize I'll be giving them the missing information, they listen more actively as they complete the **Worksheet** during class.

Another way to use **Worksheets** in class is to combine this strategy with **Case Studies** and **Group Thought.** In this combined exercise, I provide the students with the following case and a copy of a blank incident report. Students fill in the components of the incident report and learn a valuable lesson about this part of professional nursing. These paper forms may replicate agency forms that are available through their intranet.

Medication Incident/Variance Report Case Study

You are a new nurse providing care to a client. The client's name is Jack Jones. His medical record number is MR6-798543; and the unit is 6 North at Smith Hospital. Your client is ordered to receive D5/0.45 normal saline solution by peripheral IV at 75 mL/h. A physician writes an order at 0645 to include 20 mEq of potassium chloride (KCl) in each 1000-mL bag of IV fluids. This order is not transcribed by the night shift nurse.

At 1600 in your chart review, you notice the order and realize that the client has not received the KCl. The physician is called. You draw a blood sample and find that the client's potassium level is 3.0 mEq/dL. The physician orders potassium added to the IV, and a potassium rider is hung.

Four hours later, the serum potassium level is 3.9 mEq/dL. The client is asymptomatic, has suffered no long-term effects, and is told about the incident. The family is not notified, and documentation is limited to the lab results and the client's toleration of the added potassium.

Using the incident/variance report sheet, complete the demographic information on the first page. Using the data in this case study and your personal experience, discuss the outcomes, parameters (contributing factors), and potential actions that could be taken in this case.

Ideas for Use

- To make this strategy work, you need to encourage active learning. **Worksheets** may be constructed from class lectures with blanks where some content should be. By prompting students, **Worksheets** require them to fill in the blanks, complete tasks, participate in class, and look up references and any needed information.
- **Worksheet** alternatives are no-count quizzes, matching exercises, case studies with questions, and informational charts.
- Provide **Worksheets** in advance in syllabi, class workbooks, or on internet-based classroom resources.
- Ask students to prepare by completing **Worksheets** before class. Reward participation with prizes or recognition.

- Including a **Quickie Quiz** or a **Quiz That Counts** reinforces both the material and the importance of preparation for class.
- This strategy can help you construct tests because it focuses on key information that must be revisited during the course.
- For continuing education, **Worksheets** may accompany registration materials. Participants can prepare for the class, think about its content, and develop questions in advance. In classes that require testing or a competency component (e.g., critical-care classes, resuscitation classes, and skills-based teaching sessions), **Worksheets** can ensure readiness or provide a baseline for class awareness and mastery.
- If the material is complex, a **Worksheet** or handout can provide a framework for taking class notes and for studying later. If class material is difficult to understand, organizing it into **Worksheets** may enable students to grasp it more easily.
- **Worksheets** may be loaded into the LMS, and students can be asked to download and print them or download and have them available via their devices in the classroom.

All Things Being Equal

General Description. This strategy helps students learn to set priorities and to recognize signs and symptoms that may require more immediate attention. Students are given three or four different sets of signs and symptoms, lab data, or other client information. They're asked to rank the data according to level of acuity or priority and are given no additional information.

Students frequently want to know more details about the client or the circumstances of the case. This is where **All Things Being Equal** comes in. In this strategy, tell the students that you've given them the most important data and ask them to base their decisions on that data alone.

This strategy is a great help in developing test questions and enhancing critical thinking skills. Nursing students and nurses who take objective examinations often lament the need to rank four right answers to the same question. All are correct, but the test taker must identify the action of highest priority or the problem that needs the most urgent attention. **All Things Being Equal** develops the ability to make decisions based on limited amounts of information.

Preparation and Equipment. You can prepare this strategy easily while preparing a lecture or practicing your delivery. The exercises may be shown on a PowerPoint slide, a handout, or a whiteboard or blackboard.

Example of the Strategy at Work. I use **All Things Being Equal** to help students differentiate severe or life-threatening conditions from less urgent ones. During a lecture on pediatric respiration, the students needed to compare vital signs with norms, distinguish benign symptoms from more ominous ones, and interpret normal and abnormal lab data (see Box 5–2). This strategy provided a framework in which they could practice their skills.

Box 5–2.
Set Priorities for These Clients

(A) An infant with a respiratory rate of 18/min
(B) A school-age child with an expiratory wheeze
(C) A child with chronic allergies and an O_2 saturation of 90%

(A) An infant with a bobbing head
(B) An infant with peripheral cyanosis
(C) An adolescent with a barrel chest

(A) A child with bronchitis and coarse breath sounds
(B) An infant with slow, seesaw respirations
(C) A child with asthma who has an intermittent cough

Because classes can bombard them with so much material, students may find it difficult to sift through and discern the signs and symptoms that take highest priority. Years of experience have taught practicing nurses the importance of keeping an airway patent, attending to physiological and safety needs, and managing pain. In contrast, novices find it difficult to sort data into levels of severity because they lack a clinical foundation for knowledge development. This strategy provides the perspective necessary for an informed clinical judgment.

Ideas for Use

- Use **All Things Being Equal** to reinforce lab data. One difficult area for nursing students is the extent to which a lab result can deviate from the norm before it indicates a problem. For example, a practicing nurse knows the significance of a serum potassium level of 2.0 mEq/L, but a novice may not. This strategy assists students in differentiating critical values from simply abnormal values.
- You can base test questions on some of the exercises. Write a scenario for the test question and ask, "Which symptom concerns

the nurse the most?" or "Which symptom indicates a need for immediate attention?"

- Encourage students to quiz each other using **All Things Being Equal.** Making up these exercises is an excellent way for students to prepare for an examination.

- **All Things Being Equal** can be used to rank the priorities for several clients or to rank conflicting priorities in a single client. Students may be given several cases depicting clients and then consider the following questions: "Which client would you see first?" or "Which client is the highest priority?" You can also ask questions about potential nursing interventions. This allows students to link assessments with interventions and provides a valuable skill often tested on NCLEX®.

- **All Things Being Equal** reinforces the need to set priorities and answer questions with only the information at hand. The student is forced to focus on limited but adequate amounts of data.

When You Think of This, Think of That

General Description. This strategy is a matching exercise used to reinforce classroom material. The information is set up in two columns, and students are asked to match items. It's important to have several correct matches; thus, students have to think rather than simply eliminate choices. Some items will have only one match, but others will have several. Box 5–3 shows an example: the only match for rheumatic heart disease is the sequela of an untreated streptococcal infection.

Preparation and Equipment. You'll need to set up your two-column list and decide the best way to present it. It can be made into a handout, put on a PowerPoint slide, or written on the whiteboard or blackboard. You can also use it as a format for **Quickie Quizzes** or **Quizzes That Count.**

Example of the Strategy at Work. In a pediatric respiration class, I used a PowerPoint slide that the students could enlarge and use as a study aid. In class we discussed all the diagnoses in the right column and several items in the left column (see Box 5–3). We covered important concepts by focusing on the differences between gradual- and sudden-onset conditions. My version of **When You Think of This, Think of That** strategy reinforced the importance of knowing the differences, and the students were able to practice the concepts in a matching exercise.

Ideas for Use

- Use **When You Think of This, Think of That** for any subject matter in which students are asked to memorize or learn complex symptomatology or pathophysiology.

Box 5–3.
More Than One Answer Works

No intubation or throat examination	Epiglottis
"Barky" cough	Respiratory syncytial virus
Coughing, wheezing	Asthma
Pulling at ears	Bronchitis
High fever, drooling	Otitis media
Lots of nasal mucus	Tonsillitis
Sequelae—lack of strep medication	Acute nasal pharyngitis
Coarse breath sounds	Acute spasmodic laryngitis
Life-threatening situation	Acute laryngotracheal bronchitis
Medical and surgical management	Rheumatic heart disease
Bathroom shower	
Sudden onset	
Gradual onset	

- This strategy can be adapted for **Quickie Quizzes** and **Quizzes That Count.**
- You can use the strategy in a game format: keep score, promote healthy competition, and give out prizes.
- As noted by one nurse colleague "You can't think critically about things you don't know yet." This strategy is effective in learning and memorizing material for later application to higher-order thinking.
- Encourage students individually to review lists used in **When You Think of This, Think of That.** Then you can solicit answers from the class as a whole. This tactic actively involves the students rather than letting them wait passively for answers without doing any work.

Current Events

General Description. In this strategy, current world events provide a springboard for class discussion or reinforce important concepts. Using **Current Events** from the newspaper, online news sites, or television news broadcasts can inspire up-to-date application of nursing knowledge. I have often heard radio stories that have direct application to class content.

Students who are deeply embedded in schoolwork or nurses who juggle several priorities may be insulated from the goings-on of the world. However, nursing is a profession with a strong social conscience. **Current Events** introduces current affairs to the classroom and highlights the extent to which nursing can influence world situations.

Preparation and Equipment. Staying informed about **Current Events** is the only preparation needed for this strategy. Depending on the class objectives, **Current Events** may present themselves as major topics for discussion. Other news events may need to be researched by you or the students.

Example of the Strategy at Work. The following case summarizes a widely publicized event in which a family relinquished care of their disabled son. They pleaded stress and lack of respite resources. I used this case to discuss the stress of chronic illness on the family and their need for support and respite to alleviate the constant demands of their son's condition.

A Current Case

A Family in Crisis

12/26: A mother allegedly drops off her disabled son, S., at a hospital, with a note stating that the parents could no longer care for him. S., who has cerebral palsy, is admitted to the hospital.

12/27: The parents surrender to police and are charged with child abandonment and conspiracy. These are misdemeanor charges.

12/28: The parents are released on condition that they have no contact with S.

12/29: Offers are made to watch S. The state would like to return him to his parents.

1/1: The father is given leave from work.

All **Current Events** should be presented as they were reported in the news, without editorial comment. If news is local, information available to locals should not be included. On the other hand, any news disseminated in a public way is considered public record and is appropriate for classroom discussion.

I've also used **Current Events** to update pharmacological information and present medical advances. Often the lay literature portrays a medical advance as a breakthrough and claims that it abolishes a condition. If the story is based on a single research study or discovery, spirited classroom discussion may ensue. Such examples reinforce the need for a sound knowledge base before changes can be made in practice. **Current Events** is a great opportunity to teach this important principle of evidence-based practice.

Ideas for Use

- Students can be asked to provide the current event as part of a **Quick Write, Email Exercise,** or **Admit Ticket.**
- Most students remember the use of **Current Events** and will transfer their importance to higher education and the working world.
- Local health-related events also may be important to the class. Agency newsletters, community papers, or other resources may be used to access information.
- Students can use newspaper-related search engines (e.g., Lexus-Nexus) to conduct searches of **Current Events** in subscribed works.

    This strategy may be used to reinforce the importance of critiquing the validity of news and other stories read in the media. Nurses have a key role in ensuring the safety of consumers and acting as a critical consumer of news and findings related to health, pharmaceuticals, and healthcare.

Bring in the Reinforcements and In-Class Applications

General Description. This strategy requires a pause in your teaching so you can reinforce or apply concepts while they're being discussed. It's easy to gloss over material quickly without making sure the students understand it. **Bring in the Reinforcements** lets you use short class exercises to *reinforce* class material in a few moments. **In-Class Applications** allows students to *apply* information quickly after hearing it. Both strategies increase the likelihood of learning and retention.

Preparation and Equipment. Develop the exercises after preparing your class material. These exercises should be short and to the point so students can get immediate feedback about how well they've understood the concepts.

Example of the Strategy at Work. One way to use **Bring in the Reinforcements** in class is to define terms and then ask students to identify examples. I use this tactic when discussing types of change: planned, developmental, covert, and so on. Then I show a slide listing selected examples of change (see Boxes 5–4 and 5–5). Students identify the types of change each example signifies, immediately reinforcing what they've just learned. The concept that more than one type of change may be applicable to life events is difficult and better explained with a concrete example.

Box 5–4.
Types of Change

- Planned
- Unplanned
- Covert
- Overt
- Developmental
- More than one type

Box 5–5.
Types of Change

- A girl reaching puberty
- A teaching session on self-injection
- A toddler sustaining life-threatening burns by spilling scalding water
- A person gaining 50 lb
- Cancer growing in a 72-year-old woman's bones
- An 85-year-old having a cerebrovascular accident
- A nursing plan to help a client stop smoking
- A teaching session for new parents on baby care

An example of **Bring in the Reinforcements** comes from a continuing education program on assertiveness. Students were given a conflict common in their personal unit or job situation. They were asked to construct various responses: assertive, passive, aggressive, and passive-aggressive. Much as in **Invented Dialogues,** students practiced their constructed responses and also compared the outcomes of each one in the given situation.

An example of **In-Class Applications** is the use of mini-cases to apply concepts learned in class to real-life situations. One class focused on health and different individuals' reactions to illness. We discussed emotional dimensions, locus of control, external factors, and motivation.

A brief case study revealed the stark differences between two clients' reactions to a heart attack. These cases illustrate the differences in clients' responses much better than a simple description would.

Applying Health Concepts

Jerry's Case

Jerry suffered a heart attack. On his physician's advice, he started exercising, changed his diet, started stress management classes, and returned to work. He has a positive outlook and considers himself "well."

Joe's Case

After his heart attack, Joe also changed his diet and started exercising. However, he hasn't been able to quit smoking, although he wants to and has been vehemently advised to do so. Joe is often despondent and fears having another heart attack. He has not returned to work and describes himself as "ill."

Discussion Points

- Emotional dimensions
- Locus of control
- External factors
- Motivation
- Nursing interventions

Another way to use **In-Class Applications** is to develop a short illustrative scenario and ask students to identify different features. I have used this method in teaching leadership styles. We discuss laissez-faire, autocratic, charismatic, and democratic styles. Then I lay the groundwork for the exercise.

Leadership Styles

You've progressed in your career and have become nurse leader of a nurse-run community health center. You recently became aware of a problem with long waits in the clinic. Clients are complaining about waiting 1.5 hours for routine care and are starting to skip appointments. Realizing that the situation undermines the care that the clinic provides, you begin to explore solutions.

I then show slides illustrating different leadership styles and ask the students to identify them (see the following case). I also tell them that they'll be expected to demonstrate their knowledge in future examination questions.

Name That Leadership Style I

You call a meeting with your staff members. You appeal to their emotional side, reading them letters clients have written about their clinic experiences. The letters describe endless waits and sick children who go unattended. You discuss the personal impact of these long waits and suggest several solutions.

What style of leadership is this?

Name That Leadership Style II

You call a meeting with your staff members. You tell them the long waits are unacceptable. The clinic is coming up for grant renewal, and client satisfaction is an important parameter. You tell the employees they'll need to work faster, more efficiently, and with decreasing resources. You add that if conditions don't improve, heads will roll!

What style of leadership is this?

Name That Leadership Style III

You call a meeting with your staff members. You delineate the problem with long waits and ask the employees to solve it. Withholding any suggestions, you let the employees decide the best way to proceed. You ask them to come up with strategies and report back at the next meeting.

What style of leadership is this?

Name That Leadership Style IV

You call a meeting with your staff members. Using a flip chart, you summarize the factors contributing to the long waits. You separate the employees into groups to find solutions to the most significant factors. Working with you, the groups will reconvene to discuss which solutions should be tried first.

What style of leadership is this?

Ideas for Use

- **Bring in the Reinforcements** and **In-Class Applications** are great ways to review material before an examination.
- These strategies make good transitions to a different topic.
- The short cases make students aware of the importance of the material and the potential examination information.
- Experienced nurses may respond well to this strategy as a way to open class and remind them of information they've learned but perhaps forgotten. By applying basic concepts through a reinforcing strategy, you can ensure that everyone is ready to learn more advanced material.

Speak UP

General Description. Some students think of questions but don't always feel comfortable interrupting a lecture or creative strategy. That's where **Speak UP** comes in handy. If you say these two words at transitional points in the class, you give your students license to ask their questions or request that you repeat something. Simply pause at selected moments and say, "**Speak UP**—this is your opportunity to ask questions or comment." Instructors should emphasize that **Speak UP** represents the students' time for individualized learning and growth. Saying these words provides students with a voice in the classroom.

Preparation and Equipment. The only preparation for this strategy is to review your plan for the class and create opportunities for questions. You can announce the question-and-answer period informally or use slides with the words **Speak UP.**

Example of the Strategy at Work. **Speak UP** works in any class setting but is especially valuable in large classes. Sometimes students ask questions unthinkingly while taking notes; other questions demonstrate a lack of preparation for class. Sometimes such low-level questions frustrate other class participants. On the other hand, each student deserves some clarification of class material. By channeling questions to **Speak UP** periods, you give students time to reflect on other students' questions and make sure they have time to ask their own.

Ideas for Use

- **Speak UP** is a good strategy to use in large classes or when students have many questions. It allows material to flow while respecting students' needs for clarification.
- Instruct students to jot down questions as they arise and wait for the **Speak UP** moment. Sometimes students find that their

question is answered before the **Speak UP** moment or that they are able to reason it out on their own, reflecting a key learning experience.

- Many instructors don't wait long enough for students to compose their thoughts and questions. It's important to wait for a response after we say **Speak UP.** Sources indicate that we should count 5 seconds while waiting for volunteers with questions or comments. You can easily feel pressured to continue class, not allowing students a real opportunity to offer comments, questions, or observations.

- Gauge your time according to the needs of the entire class. This strategy does require you to exert some control to keep a few students from dominating the **Speak UP** time. Students with extensive needs may be invited to visit during office hours or to make an appointment to see you.

- **Speak UP** is a great test review. This strategy gives students a voice in the review session by encouraging them to ask questions and delineate areas of confusion. Rather than reverting to another lecture or teacher-led discussion, the test review focuses on the students' issues. In fact, test reviews should be based on student questions and needs.

- **Speak UP** is a great way to end a multi-session continuing education session or to segue from one class to the next. By saying **Speak UP** at the beginning or end of a class, you give participants the opportunity to seek additional information from previous classes or about current topics without interrupting the flow of the class.

- Questions that are closely aligned with class objectives can become **Think-Pair-Share, Teaching Trios,** or **Group Thought** exercises.

Quotation Pauses

General Description. I use quotations to open each chapter in this book to reinforce material and to capture attention. Quotations provoke thought in the classroom and throw in a little entertainment. In **Quotation Pauses,** the instructor pauses at appropriate times and provides a quotation to reinforce or apply classroom concepts.

Preparation and Equipment. Simply have quotations available when material comes up. As with the chapter-opening quotations, **Quotation Pauses** are meant to generate a "pause for thought" and provide a transition to new material.

Example of the Strategy at Work. I use the following quotation to begin an adolescent health class:

> "Our youth now love luxury. They have bad manners, contempt for authority; they show disrespect for their elders and love chatter in place of exercise; they no longer rise when elders enter the room; they contradict their parents; chatter before company; gobble up their food and tyrannize their teachers." —Socrates, fifth century BC

This quotation puts generational differences in perspective. It also provides some humor to begin the class.

Ideas for Use

- Quotations can be found anywhere—newspapers, the internet, social media, television, anthologies, calendars, inspirational posters, email messages, colleagues, or daily interactions.
- Be attuned to quotations in your personal reading that could reinforce material or grab the attention of an audience.
- One can search the internet for quotes related to almost any topic. Entire websites are dedicated to quotes about learning, healthcare, and just about every topic you wish to incorporate in your teaching session.

Group Thought

General Description. Group work, or **Group Thought,** is a common strategy used in classrooms, large and small, to encourage interactive learning and active thinking. With **Group Thought,** groups of various sizes are directed to certain tasks. Each group may have the same task, or each may be given a different component of the assignment to report back to the larger class. Students in academic classes often look down on group activities as a distraction from testable material. In nonacademic settings, where participants are more receptive to passive learning, **Group Thought** may be considered frivolous and "not on task." Here are some hints to help you make **Group Thought** effective, objective-driven, and productive.

Assigning Groups

For classroom activities, assigning groups is usually preferable to letting students pick their own.

- In large classes, group selection could take all day.
- Given the choice, friends tend to group together, which may not prove productive.

- Students who have a good grasp of the material tend to gravitate to others who also understand it. The reverse is also true: students who don't comprehend material choose to work with others who don't understand it.

Grouping Ideas

- Use the traditional counting-off method: "one, two, three, four; one, two, three, four," and so on.
- Pass out fake money—distribute ones, fives, tens, twenties, and fifties. Ask the students with each denomination to find each other and form a group.
- Use colored pencils, birthday months, color of shirts, randomly picked numbers, or any other differentiating method.
- Use different types of candy to set up groups, with each class member trying to find a partner or group with the same candy.
- Once groups are established, use them for one exercise or keep them together for future group work.

Preparation and Equipment. Prepare the exercise in advance. Ensure that it reinforces class content and meets your objectives. You may want to have supplies on hand to assist with group selection or prizes to hand out as rewards for participation in the exercise.

Example of the Strategy at Work. The most common **Group Thought** exercise is the case scenario with questions. All the groups are given the same questions and different cases. Students answer the questions in relation to the individual cases and then report to the class.

I've used this type of exercise to reinforce legal and ethical principles in the classroom. Using an ethical decision-making model from their text, groups of students review a case and answer these questions:

1. How would you respond?
2. What are the actual and potential legal issues?
3. What are the actual and potential impacts on ethical principles?
4. How do your values influence your thinking about this scenario?
5. What could or should a nurse do, considering this information?

Here are some case studies I have used.

Case 1

A 50-year-old woman is admitted for uterine bleeding and pain. In the assessment, you discover that her husband died 1 week ago and that she is emotionally distraught. She meets with a surgeon who recommends a hysterectomy. The surgeon reviews the informed consent form rapidly and appears hurried. The client is distracted and inattentive, signing the consent form when urged to do so by the surgeon. You have watched the client–surgeon interaction, and the surgeon asks you to witness the consent.

Case 2

A client was admitted with lumbar disk herniation and placed in pelvic traction by a new graduate nurse. Although she had not performed the procedure before, she thought she could do it and did not check the hospital procedure manual. After 3 hours in traction, the client requested pain medication and removal of the traction.

The client noted that the intramuscular (IM) injection did not hurt at all. He realized he had lost feeling in his buttocks and legs and became very agitated. He told the new nurse, who realized she had contributed to the problem. She was afraid to document the treatments and the new developments. She called the physician, who stated that disk herniation is frequently accompanied by these symptoms. The nurse was relieved and did not document the event. The client remained upset and refused traction. His numbness continued after hospitalization.

Case 3

At 7:30 a.m., a 60-year-old female postoperative client complains of pain. She states that she has not received pain medication since last night before bed. She wants to start her day with some pain medication on board. She appears alert and demonstrates signs and behaviors consistent with acute pain. When you see the medical review, you note that the narcotic pain medication was signed out at 8 p.m., 12 midnight, and 4 a.m. The client is due for medication at 8 a.m.

You wonder why the client does not remember the medication. When you look at her chart, you see no mention of medications or pain assessments. The night nurse did not mention administering pain medication, was sleepy in morning report, and expressed that she was anxious to go home.

Case 4

You are caring for a pediatric client receiving chemotherapy for leukemia. The chemotherapy is administered every 4 hours. At 8 p.m., you are very busy with a heavy client assignment, many medications, and lots of treatments. You get your tasks done and feel accomplished in your abilities. When you prepare the next dose of chemotherapy, you discover that you made a calculation error and gave an incorrect dose at 8 p.m.

Case 5

A 75-year-old man is dying of lung cancer and is in extreme pain. You are a hospice nurse, visiting the client in his home. He lives alone and is grieving the loss of his wife 1 year ago. He expresses hopelessness and helplessness to you. He is in despair about his continued anguish and lack of relief. He asks you to leave him enough narcotic pain medication to allow him to self-administer a lethal dose. He is alert and has contemplated his choices. He is not asking you to administer the medication, just to provide enough so he can leave this world.

Students are asked to review these cases and answer the questions in a group. I keep the groups to three or four people to ensure that everyone participates. Because our classes are large, we frequently have more than one group per topic.

I ask each group to report to the class. Other groups add additional findings to the discussion. All the case studies can be found in the LMS and may be used in developing test items. I instruct the students to review all the case studies and listen attentively in class in preparation for the examination.

The **Group Thought** in the following case is one that I have used with senior nursing students and practicing nurses. It involves delegation and how to decide patient assignments, which are difficult concepts to teach.

Management of Client Care: Case Study

The charge nurse is establishing the patient assignments for the shift. Here are the details of the clients and staff members:

- Number of clients: 30
- Number of Registered Nurses (RNs): 4 plus the charge nurse
- Number of Unlicensed Assistive Personnel: 3

Here is the assignment for each Registered Nurse:

RN 1: eight clients (all require routine care; one routine discharge)
RN 2: six clients (two receiving blood; one new admission)
RN 3: six clients (one complex discharge; two beginning chemotherapy)
RN 4: eight clients (two routine discharges; one recent postoperative client)
Charge Nurse: two clients (one has a tracheostomy and is on a ventilator; one needs routine care).

You are assigning the unlicensed assistive personnel (UAP) to assist in managing the unit. Here are the details for the care of some of the clients. Assign them using an assignment sheet from a local clinical agency or one made up to reflect the data in the exercise.

Client 1: This client is being cared for by the charge nurse. He has been on a ventilator for 1 year secondary to cerebral anoxia following a cerebrovascular accident. The client needs lots of suctioning. He receives percutaneous endoscopic gastrostomy tube feedings and needs total care. The UAP is a senior nursing student who has cared for complex conditions but is not as familiar with ventilators. The charge nurse has 6 years' experience on the unit and is well versed in client care and delegation. The charge nurse has had the client the last two nights. The client's status is stable. He is incontinent and has a Glasgow Coma Scale score of 5.

Client 2: This client is under the care of RN 2. He has been newly admitted directly from the doctor's office. His diagnosis is chronic obstructive pulmonary disease (COPD) with acute exacerbation and mild respiratory distress. He is 89 years old and disoriented and has difficulty in swallowing. He needs assistance with activities of daily living and ambulation; he can wash and feed himself. The UAP has been on the unit for 3 years and typically cares for clients with similar needs. The RN caring for the client has been pulled from the pediatric unit but is experienced in the care of clients with respiratory distress.

Client 3: This client is under the care of RN 3. She is postoperative, having had open-heart surgery. She was transferred yesterday from the cardiovascular intensive care unit after being treated for cardiogenic shock and ventricular dysrhythmias. She has a chest tube hooked to 20-cm wall suction through a disposable bedside collection device. She is receiving 40 percent oxygen through a Venturi mask. She is at high risk for postoperative ventricular rhythm disturbances. The RN assigned to the client has had a telemetry course and has moderate experience with cardiac rhythms and postoperative cardiac care. The UAP has recently finished orientation and has not worked with the cardiovascular surgical population.

Students are divided into groups. They're given or asked to bring a copy of the assignment sheet. Students are asked to consider the assignments of each of the RNs and the charge nurse and create a plan for delegating to the UAP. This assignment is an excellent one but does take 15 minutes to complete, potentially taking time from other activities.

Ideas for Use

- Stay in the classroom and roam among the groups. An instructor who leaves the room, checks voice mail, or does other work communicates to the class that the activity is not of much value for participants.
- When students move into groups, allow them to be comfortable. Let them sit on the floor, turn chairs, or leave the room if that's possible.
- Keep group activities short—5 to 7 minutes—and keep time carefully. Difficult or in-depth assignments may prove daunting, and the groups may spend more time complaining than working. To quote my colleague Michelle Deck again, use short periods of time so that students feel some duress in getting their task done and keep the times somewhat irregular to keep participants on task, for example, 3.5 minutes for an assigned exercise.
- Set clear time parameters for **Group Thought.** Use whistles or other attention-getting devices to call the class to order. You may want the students to stay in their positions or return to their more traditional seating patterns when the groups report or when class resumes.
- You may want to vary the size of the groups or their composition. This tactic is helpful if groups aren't staying on task or if one group appears to be struggling more than another.

- For academic classes, make sure that the students connect the group activity with class objectives and testable material.
- Listen to the volume of the group activities. Experience has taught me that the volume in the room goes up when the groups finish their task and revert to personal conversation. Give 1-minute warnings and walk around the room to ensure that groups stay on task.
- **Group Thought** is a great way to foster cooperative learning of complex material, such as setting priorities; interpreting lab, electrocardiogram (ECG), or arterial blood gas data; determining methods of conflict resolution; or focusing on important nursing interventions related to client needs, as in the perioperative period.
- **Group Thought** is an important strategy for building rapport among nurses who work together or spend time together between units. Case studies that reflect clinical skills and daily nursing practice are well received.
- Group activities are critical in nursing education and practice, although not always embraced by students. Working in teams and collaborating are key components of safe care and should be integral to creative teaching in nursing education and as nurses progress into healthcare settings.

Using Mnemonics

General Description. We use mnemonics throughout our lives to remember facts. They provide verbal cues to remembering complex or difficult information. This is an area in which students and instructors can share their memory aids with each other.

Preparation and Equipment. The only preparation for this strategy is to remind yourself about **Using Mnemonics** when covering class content. Search the internet for mnemonics and encourage students to share their own.

Example of the Strategy at Work. Students have great ideas about mnemonics, and experience allows us all to accumulate them as we go along. Here are a few I enjoy:

> In a class on neurological deterioration I explain decorticate and decerebrate posturing. I tell the class that in decorticate posturing the client brings the upper extremities "toward the core." The word *decerebrate* has more Es, indicating extension of the arms.
> When we discuss the uses of different antigout medications, students learn about allopurinol and colchicine. Allopurinol is given for

chronic gout and colchicine for acute gout, so I tell the students that the As and Cs don't match up.

In the class on diabetes, I tell students that hypoglycemia is the "wet one," marked by diaphoresis, and that hyperglycemia is the "dry one," with symptoms of dehydration.

The ABCs of the alphabet are used to reinforce airway– breathing– circulation concepts in cardiopulmonary resuscitation. When memorizing the steps of the nursing process, students are taught to think of "A Delicious Apple PIE" to remember assessment, diagnosis–analysis, planning, implementation, and evaluation.

The potential list is endless. The importance of this strategy is the ability of students to make their own connections and to understand and **Use Mnemonics** consistently.

Ideas for Use

- Try to **Use Mnemonics** any time a complex process requires some level of memorization.
- Several published memorization resources can provide additional ideas. Go to www.medicalmnemonics.com to access additional mnemonics for nursing education.
- Have students post their memory aids on the class website, LMS, or in **Online Discussions.**
- Make sure students understand that mnemonics are memory devices and that they'll eventually need to step beyond retention to critical thinking. Memorization allows students to move on and think more analytically and critically about memorized material.
- Use the strategy of metaphor much as you would use mnemonics. One instructor based the entire class on a "recipe for success" and referred frequently to cooking, ingredients, time, and the product to build a story for the class participants.

Keep 'Em Awake Quizzes, Quickie Quizzes, Quizzes That Count

General Description. Just the mention of the word *quiz* makes students sit up straighter, complain, and panic. From the perspective of the instructor, quizzes provide a valuable way to assess understanding, document class attendance, and get a continuous measure of preparation and knowledge acquisition. Not all quizzes have to count, but quizzes interspersed with classroom presentations may provide a useful way to assess learning.

Keep 'Em Awake Quizzes are simply two or three questions asked in the middle of class. They let you assess understanding and get a "read" on the class. **Quickie Quizzes** can be used as an opener to refresh previously learned material or reinforce preparation for that day's class. These two types of quizzes don't count toward the course grade and can be used effectively in continuing education and staff development.

Quizzes That Count can assess class knowledge, encourage participation and preparation, and offer another chance to students whose test grades are low because of anxiety or poor performance. For our purposes, quizzes consist of three to eight questions and take less than 10 minutes of class time.

Preparation and Equipment. Write the quiz and the answer key before class. Set aside class time for the quiz—you may provide the answers right after the quiz or later. For **Quizzes That Count,** make sure the quiz policy is clear in the class syllabus and that there are guidelines for quiz makeups and grading. You can hand out quizzes or put them on PowerPoint slides. For quiz handouts, use colored paper to set the papers apart from other white papers in their notebooks, or half sheets to conserve paper.

Example of the Strategy at Work.

Quickie Quiz

For a class opener, and as a way to remind students about what they have already learned, I've asked students to complete the following quiz at the start of class. (Our curriculum teaches pathophysiology separately from nursing interventions.) The students are always told that the quiz doesn't count.

Quickie Quiz

Cystic Fibrosis (CF) Quiz—IT DOESN'T COUNT!

1. CF is marked by _____ gland dysfunction.

2. CF is inherited as a(n) _____ trait.

3. The mucus produced in CF can be described as _____ and _____.

4. Stagnant respiratory mucus leads to _____, _____, and _____.

5. Fibrotic changes in the pancreas prevent the release of _____ into the _____.

6. Stools containing fat (_____) and protein (_____) are found in clients with CF.

7. Respiratory assessment of a client with CF and significant pulmonary involvement would show _____.

8. Respiratory care includes _____.

Keep 'Em Awake Quizzes

In the middle of class, I show a few questions on slides to determine how well the students comprehend the material (see the following quiz).

Keep 'Em Awake Quiz

The nurse is caring for a client with a laryngectomy for whom all of the following actions are necessary. Which action should take priority?
A. Bathing and hygiene
B. Assisting with breakfast
C. Suctioning the airway
D. Ambulating to the bathroom

Which of the following is an intervention to prevent the most common complication of a splenectomy?
A. Ambulation
B. Coughing and deep breathing
C. Maintaining IV fluids
D. Isolation precautions

Asking these questions allows students to apply material immediately and show whether or not they understand it.

Quizzes That Count

This strategy was shared with me by a colleague who attended a conference on student evaluation. Nursing education participants had complained about poor class attendance, lack of preparation, and lack of attentiveness. **Quizzes That Count** was developed as a result of these frustrations. The quizzes consist of three questions: the student's name (as a way to take attendance), one about the class readings, and one about the class discussion.

Following is the quiz I give in the middle of the class on cleft lip and palate. At the time that I give the quiz, I have discussed cleft lip but not cleft palate. Thus, the second question assesses attentiveness and the third question assesses the level of class preparation.

A Quiz That Counts

1. Name: _____
2. Name one nursing intervention to protect the incision after a cleft lip repair.
3. Name one nursing intervention to protect the incision after a cleft palate repair.

We allot points in each student's grade for these quizzes. They're given randomly throughout the semester and are unannounced. It's best to vary the time to ensure that the class attends the entire session.

Our instructors have embraced these quizzes with some controversy. Many believe that class attendance and preparation are a personal choice and a component of adult learning. For more junior students, however, quizzes provide structure and incentive to attend, and they illustrate the importance of class readiness. We drop one quiz per semester from the grade to allow for unexcused absences. Our policy is conservative in what we consider an excused absence.

Ideas for Use

- Develop a **Keep 'Em Awake Quiz** in a class with complex material before moving on to the next topic. Students may not admit that they don't know something—or haven't even thought about it yet. A small quiz highlights the material and allows students to figure out whether they understand it or have any questions.
- These **Quizzes** may be used for extra credit when student interest is waning, and before breaks or at the end of the semester.
- **Quizzes** may be used in continuing education programs, such as critical care or other classes in which students are expected to review before attending.
- Use **Quizzes** to focus studying for examinations, or give them before class to ensure that students are prepared. You'll reward their preparation by just going over the answers in class or in a review session.
- **Quizzes** are a great way to keep attention in a continuing education or staff development class. Prizes or other incentives can make them even more interesting.

- Use old examination questions for **Quizzes** to get students comfortable with the level of difficulty and the test question format. You can recycle old quiz questions for subsequent examinations. Doing this reinforces the importance of class attendance.
- Frequent quizzing, as noted in Chapter 3, is a way to help students practice retrieval of forgotten material, calibrate their own knowledge, and assess their future study needs.
- Using **Quickie Quizzes** at the beginning of class encourages students to be on time and settle in quickly.
- One strategy noted in the literature is a **Concept Map Quiz.**[11] Students are charged with developing a concept map based on instructions, and quizzes are graded on depth of knowledge and demonstrated thinking, creativity, and originality.

Feedback Lecture

General Description. The **Feedback Lecture** is a well-documented strategy used to complement traditional lectures and as a means of combining lecture with performance-based instruction.[14] In this way, feedback becomes reciprocal, with both students and teachers learning throughout the process.

As originally designed, the **Feedback Lecture** includes procedures, an introduction, objectives, a pretest, an outline, discussion questions, feedback on discussion questions, warmup activities, and a posttest. Because I've adapted this method to allow for quick feedback, my method includes a pretest, the standard test outline, and a posttest. I encourage you to research the **Feedback Lecture** and use it in any form useful for your own teaching needs.

Preparation and Equipment. As originally designed, this method takes a fair amount of preparation. Even for the abridged version, you need to develop the pretest, outline the lecture (usually done anyway), write the lecture (necessary), and develop the posttest. Once the work is done, however, the **Feedback Lecture** can be used repeatedly in classes.

Example of the Strategy at Work

Pretest

1. Name three components of the preoperative check that the nurse is responsible for completing before sending a client into surgery.
2. Name three components of preoperative teaching and three common postoperative complications that can be prevented through preoperative teaching.

3. Name one way to confirm a client's identity before a surgical procedure.
4. Discuss three differences between the scrub nurse and the circulating nurse.

Discussion Questions

1. How do you respond when you believe a client does not comprehend his or her preoperative teaching?
2. How would you react in the operating room if you were in a situation where a client's condition deteriorated?
3. What safety factors are in place to ensure that the correct surgery is done on a client?
4. How would you react to an immediately postoperative client who refuses pain medication?

Class Outline

I. The role of the nurse in the care of the preoperative client
   A. Preoperative assessments
   B. Preoperative teaching
   C. Safety and risk management
II. The role of the nurse in the care of the intraoperative client
   A. The circulating nurse and the scrub nurse
   B. Anesthesia agents, stages, and client responses
   C. Estimated blood loss; estimated blood replaced
III. The role of the nurse in caring for the postoperative client
   A. Assessments and monitoring
   B. Postanesthesia care unit parameters
   C. Postoperative complications and prevention
   D. Pain and pain management
   E. Diet and activity progression
   F. Dressings and drains
   G. IV therapy
   H. Transfer to the unit or discharge
   I. Discharge teaching

I have used this method to teach difficult topics with many different facets, such as perioperative nursing. I provide the pretest, give the short lecture, allow group discussion on several questions, and then give the posttest. I use the same pre- and posttest for this exercise, but you can make up different ones. I allot significant time to the lecture and discussion portions, encouraging the students to do the pretest before class and the posttest as an **Email Exercise.**

Ideas for Use

- Intersperse **Group Thought** with the **Feedback Lecture** to combine lecture content with interactive learning.
- Use the **Feedback Lecture** with **Admit Ticket** and allow the pretest to be the student's "entrance fee" into class.
- Develop the **Feedback Lecture** format for each class so students get into the habit of being prepared and completing the pretest before class. Build on the pretest questions to construct examination questions.
- For small classes, have individuals or groups develop classes, class outlines, and pretests and posttests. They can present class content to each other while you reinforce or clarify information.
- Use textbook resources to develop pretest and posttest questions and class outlines.

References

1. Herrman J. Using film clips to enhance nursing education. Nurse Educator 31(6):264–269, 2006.
2. Weeks CS. Text-Book for Nursing. Appleton & Co, 1885.
3. Chenovert M. What Do Nurses Do? Pro-Nurse, 2000.
4. Buscaglia L. The Fall of Freddy the Leaf. Holt Rinehart & Winston, 1983.
5. Moss J. Bob and Jack: A Boy and His Yak. Bantam, 1992.
6. Scieszka J. The True Story of the Three Little Pigs. Scholastic, 1989.
7. Jackson K. Nurse Nancy. Golden Books, 1952.
8. Gaspard H. Doctor Dan the Bandage Man. Golden Books, 1950.
9. Applegate K. The One and Only Ivan. HarperCollins, 2015.
10. Smith C. The wonky donkey. Scholastic Paperbacks, 2010.
11. Breytenbach C, Ham-Baloyi W, and Jordan P. An integrative literature review of evidence-based teaching strategies for nurse educators. Nursing Education Perspective 38(4), 193–197, 2017.
12. Glendon KJ and Ulrich DL. Unfolding Case Studies: Experiencing the Realities of Clinical Nursing Practice. Prentice-Hall, 2001.
13. Beyer DA. Reverse case study: To think like a nurse. Journal of Nursing Education 50(1), 48–50, 2011.
14. Flinders University: Using feedback lectures with large classes. www.flinders.edu.au, 2018.

Chapter 6

Strategies for Small Classes

Challenges

> *"Implementing creative teaching strategies that will change a classroom from a four-walled room with educational hopes into an environment that is infused with excitement, curiosity, and genuine student learning."*—Joseph S. C. Simplicio

- Small classes are usually the most enjoyable to teach. Many instructors feel they are most effective when working with smaller groups. Small classes do present challenges in reaching all the students. In some situations, a class of 10 is considered small; in others, a small class can comprise as many as 50 students. The strategies in this chapter are generally useful for groups of 20 to 30, although subtle adaptations can make them applicable to bigger or smaller classes.
- Some students are reluctant to participate and may feel conspicuous in the smaller classroom because it lacks the anonymity of larger classes.
- Smaller classes may be graded for participation. Some contributions are more valuable than others, and some students do not actively participate in class. Therefore, assessing a student's participation creates special challenges for the instructor.
- Small classrooms are especially vulnerable to group dynamics. The personality of the class may encourage a spirit of inquiry or its negative counterpart, a spirit of disdain. Group cohesiveness, or its lack, may challenge instructors who wish to engage students in active strategies.
- Smaller classes may need considerable teaching energy to maintain a high pace of learning and zest for more information.

Small classes offer a great environment for cooperative learning, problem-based formats, and group learning strategies. Creative teaching strategies can enhance an already fertile ground for learning. Innovative teaching gives the instructor a chance to assess group attitudes and needs and improve group functioning. If you're teaching a small class, you can use creative strategies to provide one of the most pleasurable learning experiences for yourself and your students.

IDEAS

Six Hats Exercise

General Description. The **Six Hats Exercise** is used frequently in nursing education and management.[1] It was originally developed by deBono[2] as a way to encourage team building and conflict resolution. Gross[3] has used this tool with nurses and healthcare workers to cultivate decision making, teamwork, and empathy.

In this exercise, hats of different colors represent different ways of looking at an issue. Participants are given hats, each representing a different perspective on an issue. Each student is asked to view a situation through the assigned color. Gross[3] uses the colored hats to represent different perspectives, including red (emotional), green (creative), black (pessimistic), white (logical), yellow (optimistic), and blue (overarching values). Fig. 6–1 shows possible interpretations of the six hats and the perspective each represents.

Preparation and Equipment. If you wish to use this technique, you'll need a situation that lends itself to debate and different perspectives. Look for color-appropriate party hats or other toy hats to pass out to each member of the team. If class size permits, each group should have six members.

Example of the Strategy at Work. I've used this strategy to work on problem-solving skills in two different situations. In the first, a nursing clinical group had just met each other several days before. They encountered a client in circumstances similar to those described in Box 6–1. The students, seeing an ethical issue firsthand, were having a difficult time resolving it both within and among themselves. I used the **Six Hats Exercise** to get them thinking about their own personal views and the perspectives of others, and how to use problem-solving skills in a true dilemma.

I passed out six sheets of colored paper, corresponding to the colors of the hats. My group had seven people, so I gave two people a blue sheet. One person acted as recorder and another as moderator. I set the ground rules for the discussion and the exercise began.

The "blue hat" started the conversation and asked each "hat" to address the situation from its perspective. After each member contributed to the

THE SIX HATS

Emotional RED	Overarching Values BLUE	Logical WHITE
Creative GREEN	Optimistic YELLOW	Pessimistic GREY

Fig. 6–1.   Different perspectives provide a forum for discussion.

conversation, the entire group discussed the ethical problem. The students analyzed the issue using their new understanding and perspectives.

During an in-service training for faculty members, I used the exercise shown in Box 6–2. In this setting, the point of the exercise was to demonstrate its versatility and its possible use in many conflict situations. It's a great decision-making guide and an effective icebreaker. You can use it

---

Box 6–1.
Six Hats for Clinical Nursing Students

Your group has been caring for a client with a ventilator for 1 month. Each member of your group has cared for the client at least once. The client is unresponsive except to painful stimuli and is displaying decerebrate posturing. Sustenance is maintained by the ventilator, hydration, and nasogastric tube feedings.

The students are feeling conflicted, especially because the family keeps asking when the client will be better and will be able to go home. The medical ethics committee has recommended discontinuing the ventilator. Use the six hats to address this issue.

Box 6–2.
Six Hats for Faculty Members

You have a clinical group with eight juniors. Three have worked as hospital aides and two are second-career adult learners. The group has a considerable amount of discord, poor teamwork skills, and a low level of motivation. They bicker and compete with each other. As the instructor, you realize something has to be done. As a group of instructors, use the six hats to think of potential solutions for resolving the group dysfunction.

in leadership training as a strategy for dealing with difficult situations and understanding other perspectives.

Ideas for Use

- Faculty may find the **Six Hats Exercise** a great strategy to use in legal and ethical discussions, with clinical groups, or any time a sensitive issue needs to be addressed.
- Instead of hats, you can give students color-coded name tags or colored paper.
- Use the **Six Hats Exercise** to resolve conflicts or when teamwork is otherwise a challenge. This exercise builds rapport and collegiality. It also develops empathy skills by challenging participants to understand points of view different from their own.
- If time permits, have participants wear more than one hat so they can view a situation from multiple perspectives.
- If you know the group well, assign colors that don't fit the participants' characteristic personalities. For example, give the eternal pessimist a yellow hat and the unemotional person a red one. Arguing from an unaccustomed position fosters critical thinking skills.
- After all the participants have expressed their views, use the discussion time for debriefing. Analyze not only the situation but also the group process. Talk about the emotions and the knowledge participants glean from "walking in each other's moccasins."
- Combine **In-Class Debate** with the **Six Hats Exercise.** Your students will combine research with the perspectives of others to address common issues and arrive at workable conclusions.

In-Basket Exercise

General Description. The **In-Basket Exercise,** first described by Sweeney and Moeller,[4] gives students a task, a time frame, and a limited amount of information. This strategy is a lot like getting an assignment in the in-basket of your computer. Decisions need to be made based on this information because it comes to the in-basket alone, potentially without giving you the opportunity to solicit additional information or view the situation from a variety of perspectives.[5] These exercises are effective in developing group cohesiveness, as early group activities, and in helping students solve problems with incomplete information.

Preparation and Equipment. You need to develop case scenarios that relate to class objectives. The **In-Basket Exercise** works on priority setting, group process, and conflict resolution. The group solves a problem using only the data presented. Each group receives a case study that articulates the client's needs. The case study provides just enough information to ensure resolution but not enough to allow for significant deliberation about the work. Case scenarios may be tailored to specific class content and class objectives.

Example of the Strategy at Work. Here is the exercise I give in class. The students need to base decisions on the information given to them— no extraneous information will be provided—so I issue the following warning:

> This exercise will assist you in analyzing group process. You will have 10 minutes to work in groups of six. All groups will work on the same issue, so it will be interesting to see how different groups think. We will reconvene for 5 minutes to discuss your results and rationales. I'll ask you then to consider the group process information we have discussed in class. We'll assess how your group functioned, the patterns of decision making, and the leadership styles.

The exercise follows.

Stuck

You work in a building with 10 floors. The six group members are on an elevator going up when the elevator stops. When you call for help, you find that all six passengers must be stuck on the elevator for 24 hours. There is no immediate threat to your safety, but you will not be able to get out.

The security manager is able to send down one small plastic grocery bag of supplies for your group to use in those 24 hours. This is all you are allowed. The elevator has ample room and there is enough oxygen, light, and heat for the duration. The security manager will contact you in 10 minutes to determine your requests. Please include a brief rationale for each supply item.

After the group work, it's beneficial to share findings within the class. Repeated use of this strategy teaches the common needs of existence (a great way to reinforce Maslow's Hierarchy of Needs[6]) but also highlights the individuality of human needs. Hygiene, water, food, and diversional activities are paramount. More technical needs—medication, blood glucose monitors, or sedation for people with claustrophobia—enlighten group members to the varied needs of others. This exercise also highlights the complexities of disaster and emergency management.

I used the strategy in a continuing education seminar as a lighthearted exercise for determining the contents of an emergency code bag. Participants in an advanced life-support conference were given the following task:

> You are a transport person who is asked to stock a box with the supplies needed for emergency resuscitation and transport. Unfortunately you can only take enough supplies to fit a 10-in × 18-in × 24-in bag. Spend the next 10 minutes deciding on the integral components for that emergency response bag.

As you can imagine, a spirited discussion followed this assignment.

Ideas for Use

- Subjects for **In-Basket Exercises** may come from clinical situations, legal and ethical conflicts, priority setting, conflicts, and other nursing situations.
- For this strategy to succeed, group members must understand that no more information is available. Like a computer in-basket, these exercises provide only what's there without the luxury of other details.
- You can follow the **In-Basket Exercise** with a class discussion or use a **Write to Learn** or **Quick Write** as an opportunity to comment. **Ah-Ha Journals** may also be used to reflect on the exercise.
- In completing the feature STUCK, mentioned earlier in this chapter, you can ask participants to think of a list of 10 supplies. Then announce they are only allowed three things. This further hones their priority-setting skills.
- **In-Basket Exercises** can keep pace with the increasing knowledge base of a student or novice nurse. You can make the strategy more complex by including more detail about client conditions and clinical situations. This strategy is feasible at many levels of practice. You simply need to design it so students can answer the questions while continuing to feel challenged.
- Community concepts can be reinforced by discussing packing a bag in a disaster, gathering first aid supplies for a mission trip, or caring for a client at home who needs certain supplies and equipment.

- Carefully constructed **In-Basket Exercises** provide a great vehicle for any nursing lesson involving selected data, conflicting priorities, and the establishment of key concerns. I have used it with caring for a client with type 1 diabetes mellitus, a woman in labor at 41 weeks gestation, and a client with bipolar disorder on lithium therapy.
- Orientees may do an **In-Basket Exercise** to learn to deal with nurse-physician conflicts, reacting in sensitive situations, delegating, and other simulated situations.

The Right Thing to Do

General Description. **The Right Thing to Do** is a particularly good way to introduce legal and ethical issues (additional legal case studies are found in Chapter 5). This strategy helps to socialize beginning nurses and nursing students. Hypothetical cases, real issues, and potential dilemmas are presented in class. Students are then asked, "What is **The Right Thing to Do**?"

Preparation and Equipment. Anticipate when legal and ethical issues will come into the foreground of class discussion. Make notations in your lecture notes to set time aside for these issues.

Example of the Strategy at Work. In a discussion about the rights associated with participation in research, such as informed consent, justice, autonomy, and risks versus benefits, I presented several ethical questions to the students (see the list in the feature below). After reading each one I asked, "What is **The Right Thing to Do**?"

Asking individual students "What is **The Right Thing to Do**?" encourages the entire class to stay involved in the process. Applying the question in different circumstances stimulates the development of both critical thinking and professional valuing. I presented the following situations.

- You discover that a colleague has been taking supplies from the unit closet and taking them home for personal use. What is **The Right Thing to Do?**
- A client is very worried that she will undergo the wrong surgical procedure. What is **The Right Thing to Do?**
- A colleague comes to work dressed unprofessionally. What is **The Right Thing to Do?**
- You are caring for a child in the hospital. Walking into the room, you find the child's mother hitting the child repeatedly. What is **The Right Thing to Do?**
- The wife of your client's roommate asks you about the health status of your client. What is **The Right Thing to Do?**

This strategy can promote discussion of some of the general knowledge aspects of nursing. Ask students to reflect on interventions from the commonsense viewpoint inherent in nursing care. Nursing instructors have been accused of stripping innate knowledge from people with common sense, then filling their brains with "nursing knowledge." At any level, this exercise helps instructors recapture the students' common sense and encourages the students to think before acting.

A good example happened with a student I taught early in my educational career. The student had four children; I had none and was fresh out of my graduate program. One evening in clinical, the student rushed toward me in a panic. A child she was taking care of had a temperature of 39.5 degrees Celsius.

The student asked, "What do we do?" in a panicked voice. I replied, "What would you do if you were home and one of your children had that body temperature?" In essence I was asking her, "What is **The Right Thing to Do?**" She answered that she would force fluids, take off excess blankets, give an antipyretic, and call the doctor. I responded, "That's what we do here," indicating that we used the same measures in the clinical area to address a fever.

A component of nursing education is the license to use thinking skills and common sense in solving problems. **The Right Thing to Do** provides that opportunity.

Ideas for Use

- Use a legal and ethical decision-making framework to expand the strategy. You can share this strategy with the students in class. Then provide students with legal or ethical case studies such as those that follow and then simply ask, "What is **The Right Thing to Do?**"

Case 1

A 20-year-old male client reveals during a database completion that he has been a prostitute for 4 years and has engaged in homosexual and heterosexual relationships. He is admitted with signs of respiratory and gastrointestinal infections and is undergoing diagnostic procedures to pinpoint the origin of the infections. He asks you not to tell anyone and becomes angry and anxious about divulging this information.

Case 2

An 18-year-old female client was given general anesthesia for the reduction and casting of fractures of her tibia and fibula. As she was waking up from anesthesia, the nurse explained her care following discharge while her friend went to get the car for the trip home. The nurse wrote in the chart, "Client was instructed and discharged in a wheelchair with her friend." The client went home to bed, took her pain medication, and fell asleep. She awoke finding her foot swollen, cold, and bluish. She attributed these signs and her increasing pain to the fall that caused the fractures. Three days later, she was admitted to the hospital and required a below-the-knee amputation.

Case 3

A 76-year-old woman from a nursing home is admitted to an acute-care facility in acute dehydration. The woman's usual mentation is disorganized but alert. The dehydration has caused her to be disoriented and combative. Restraints are applied to maintain her safety and prevent her from pulling out her intravenous lines. She is visited by her daughter, who is very upset about the restraints. The daughter contends that her mother's nursing home is a restraint-free environment and asks that the restraints be removed.

Case 4

You are an RN who supervises nursing assistants. At the beginning of your shift, you discover that one of the clients has been experiencing dizziness and complaining of lightheadedness. When you delegate tasks to the nursing assistant, you instruct her to be cautious when helping the client to walk. You encourage her to seek help if needed. At 10 p.m. the nursing assistant comes to tell you that she found the client on the bathroom floor. She states that she left the client at the sink to brush her teeth while she saw to another client's needs. The client is sitting on the bathroom floor holding her head when you arrive.

Case 5

A 45-year-old man is a client in your community clinic. He has a known history of drug abuse and has been treated recently for a fractured femur. He arrives at the clinic complaining of continued pain. The healthcare provider prescribes that you dispense a placebo medication, arguing that the client is addicted to the drugs and is not experiencing real pain.

Case 6

You work in a family planning clinic. You are completing the database for a 16-year-old girl who believes she is pregnant. You find that she has one 3-year-old child and has had two abortion procedures since the birth of that child. Her pregnancy test is negative, but you find that she has been forced to have sexual relations with her older brother's friends.

- Asking "What is **The Right Thing to Do?**" encourages students to use common sense and basic principles to reason through a situation.
- Bowles[5] proposed a game entitled "Find the Error." In this exercise, instructors provide statements with incorrect components. Students correct the statements using critical thinking skills. These statements are meant to challenge analytical skills rather than simple recall of facts.
- This strategy may be used to discuss any legal or ethical dilemma, such as substance abuse, access to care, and much more.
- Discussing **The Right Thing to Do** is a great way to spark conversation in the clinical area. Students frequently feel pulled between the priorities of clinical work, the needs of the client, and whatever conflicts their classes have taught them to anticipate. The strategy challenges students to consider several perspectives and come to some conclusion about what may and may not be right in specific situations.
- Clinical groups may discuss nursing practices different from the ones they've learned previously. This exercise helps them judge the merits and the correctness of unfamiliar practices.
- Students have trouble accepting the fact that different methods can produce the same result. They want to learn the one right method and are frustrated by multiple perspectives. **The Right**

Thing to Do emphasizes that many things can be done in more than one way.

- The strategy reminds nurses of their responsibility for ensuring the basic principles of asepsis, safety, and client respect. Any alternative method must adhere to these principles. The old adage "There's more than one way to skin a cat" reinforces the reality of pluralist, multiple approaches in many nursing processes. A discussion of basic principles can go a long way toward allaying fears and clarifying procedures, and may generate research questions about clinical practice.

Gaming

General Description. Any nursing class content can be put into game format. You can choose a marketed game, adapt a game show, or devise your own games at home. Computer-based games have also been documented in the literature as effective in reinforcing key concepts and are easy to implement in today's classroom.[7] The use of avatars, software packages, and computer simulation provide opportunities for bringing gaming into students' learning experiences.

Preparation and Equipment When planning a game, keep in mind the class objectives, group size, and volume of content. Games can last 10 minutes or the entire class period. You can use games to test knowledge or provide an unusual out-of-class study. You may want to clarify the purpose of the game—teaching information, reinforcing content, assessing knowledge level, summarizing a class, or reviewing for an examination.

In smaller classes you can use board games to teach concepts. These games can be purchased or you can make your own. You can also adapt a game show to assist with course-specific content. Students enjoy the competition, creativity, and fun associated with gaming in the classroom, but the games do take a lot of preparation and time in the classroom.

One game show popular in the classroom is *Jeopardy.* You need to pick the topic for *Jeopardy* and find five categories for answers. You compose five answers for each category in which questions are progressively more difficult as the money amount increases on the chart. Some instructors choose to develop a Daily Double to add an extra challenge. Search the internet for digital, PowerPoint jeopardy setups that include the jingle, the host, and Daily Double, and other highlight in the templates.

Example of the Strategy at Work. Table 6–1 shows my game board for Developmental Jeopardy. I use this game to teach the developmental aspects of caring for a client with diabetes. PowerPoint lets me use animation in my game boards, and I can make answers emerge with a mouse click. The more real you can make the game, the better.

Table 6–1.   Developmental Jeopardy

Psychomotor Skills	Psychoemotional Characteristics	Cognitive Understanding	Teaching Strategies	Name That Stage
100	100	100	100	100
200	200	200	200	200
300	300	300	300	300
400	400	400	400	400
500	500	500	500	500

Developmental Jeopardy

In Developmental Jeopardy, I use some of the following questions for the Cognitive Understanding category:

100 This developmental skill allows children to use literature, check doses, and use lists.
(What is reading?)

200 This developmental skill allows school-age children to categorize the symptoms of hyperglycemia and hypoglycemia.
(What is classification?)

300 This developmental skill allows school-age children to know when to get injections, snacks, and meals.
(What is the concept of time?)

400 An adolescent girl needs to know that during her menses, insulin needs may _____.
(What is increase?)

500 This form of reasoning allows children to make the leap from signs and symptoms of hypoglycemia to action steps.
(What is inductive?)

Here's an example of the questions I use for the Teaching Principles category:

100 Doing an activity over and over adheres to this principle of teaching skills.
(What is repetition?)

200 Using a doll could assist in teaching these skills.
(What are insulin administration and blood glucose monitoring?)

300 These strategies may be effective in teaching diet planning to school-age children.
(What are meal planning and 24-hour diet recall?)

400 Including the family is an effective teaching strategy because diabetes is this kind of disease.
(What is a family disease?)

500 Role playing may be effective in addressing emotional issues because it does this.
(What is provides practice or develops empathy?)

In this class, Jeopardy is used to introduce the content. When you use a game to teach a topic for the first time, make sure the content is easily understood or that it synthesizes existing knowledge. You can also provide a **Worksheet** or handout for students who need more comprehensive and organized coverage of the topic.

My favorite use of Jeopardy is in test reviews. Students seem to especially enjoy Pharmacology Jeopardy as a way to prepare for the final examination. I bring bells for the students to ring when they have an answer and give prizes to everyone. I'm always surprised at the level of competition these games create, even though no real rewards or consequences are associated with them.

Gaming doesn't have to get this elaborate to be fun and thought-provoking. Puzzles and simple games make great brain teasers and icebreakers. On the first day of clinical rotation, they help to allay fears and encourage teamwork. Here is one inspired by a common household magazine.

Rhyming Puzzlers

Think of a three-word common phrase to rhyme with the Puzzler.

Puzzler	Answers
1. Took, Sign, Blinker	Hook, Line, Sinker
2. Flop, Cook, Glisten	Stop, Look, Listen
3. Leg, Sorrow, Wheel	Beg, Borrow, Steal
4. Trap, Shackle, Top	Snap, Crackle, Pop
5. Mud, Fret, Cheers	Blood, Sweat, Tears
6. Sprawl, Tedium, Barge	Small, Medium, Large
7. Ball, Stark, Ransom	Tall, Dark, Handsome
8. Versed, Beckoned, Heard	First, Second, Third
9. Wife, Pork, Croon	Knife, Fork, Spoon
10. Head, Fright, Crew	Red, White, Blue

Box 6–3.
Match Game

"Sunsetting" eyes, bulging fontanel	Increased intracranial pressure
Sunken fontanel, dry mucous membranes	Dehydration
No stools, can't pass rectal thermometer	Imperforate anus
Positive Barlow's and Ortolani's signs	Developmental hip dysplasia
Respiratory distress, formula from nose	Cleft palate
Tremors, lethargy	Hypoglycemia
Machine-like heart murmur	Patent ductus arteriosus
Small pustular rash	Milia
Cheeselike substance on skin	Vernix caseosa
Meatus under penis	Hypospadias

Match Game

Another game I have used is much simpler and makes a good icebreaker. I gave each student an index card. Half the cards listed the major signs and symptoms of a disease or condition; the other half had the names of those diseases or conditions. Students had to travel around the room to find the card that matched theirs. The game took only 5 minutes, but it provided a rapid review of class content. Box 6–3 shows some of the Match Game cards I used when teaching newborn assessment.

Ideas for Use

- **Gaming** is a great way for both you and your students to assess knowledge before class discussion or in preparation for an examination.
- Use **Gaming** at the end of the semester, or the end of the course, as an examination review or to encourage cumulative learning.
- Several marketed games have been developed by entrepreneurial nurses to foster learning. One such person is Kathleen Walsh Free,[8] who developed a game called What If? What Else? What Then? Free has developed more than eight games to reinforce critical thinking skills, prioritization, data analysis methods, problem solving, and nursing interventions. Games are specialty specific; I've used the pediatric edition in pediatric clinical post-conferences. A new game called What Next? provides unfolding

case studies that reflect complex, dynamic client conditions. These games are valuable in nursing orientation groups and classes on decision making. For more information, see www.whatifgame .homestead.com.

- Technology has greatly advanced our **Gaming** opportunities. Many websites are available to assist with game construction and development. Just a word of caution: games take a lot of class time. Always keep class objectives in mind to ensure that **Gaming** stays on task.

- Paul and Elder[9] proposed a game entitled Deck of Events. Instructors use a deck of index cards, each with a critical thinking exercise or clinical question. The authors propose that instructors design their own clinical question deck and use it to challenge students during free time in the clinical area or at postconference.

- If you are using **Gaming** as a test review, make a **Worksheet** of the major concepts and allow students to fill in the blanks. This technique allows the game to proceed in a more controlled fashion.

- Imitating the television show *What's My Line?,* Bowles[10] proposed forming panels of students who represent specific diseases, diagnoses, or procedures. Other students question the panel in order to guess their identities. Bowles also cites a game entitled Reverse Bingo as a means to review class material. The instructor prepares a bingo card for each student. Only one card has the answers to all 25 questions in the game. The instructor calls out the 25 questions, and students cover each answer as the matching question is asked. The winning student fills the bingo card and correctly answers the 25 questions.

Imagine and Remember When

General Description. Teaching empathy to new nurses can be a challenge. Asking students to **Imagine** living through an ordeal and using personal imagery to describe the emotions evoked is a valuable way to enhance sensitivity. Sources document the use of imagery as a means to let students develop mental models of learned material, and then practice it to master skills and acquire knowledge.[11]

Remember When asks students to step back in time to remember a situation in their own lives similar to the one being discussed in class. Again, empathic understanding is the key lesson in this exercise.

Preparation and Equipment. There is little preparation for this exercise. Consider class content for which these strategies may be appropriate. You

> ## Box 6–4.
> ## Imagine
>
> You are 6 years old. You've been admitted to the hospital for a tonsillectomy. You're having significant pain at the surgical site. Your mother is staying with you in the hospital. Your roommate is a 1-year-old with "a bad cold."
>
> You don't want to express your pain because the nurse will make you swallow yucky medicine. The nurse tells your mom, with you listening, that you can't go home until you drink and pee. You don't like strange potties. It hurts to drink.
>
> Now it's getting dark and you're afraid. Your mom has gone to the bathroom. The IV pump at your bedside starts to beep. People are talking in the hall, but you're lonely. You want to go home. You feel a tear fall down your cheek. You wipe it away and the IV board on your hand scratches you.
>
> The nurse comes in and says hi, smiles, and turns on the bright lights. He's holding a drink, an electric thermometer, and a chart. You can tell he means business. Your mom isn't back yet, and you're really scared!

may want to create slides to formalize the exercise and encourage students to see its value.

Example of the Strategy at Work. In a class about children's responses to surgery and hospitalization, I used an imagery exercise slide to help my students **Imagine** (Box 6–4). We then discussed the developmental considerations of caring for pediatric clients, the fears children have in the clinical area, and the nurse's role in helping children cope with these stressors. I applied **Remember When** in a course on adolescent health behavior, asking students to think back to some of the struggles associated with the adolescent years (Box 6–5).

In a class on change theory, I asked students to **Remember When** they changed a personal behavior or habit. After they have identified the habit, such as biting nails, unhealthy eating, beginning an exercise routine, or adhering to a budget, they then explore the facilitating factors, the barriers to change, and the benefits of making the change.

For many students, the illness, pain, and injury they witness in the clinical area are foreign to their personal experience. **Imagine** helps these students contemplate the impact such stressors may have on their personal lives.

In contrast, many students can draw on personal or familial events to develop or enhance empathy skills. **Remember When** allows students

Box 6–5.
Remember When

Remember your adolescent years:
- Your level of self-esteem
- Your peer pressures
- Your parents' expectations
- Your own concerns and expectations
- Societal issues and pressures

to share these personal experiences in class. For life skills classes, such as assertiveness, conflict resolution, or stress management, **Remember When** is a great way to uncover previous experiences and discuss how they were resolved. Thinking of alternative resolutions and discussing consequences foster problem-solving skills.

Ideas for Use

- Many people enter nursing because of personal experiences with healthcare or illness. **Remember When** provides a mechanism for catharsis and vicarious learning. You may need to guide this discussion if it gets off track or more detailed than class time will allow.
- **Imagine** may be used as a personal role-play exercise. Students build empathy by picturing what it would be like to experience any of the conditions discussed in class. Some **Imagine** exercises may be so realistic that they stimulate significant emotional responses. Instructors need to assess classes and provide debriefing or personal attention as needed.[11]
- Many athletes use **Imagine** or some other type of imagery to mentally accomplish a task, win a race, or reach a goal. Have your students **Imagine** changing a dressing, inserting a nasogastric tube, providing tracheostomy care, or administering an injection so that they may master these skills more easily. Newer research is examining the value of **Imagine** for teaching psychomotor skills, approaches to care situations, and ways to handle unexpected circumstances.[12]
- Combine **Imagine** or **Remember When** with **Write to Learn** or **Quick Writes** to let students reflect on these exercises.
- In both **Imagine** and **Remember When**, ask students to focus on the emotions evoked during the scenarios. Have the class discuss these emotions and the role they play in fostering empathy. Ask the students to consider the client's reactions to the nonempathic nurse.

- One creative colleague assigns freshmen students the first *Harry Potter* novel, in which Harry arrives at his new school.[13] The instructor then asks students to **Imagine** their new lives as college students. How are their experiences similar to Harry's? How are they different? What a great way to help new students examine their personal lives and emotions!
- Construct an **Email Exercise** asking students to **Remember When** and discuss a time when they confronted a challenge or obstacle. Ask them to compare and contrast this event with the challenge a client faces when receiving a new medical diagnosis.
- Foster relationships by asking practicing nurses to **Remember When** they were students or novice nurses.

Twosies

General Description. In this strategy, students pair up to accomplish a task. This exercise may be very brief or more involved. Pairs can stay together for a single exercise or throughout the session or even longer. The small size of the group helps students get comfortable with the exercise. This strategy is less elaborate than **Think-Pair-Share.** In **Twosies**, students simply pair up for the exercise and complete the task.

Preparation and Equipment. Little preparation or equipment is needed, but you must plan when to use **Twosies** and how to make it work in class.

Example of the Strategy at Work. I have used this strategy in several ways. When discussing how nonverbal gestures and facial expressions affect communication, I ask the **Twosie** partners to say to each other, "I like your shirt," twice. The first time they use positive nonverbal signals: a pleasant tone and expression convey sincerity. The second time they frown and speak in a disdainful tone, their insincerity obvious. The students quickly get the importance of nonverbal communication and understand why a nurse must assess both verbal and nonverbal modes when "reading" a client. In addition, students are encouraged to consider their own nonverbal messages to which clients may be exposed. In the same class, the students showed each other expressions of happiness, anger, sadness, and fear, reinforcing the role of facial expressions in communication and client assessment. I used **Twosies** again in a class on pain assessment, emphasizing the need to evaluate facial grimacing as a nonverbal sign of pain.

Students in my assessment class paired up and looked at each other's shoes. I asked them to come up with 10 words to describe those shoes— *old, new, dirty, clean, big, little,* the color, and so on. I pointed out that they'd just done an assessment. We discussed the words they would use and the things they would look for when assessing clients, families, and communities. Used this way, **Twosies** brings home the nature of assessment and the need for assessment skills in comprehensive care. Students realized the need to learn both the techniques and the terminology of assessment. In **Twosies**, students can count each other's respirations, auscultate breath sounds, assess muscle tone or other aspects of physical assessment.

Brain teasers, games, and activities may be used in **Twosie** pairs. Here's a game I participated in at a conference. It's best done with students who are experienced travelers. You can use it as an icebreaker or as a **Twosie** to build rapport. Pairs work together to identify the following airport abbreviations. This is a stumper for even the most seasoned traveler. Answers follow, and some will surprise you.

Name That Airport

United States
1. LAS _____
2. SMF _____
3. RSW _____
4. HNL _____
5. LAX _____
6. MCO _____
7. AUS _____
8. TPA _____
9. JAX _____
10. MSP _____

International
11. HKG _____
12. CDG _____
13. ATH _____
14. TXL _____
15. PEK _____
16. VCE _____
17. YYZ _____
18. SYD _____
19. FCO _____
20. SVO _____

Answers
1. Las Vegas
2. Sacramento
3. Fort Myers
4. Honolulu
5. Los Angeles
6. Orlando
7. Austin
8. Tampa
9. Jacksonville
10. Minneapolis

Answers
11. Hong Kong
12. Paris
13. Athens
14. Berlin
15. Beijing
16. Venice
17. Toronto
18. Sydney
19. Rome
20. Moscow

Ideas for Use

- **Twosies** is an excellent strategy to use in large classes where students don't know each other or where group work may become too cumbersome.
- **Twosie** pairs can address any exercise, assignment, or question.
- Use tavern and children's puzzles, **Clinical Decision-Making Exercises,** and other creative strategies to develop **Twosie** activities.
- **Twosie** exercises are great ways to learn technical clinical information. Have pairs work on interpreting electrocardiogram strips, deciphering lab results, interpreting blood gas values, calculating medication dosages, troubleshooting equipment, answering complex questions, or wading through the **Muddiest Part** of class content.

What's the Point? or What's the Big Deal?

General Description. This strategy is named after one of my personal experiences in nursing school. After making a grave but not life-threatening medication error, I said to my clinical instructor, "Well, what's the big deal?" That phrase has haunted me throughout my years as nurse and educator—I didn't know, but should have, what the big deal was. Now my role as nurse educator is to teach students **What's the Big Deal?**

Practicing nurses usually know what the priorities are and **What's the Big Deal?** Novices may need some guidance in discerning priorities, especially in complex situations. This strategy provides that guidance. After presenting content or a client case, ask students, **What's the Point?** or **What's the Big Deal?** Grounding content and emphasizing priorities are vital not only in nursing care but also for passing the NCLEX® examination.

Preparation and Equipment. Consider the right time to ask these questions in class. The timing depends on the level of your students, the course content, and the priorities you wish to emphasize. Priority setting requires subtle thinking and may be difficult at first—students must differentiate between intricate datasets to discover which priorities are highest. Experienced nurses may practice this skill intuitively, but new nurses and students benefit greatly from practice.

Example of the Strategy at Work. I use this strategy in many of the lectures I present. It's a great way to get attention. Sometimes, when the class is writing notes with heads bowed, I ask, **"What's the Big Deal?"** or **"What's the Point?"** It usually surprises me to see heads pop up. Suddenly the students are all ears—they want to know the answers. They may just be curious. They may also realize these cue questions mean "This is important and may be on the test."

Simply asking these questions starts the students thinking. For example, in a pharmacology class we were discussing nitroglycerine and its actions in relieving angina. We discussed client education and the side effects of the medication. Sildenafil (Viagra) is contraindicated with nitroglycerine. By simply asking, **"What's the Big Deal?,"** I helped students realize that potentially life-threatening hypotension could result from an interaction. My question brought home the importance of this issue in clinical assessment.

In another class, we were discussing sickle cell crisis and the significance of abdominal distention. I presented a **Quickie Case Study** in which the nurse notes that the client's blood pressure is lower than previous values. I asked, **"What's the Point?"** The class discussed the implications of abdominal distention and falling blood pressure: possible sequestration crisis, splenic rupture, and shock. When I placed the situation in this framework, the students understood its gravity.

In a seminar for senior students, we discussed their progress through nursing school and their ability to now "think like a nurse." In that discussion, we talked of the following client picture: A 4-year-old client enters the emergency department with a high fever, nuchal rigidity, a decreased level of consciousness, and a rash on her entire torso—**What's the Big Deal?** Students were asked to consider what their concerns would have been freshman year as novices and now as graduating seniors. To the novice student, a fever and rash do not seem serious. The stiff neck is from "sleeping the wrong way." In contrast, experienced nurses know the signs of bacterial meningitis with potentially life-threatening outcomes and find this situation a grave one needing immediate nursing and medical care.

Ideas for Use

- Use these questions—**"What's the Big Deal?"** and **"What's the Point?"**—any time you want to convey the seriousness of a condition or the importance of a nursing intervention. If you use them often, students will soon recognize these questions as a signal designating important information.
- These questions enhance test-taking skills. Here's a common student frustration with multiple-choice nursing examinations: often all four answers are correct. Students are expected to pick the *best* answer. This strategy helps them discriminate enough to choose the highest priority.
- Use **Case Studies** to set the climate for these questions. Have students sift through to find the most significant data by asking, **"What's the Big Deal?"**

- Use these questions to ask students to relate class content to their personal or clinical experiences.
- You can also ask experienced students to differentiate priorities between clients, asking **"What's the Big Deal?"** when seeking priorities of care.
- For a lesson in diversity, ask, **"What's the Point?"** when discussing cultural or spiritual priorities. Students are often surprised to discover the variety of their classmates' attitudes toward these issues. This strategy provides insight into the importance of assessing and respecting the cultural or spiritual aspects of a client's life.

Jigsaw

General Description. As the title suggests, this strategy is designed like a jigsaw puzzle. Each piece represents information that contributes to the whole picture but may not mean much in itself. Students learn that their piece of the puzzle—their contribution—is an important part of the whole; as systems theory tells us, the whole is greater than the sum of its parts. This strategy, first described by Aronson et al.,[14] has been used extensively in nursing, education, and medicine to teach group problem solving and course content.[15]

Preparation and Equipment. In **Jigsaw** you need to break the class content or objectives into manageable chunks. These chunks represent the pieces of the puzzle, which can be completed by a group, pair, or individual. You then give each group the assignment and a time frame for the task. You must also allot time for sharing in the classroom or think of a way to communicate findings to all the students.

Example of the Strategy at Work. I used this exercise in a class on pediatric orthopedic anomalies. The class was designed to discuss five or six diagnoses. There were significant commonalities among the different conditions. I decided to form groups to work on each diagnosis so we could discuss these similarities in class, which included pain control, postsurgical care, neurovascular assessment, skin care, immobility, and developmental care.

In preparation for the class I assembled a list of conditions from the course objectives. They included developmental dysplasia of the hip, scoliosis, Legg-Calvé-Perthes disease, slipped capital femoral epiphysis, and talipes equinovarus (clubfoot). Each group was assigned a diagnosis. I asked the students to bring their pediatric text and be ready to work. To give each group its assignment, I used a colorful slide (see Fig. 6–2).

TODAY'S ACTIVITY FOR EACH DISORDER

- **Organic Changes**
  (Define the disorder and
  the pathophysiology)

- **Assessment**
  (Identify 5–6 assessments
  and diagnostic tests to
  detect/differentiate
  this disorder)

- **List 5–6 Management
  Strategies**

- **List 5–6 Nursing
  Considerations**
  (Consider nursing role
  with treatments)

Fig. 6–2. Jigsaw exercise for a class on pediatric orthopedic abnormalities.

For each disorder, the group had the following responsibilities:

- Define the disorder and the pathophysiology (identify organic changes).
- Identify five to six assessments and diagnostic tests to detect and differentiate this disorder.
- List five to six management strategies.
- Identify five to six nursing considerations—consider the nurse's role in each treatment.

I printed out the slides I'd created for each diagnosis and gave each group the appropriate printout as a **Worksheet.** We then reconvened to discuss the exercise and the common components of care. Students discussed the surgical procedures, pain issues, assessments, and the role of the nurse in the care of these children. Students were encouraged to take notes on each other's presentations. The **Worksheets** were posted outside the classroom. Test questions were derived from the content of the **Worksheets** and from the notes.

Ideas for Use

- This strategy requires significant student buy-in. The first time I used it, only two of more than 100 students remembered to bring their text. As a result, the exercise was so devalued that I ended up delivering a traditional lecture. The next time this class came around, I emphasized the students' need to bring their pediatric texts and assured them that test questions would be derived from the exercise.
- You may wish to do a smaller version of **Jigsaw** in a discussion group or clinical group (see **Clinical Puzzle**).
- Use **Case studies** to develop a **Jigsaw** exercise. In this exercise, it's necessary to show that each group member's contribution is integral to the whole.
- Make sure to set specific and realistic time limits so students use their time well.
- Circulate in the classroom to answer questions and keep the class on track.
- Post the **Worksheets** and the groups' conclusions on the learning management system (LMS).
- Groups can give miniseminars in class. Encourage students to take notes on their classmates' findings.
- Use **Jigsaw** as a way to teach project management, group process, and other exercises that foster teamwork.

Clinical Decision-Making Exercises

General Description. **Clinical Decision-Making Exercises** help students learn critical thinking and problem-solving skills. Resolution of conflicts and other problems is based on case studies and interviews. Each case study is developed to coincide with class content and objectives, and students apply the decision-making strategies they've discussed in class. In addition to these skills, they can draw on personal experience and clinical information.

Preparation and Equipment. You need to develop the case study and questions in advance. Consider the decision-making strategies you've taught in class, and design cases to challenge the students' problem-solving skills.

Continuing education and staff development instructors can use a single case study for a needed break during class or in-services. It's an effective way to reinforce points of interest. Academic instructors need to develop a grading system and explain it in the class syllabus. One downside of these assignments is that they can take a long time to correct and log in. (What better opportunity to put teaching assistants or graduate students to work?)

It's rewarding to read the students' answers, which generally demonstrate insight and thought. Here are the grading system and instructions I use with this assignment:

Students will read cases, interviews, and scenarios (see the LMS). Students will answer questions and provide reflections via email responses. Emails must be sent to class teaching assistants via the LMS. They are sent using the email assignment/mailbox icon on the course home page. No emails are accepted if they are received via other email routes.

Clinical decision-making assignments are due by 5:00 p.m. on the date given in the class schedule. No assignments are accepted late!

GRADING RUBRIC

2 points: Submission meets assignment objectives, was on time.
1 point: Submission does not fully meet assignment objectives, was on time.
0 points: Submission was not on time, was not done, or did not meet assignment objectives.

Example of the Strategy at Work. Here are some of the assignments I used in an introductory nursing class. You can see how easily this assignment may be adapted for the content of your class.

Clinical Decision Making: Assignment 1

Hello. My name is Margaret Sanger. I am best known for my work in advocating for birth control to provide women with choices about their fertility. I am a nurse, but I found the occupation somewhat confining and decided to work as both a nurse and a socially conscious citizen.

Early in my career as a public health nurse, I saw women who were forced to bear many children because they lacked family planning resources and information. I was present at the death of a woman who had had several children in a few years, had no healthcare resources, and was financially unable to support her growing family. When I was taken to her third-floor apartment,

I noted the dirty, poverty-ridden environment. The client later died of hemorrhage and infection. I vowed I would devote my life work to affording every woman the right to control conception.

I found that rich women had access to information and birth control methods from Europe. Poor women, who had an even greater reason to control conceptions, were lacking in such resources. My efforts in providing birth control information included writing documents about family planning, traveling to other countries to research their contraceptive practices, and lobbying for the provision of birth control to the public. I was scorned for my work, arrested in several states because of the information I had disseminated, and criticized for my stance on women's rights and choices.

At the time, women had just been granted the right to vote. Many legislators and other men in the United States still believed that entitlement to be wrong. Birth control was considered a private, "non-discussed" issues among many policy makers—who were, of course, male. Yet I challenge each of them to consider their own sexual practices. I challenge them also to think of their own children, and to consider childbearing and childrearing from the perspective of a woman. If they were not wearing the cloak of denial, they might feel very differently and might change their belief that birth control is only a woman's concern.

Many people accused me of wanting to control births among the poorer lower classes because I wanted to create a superior race. I must defend my efforts by saying that it is the poor who most direly need access to and information about birth control. I in no way wish to create another segment of society. In contrast, I want to let women enjoy sexual activity without the constant fear of pregnancy. I want to let families grow to their desired, affordable, and optimal size. I want to give women a way to function in the workforce and the public world in an arena of choice and autonomy.

These beliefs are rooted in my background as a nurse and in my philosophy about human rights. I do not regret the years I devoted to these initiatives. In fact, these early accomplishments led to the development of the Planned Parenthood Foundation, later known as the International Planned Parenthood Foundation. I hope these words provide insight into the decision making that was once required of nurses, and the impact of those nurses on today's practice.

1. Cite one aspect of Margaret Sanger's life that exemplifies clinical decision making.
2. Name one social, gender, or historical factor that may have influenced Margaret Sanger's efforts.

3. Name one way you might generalize the key points of this
    scenario to your own nursing values and practice in clinical
    decision making.

Clinical Decision Making: Assignment 2

Hello. My name is John James. I am the nurse manager of an oncology unit at a major hospital center. I deal with many staff issues
relating to professionalism and the image of nursing as a profession.

Nursing has given me the opportunity to practice nursing science
independently and use my clinical decision-making skills every day. I
work in collaboration with many other health professionals, but I feel
self-directed and independent in my practice. Many people ask me
why, as a man, I went into nursing. I'd always wanted to help people
and provide a service to the community. I also felt that people look
up to nurses for their knowledge. People who need care trust nurses.

When I got out of high school I wasn't sure what I wanted to do.
I worked in a restaurant for a while. Then I had to have my appendix
out. I watched the nurses and thought, "I can do that!" I decided to
go to a university to get a BSN.

I belong to two nursing organizations: the American Nurses
Association (ANA) and the Oncology Nursing Society. In these
groups I can actively advocate for my clients. The ANA, for example,
wrote the *Nursing Code of Ethics*, which guides me in providing safe,
confident, and respectful care. I participate in nursing research. Our
unit is studying pain management in cancer clients and is researching
ways to help families with the grieving process.

Nursing research helps with the many questions I want answered.
One problem I'd like to work on is the best way to take blood pressures. Nurses do that assessment all the time and don't realize how
important it is. On my unit we've been discussing whether a blood
pressure in the forearm will be the same as one in the upper arm.
The results of that research may change my nursing assessments
and the way I practice.

1. Cite five criteria of professionalism noted in this scenario.
2. Name one way in which these criteria can influence clinical
    decision making.
3. Without looking at any research, describe in one sentence
    what you think about using the forearm instead of the upper
    arm to assess blood pressure.

Clinical Decision Making: Assignment 3

Mr. Truman was admitted to the hospital on November 1, after experiencing chest pain and shortness of breath. He had undergone cardiac surgery about 10 years before and was beginning to have symptoms again. He was scheduled for a cardiac catheterization, but it was delayed until November 3 because of technical problems. The physician also referred Mr. Truman to a diet counselor for a low-cholesterol diet.

The cardiac catheterization was done without complications and no surgery was indicated. Mr. Truman was hospitalized overnight for observation. On November 4, it was noted that he had a low-grade fever. He was treated with acetaminophen and given three doses of IV antibiotics. His temperature returned to normal and he was discharged on November 5.

Principal diagnosis: Ischemia, heart disease
Secondary diagnosis: Disturbances heart, functional—long-term effect of cardiac surgery
Diagnosis-related group (DRG) assigned: DRG 125; circulatory disorders except acute myocardial infarction with cardiac catheterization without complex diagnosis.
Allowed length of stay: 2.2 days
Actual length of stay: 4.1 days
DRG payment per discharge = $6,800.00
Actual hospital costs = $10,348.00
Loss for hospital = $3,548.00

1. How did the technical problems and Mr. Truman's temperature affect the length of his hospital stay and the hospital costs?
2. How can a hospital make up the lost funds?
3. State one impact of healthcare financing on clinical decision making.

Clinical Decision Making: Assignment 4

Hello. My name is Joe Jones. I am 38 years old. About 10 years ago, I was a wild guy. I was drinking and riding a motorcycle without a helmet. I hit a wet spot in the road and slid. My bike went out from under me and I fell head first into the road. Witnesses said I took a dive into the ground.

After the accident I was unable to move anything from the waist down. I was taken by helicopter to a trauma center, put on a ventilator, and supported through IV fluids and nutrition. I was eventually able to breathe on my own and eat real food. I spent 3 months in a hospital rehabilitation unit learning to take care of myself. I learned how to do my own activities of daily living, live within my environment, and relate to others with my new abilities and disabilities. I've become quite independent.

Nurses took care of me in the period right after my injury, monitoring vital signs, assessing my status, and providing lots of physical care. As I progressed, nurses helped me learn how to lead a fulfilling life. I am married, we have one child, and I work at a library. I'm sad that I can't walk, but in many ways my life is better because of my life-changing accident.

1. After reviewing Neuman's systems theory or the school of nursing organizational framework, state how each defines each component of the metaparadigm: nurse, client, environment, and health.
2. State one way in which either theory can influence clinical decision making.
3. After reading the scenario, state two ways in which either theory may be used to interpret this situation.

Clinical Decision Making: Assignment 5

I'll tell you a story from when I was a new nurse. On my first weekend as an RN, I was in the middle of admitting a client who had sustained a hip fracture. The client was 75 years old and had fallen while going to the bathroom. In my opinion, a person that old should be in a nursing home anyway.

So, the client fell and I was assigned to take care of him. I knew he was alert and oriented, but I would have felt better getting a history from someone who wasn't so old and feeble. I finished the admission, and traction was ordered for the client. As a new nurse, I wasn't skilled at doing traction. I never learned how to set up traction in school or in hospital orientation, but I decided to do my best.

I put the client in traction and moved on to my other clients. The client complained of pain about 1 hour later, and I gave him a shot of analgesic in the right buttock. He jumped a little at the injection, but later expressed pain relief. I checked the traction and took the vital signs; everything appeared to be fine. I moved on to care for my other six clients.

About 4 hours later, the client again complained of pain. I prepared and administered the pain medication in the left buttock. The client exclaimed that he didn't even feel the injection. I thought, "I must be getting better!" I checked the traction and moved on to my other duties. Then I reported to the next shift and left for the day.

When I returned the next day, I found to my surprise that all was not well. The traction had been improperly applied, and the client had suffered permanent nerve damage. The client required surgery, sustained tissue destruction, and was very angry with his nursing care. I felt frustrated—after all, I'd done the best I could. These old folks can be so unreasonable! I felt angry with nursing, my agency, and this client. What else could I have done?

1. Name one legal principle violated in this scenario.
2. Name one ethical principle violated in this scenario.
3. Name one way these violations may affect clinical decision making.
4. Using sound clinical decision-making skills, state what else could have been done.

Clinical Decision Making: Assignment 6

Use Lewin's theory of change to reflect on clinical decision-making skills. How do the concepts of unfreezing, moving, and refreezing relate to your personal development of clinical decision-making skills throughout the semester?

Clinical Decision-Making: Assignment 7

After your field experience, answer the following questions:

1. How did you prepare for this experience?
2. State the values of any screening results not within normal limits. Use your clinical decision-making skills.
3. What recommendations did you make, or could you have made, based on these values?

Ideas for Use

- Use **Clinical Decision-Making Exercises** to evaluate understanding of class content. Reinforce concepts as needed. If assignments are done weekly or biweekly, you can routinely assess the students' understanding and need for additional practice.

- Have students document **Clinical Decision-Making Exercises** in an **Ah-Ha Journal** and hand it in at the end of the semester or rotation.

- For new nurses, use a **Clinical Decision-Making Exercise** each day of nursing orientation. This reinforces critical thinking skills and helps staff members get to know the clients most commonly cared for in their clinical environment.

- Students can complete **Clinical Decision-Making Exercises** in pairs or trios as part of a classroom activity.

- Students may write these exercises, post them in an **Online Discussion**, or send them as an **Email Exercise.** They are also valuable as a way to prepare prior to class discussion.

- Make sure that class examinations reflect the concepts discussed in **Clinical Decision-Making Exercises.**

- Consider peer grading: have students evaluate each other's exercises using instructor-developed criteria and/or rubrics.

- Nursing specialty classes and specialty unit orientations are rich in nursing decisions. Use **Clinical Decision-Making Exercises** as an entertaining way to review class content.

Reality Check

General Description. The term *reality check* can frame a theoretical discussion in the context of real nursing practice. Clinical examples provide a mechanism for discussion. This strategy is an excellent way for students to differentiate between real-life healthcare issues and those they see on television and read about in fiction.

In **Reality Check,** material is introduced theoretically and then given a real context. The instructor centers class topics on actual evidence and true events. **Reality Check** may be based on real clinical cases (with names omitted). Physical evidence can include hospital bills, replications of clinical records, or simulated charting. Just by saying **"Reality Check,"** you'll prompt your students to consider some of the issues that affect healthcare and their role in safe nursing practice.

Preparation and Equipment. Use your clinical practice affiliations to obtain real hospital costs, documentation samples, and other evidence (see Fig. 6–3). This exercise is a great opportunity to discuss the financial side of healthcare and demonstrate the burden it places on individuals, industry, and public resources.

REALITY CHECK

CPT: 99211 OV LEVEL 1	36.00
CPT: 90780 IV THERAPY 1ST HR	118.00
CPT: J1642 HEPARIN FLUSH, PER 10 UNITS	4.00
CPT: 96530 REFILL/MAINT INPLANT PUMP	68.00
CPT: J7030 1000CC NORMAL SALINE	22.50
CPT: J7050 NORMAL SALINE 250 ML	22.50
CPT: 96410 CHEMO INF TO 1 HR	198.00
CPT: 96410ST TRAY FEE	75.00
CPT: J9214 INTERFERON ALFA, 1MIL	746.24

This is the cost/treatment. Treatments are 5×/week for 12 months: 1,300 × 5 × 52 = **$338,000.00!** This does not include lab work, other medications, other health visits, transportation to treatments, other health concerns, durable medical supplies, nutritional supplements, diagnostics, radiation/chemo/surgery expenses, and so on.

Fig. 6–3. Reality check: five treatments per week for 12 months.

Example of the Strategy at Work. I use a slide on the idea of Fig. 6–3 as a **Reality Check** in a pharmacology class. It is easy for us to say, "Medications cost a lot." Instead, we can provide physical evidence of these costs from a real client experience to drive home these points.

After viewing the slide, we discuss the impact of healthcare costs on someone without insurance or adequate financial resources. Seeing the physical evidence brings home the reality to students. The fiscal aspects of nursing and healthcare are key parts of the **Reality Check** that nurses need to practice responsibly and safely.

Ideas for Use

- Instead of using physical evidence, just say, **"Reality Check,"** when it's time to think about putting a theory into action. You can use some questions to stimulate discussions:
  - How does this information relate to the real world?
  - How often does a nurse have time to sit down and talk with a client the way we discussed in this chapter?
  - How does a nurse care for several acutely ill clients at one time?
  - How does a nurse juggle several priorities at once?
- This strategy can highlight legal and ethical issues. It can also illustrate the workforce issues associated with nursing, such as

nurse-to-client ratios, delegation, unionization, pulling or reassigning (sending nurses to other units), cross-training (orienting nurses to multiple specialties), and professional issues.

- Hunt[16] provides a great resource for making client care more realistic. This **Reality Check** exercise is called "Armchair Shopper." Clients are given a list of questions and asked for solutions. I'm sure you'll agree that these questions, inspired by the "Armchair Shopper," are also great **Reality Checks** for new nurses and nursing students:
  - How would you navigate your snowy yard in a wheelchair?
  - How would you plan your daily diet to keep your sodium restricted?
  - How would you change your father's diaper in a public restroom?
  - How would you transfer your mother, with right-sided hemiplegia, into and out of the passenger side of the car?
  - Looking at a restaurant menu, what selections would you make to adhere to your prescribed diet?
  - Your medication must be kept cold at all times. How would you transport it on vacation?
  - What would you do if you dropped and broke your last vial of insulin on a weekend?
  - What would you do if a client suffered a cardiac arrest on an elevator and you were the only person there?
  - How would you respond if a client said he was leaving the hospital even though he had not been discharged?
  - What resources would you need to change a dressing for a client you were caring for?
  - What would you do if an IV bag ran dry and there were no other bags of that solution on the floor?

You can adapt the questions, as I have here, for inpatient care or keep them home-based for client education.

Muddiest Part

General Description. This strategy was shared with me at a class I taught about creative teaching strategies. After some research, I discovered that **Muddiest Part** was developed by Mosteller as a means to assess class learning and that it was originally called "Muddiest Point."[17] The term denotes the part of a class that students, instructors, or both consider the most confusing or complex.[18]

In nursing education, we can often tell when we've reached the **Muddiest Part.** Students shake their heads or look frustrated. You may hear a murmur in the crowd or see students craning their necks to find out whether their neighbor understood something better than they did.

These are sure signs that you've reached a **Muddiest Part.** The next step is to clarify the material. You can do this either through class discussion or by using another creative teaching strategy to present the topic differently.

Preparation and Equipment. The only preparation needed is a sensitivity to the **Muddiest Parts** of a prepared class. Usually instructors can predict them and can build in additional time or plan a teaching strategy to allay fears. Sometimes, however, students may encounter a **Muddiest Part** when the instructor least expects it. Teachers need to be vigilant for signs of frustration and confusion.

Example of the Strategy at Work. It's a good idea to peruse your lecture material and try to determine the **Muddiest Parts.** You can trudge through the mud in advance by planning a creative strategy to reinforce material. Most experienced nurses and nurse educators remember the usual areas of confusion: the neuroendocrine system, ventilator settings, interpreting arterial blood gases, calculating vasopressor drips, using chest tubes to treat a pneumothorax. These are just a few examples.

When you see that students are confused by a **Muddiest Part**, or an area of complexity emerges over the classroom, step back and clarify. Provide additional information or suggest additional resources to clear up the confusion. To assess the **Muddiest Part** by watching the class, I look for both verbal and nonverbal cues when discussing complex information.

Ideas for Use

- Students often feel relieved when they realize that a **Muddiest Part** also confuses other people.
- Ask students to identify the **Muddiest Part** in a class as an assessment technique. Use **Admit Tickets** or **Exit Tickets, Email Exercises, Ah-Ha Journals,** or **Online Discussion Groups** to collect these responses. Provide support in subsequent classes by contributing to **Online Discussion Groups,** posting information to Web-based bulletin boards, or using other innovative strategies.
- If you teach the same content repeatedly, use **Muddiest Parts** to provide insight for future teaching experiences.

In-Class Test Questions

General Description. Nursing students, especially seniors preparing for NCLEX®, are very responsive to test questions scattered throughout a lecture. New nurses in orientation groups benefit from intermittent testing of skills. Experienced nurses—especially those taking objective examinations for certification or course completion—appreciate revisiting multiple-choice test items. What better way to brush up on test-taking skills? In this strategy, the instructor inserts appropriate test questions in the lecture. **In-Class Test Questions** help you assess the class, help the students determine what they know, and provide an opportunity to practice testing skills.

Preparation and Equipment. All you need to do is develop test questions based on the lecture or discussion material. Questions may be placed in PowerPoint format. Animation may be added—for example, you can use an arrow to pinpoint, enlarge, or highlight the correct answer. It's important to remove the arrows, or anything else that gives away the correct answer, before providing handouts. The students aren't supposed to have the answers in their notes! Present a question every 15 minutes or so to coincide with learners' usual attention span.

Example of the Strategy at Work. This strategy is one of the most common ones I use for brief diversions during class. **In-Class Test Questions** also provide transition points to new topics of discussion. Box 6–6 shows a sample question I use to demonstrate the strategy to groups of nurse educators.

In-Class Test Questions are a great way to reinforce material and provide breaks in a lecture or discussion. This strategy comes with some cautions:

- Make sure the **In-Class Test Questions** match the difficulty level of the examination questions. Students will feel overconfident and be misled if the questions are too easy. Overly difficult questions will frustrate and intimidate them.
- Use questions from previous examinations to show the students what your testing style is like and what level of difficulty to expect.
- Use as many application and analysis questions as possible. You'll be asking students to make a leap from simple retention to actual use of their knowledge. For example, here is a retention question:

Box 6–6.
In-Class Test Question

Active learning is effective for young people because:
1. They are all hyperactive and have short attention spans.
2. They suffer the effects of immobility, such as pressure areas on bony prominences.
3. They have the same learning styles.
4. They learn best when participating in the teaching-learning process.

Which of the following is a common complication after a splenectomy?

1. Infection
2. Venous thrombosis
3. **Pneumonia**
4. Dehydration

This first question asks students to recall the most common complication of splenectomy: pneumonia caused by the location of the incision and the resulting postoperative pain, which limits the depth of respirations. Now it's time to leap from retention to application. Ask the students how to assess for that complication or prevent it. See the subtle differences in this question:

Which of the following nursing interventions would prevent the most common complication following a splenectomy?

1. Antibiotic therapy and wound cultures
2. Leg exercises and pneumatic compression boots
3. **Coughing and deep breathing exercises**
4. IV hydration and oral fluids

You can even take that question one step further, asking the students to evaluate the effectiveness of the intervention, as in this question:

A client you are caring for is postsplenectomy. Which of the following assessments would indicate that interventions to prevent the most common complication of this surgery were effective?

1. Client is afebrile and incision is dry and intact
2. Negative Homans' sign and lack of extremity pain
3. **Clear breath sounds and normal work of breathing**
4. Good skin turgor and adequate urine output

For this question, students must first determine the complication and then identify the prevention strategy. Although antibiotics may be used to treat the pneumonia, a better answer is to prevent it with pulmonary hygiene.

- Adhere to the standards of test construction. Don't include personal names in questions. Limit the length of questions and cases to necessary information. Don't ask all-of-the-above or none-of-the-above questions. Make sure answers are correct and similar in format and length. Distribute correct answers evenly among the four letters or numbers assigned to answer choices. Make sure the questions adequately represent testable material.
- When showing a test question in class, ask students to read it quietly and await your signal to call out the response. Nothing is

more frustrating for slower readers than to have someone call out an answer before they've even finished reading the question and the answer choices.

Ideas for Use

- Have students develop their own test questions. Composing questions is a great way to study and brings home the difficulty of test construction. Use a **Twosies** exercise—have students develop questions and switch with their partners. Ask students to post their questions to an **Online Discussion.**

- Alternatively, have students hand in questions as **Admit Tickets** and tell them you might use their questions on the examination. You'll be giving the class a way to prepare and to participate in evaluation. These questions may also be useful for test review and study sessions. Encourage students to use them in study groups (see **Learning from Each Other**). Experience has taught me that students develop hard test questions! You may need to revise them for the examination.

- During **Student-Led Seminars,** have students compose test questions and write them on an index card. You can ask these questions after the seminar to evaluate class participation and attentiveness. Again, you may find yourself selecting questions to use on an examination.

- Have students post their questions and answers with rationales to an **Online Discussion.** Not only can you use the questions for test development, but students can also use them to study for the examination. A colleague provides extra credit to students whose questions were actually used for the examination.

- Hand out electronic clickers (or ask students to purchase them) to use in answering questions. Clickers are also good for taking attendance, conducting quizzes, and assessing knowledge. Personal response systems or clickers allow students to answer questions in PowerPoint and provide the instructor with some assessment of the students' level of comprehension. Handmade or commercially made voting cards are a lower technology alternative to personal response systems.

- **In-Class Test Questions** can come from textbooks, test banks, and nursing examination review books.

- Give the class a solid foundation for the NCLEX® examination. One student told me about "NCLEX® World," where nurses have endless amounts of time, money, assistance, and resources to accomplish their tasks. This concept helps students select the correct action without considering constraints. Of course, in real clinical practice, resources are finite and nurses must often make some changes in their nursing care while staying within the basic parameters of client safety, benefit, and respect.

- Nursing examinations typically offer four correct answers. Students often find it frustrating to have to select the best, first, or highest nursing priority. **In-Class Test Questions** help them practice these skills in the classroom.
- When using **In-Class Test Questions,** make sure you cover the correct answer with rationales and discuss the reasons the others are incorrect. Students often find review of the incorrect answers a great learning experience.
- Encourage the question "What do you think they'll ask about this topic on the examination?" Students often have a difficult time anticipating and differentiating priorities. Using questions on a regular basis will foster those skills.
- Give your students a test blueprint or guide. If they know the number of questions per topic, class objective, or hour of class, they can study according to those parameters.
- One seasoned nursing instructor recommends posting a test question on the board during a class break. Whether written or in PowerPoint, the questions are reviewed when the class reconvenes. Because these questions may or may not appear on an examination, students are encouraged to return from the class break promptly.
- For more information on test construction and administration, see Oermann and Gaberson.[15]

Email Exercises

General Description. This strategy is effective in assessing knowledge level and in helping students keep up with class information. It's also a convenient way to distribute **Quick Write** or **Write to Learn** exercises. In **Email Exercises,** students email the instructor or teaching assistants with brief assignments or answers to questions. If you have an LMS, these assignments can be loaded into the assignment functions and graded within that system.

Preparation and Equipment. You'll need to compose the **Email Exercises** and establish both an evaluation mechanism and a policy regarding these assignments. Guidelines should be set out in the course syllabus.

Example of the Strategy at Work. I used **Email Exercises** throughout a pharmacology course as a key teaching and assessment strategy. Here are the syllabus guidelines for **Email Exercises:**

Email Assignments

Eleven LMS assignments are scheduled throughout the semester. See class schedules for the directions. Each assignment must be received by 5:00 p.m. on the due date. A maximum of 5 points is available; one extra assignment is included to provide flexibility when needed. Assignments received by the due date and time will receive ½ point; assignments received late or not at all will receive 0 points. LMS exercises make up 5 percent of the grade in this course.

Exercise 1

You are asked to participate in a double-blind research study. All clients will be asked to take daily medication to treat their severe, uncomfortable, chronic disease. Half of the sample will be randomly designated to receive a medication with an excellent chance of curing the illness. The other half will be assigned to a control group and will receive a placebo. This experimental treatment is the only one known for the illness. There is an informed consent procedure, and identities will be kept confidential. The subjects will receive $1,000 to participate in the study for 6 months.

State two ways in which the principle of autonomy is respected in this study. State two ways in which autonomy is threatened.

Exercise 2

A client is to be discharged with a prescription for 10 mg of oral morphine. The oral morphine is available in a solution of 2 mg/mL. Calculate how much morphine the client should receive. While in the hospital he was receiving 3 mg of morphine by IV. In two to three sentences, explain to the client why the oral dose is higher than the parenteral dose. Use your knowledge from the last few weeks to build your answer.

Exercise 3

A client with seizures is admitted to the hospital. He routinely takes phenytoin (Dilantin) as an anticonvulsant. His seizures were controlled until last night, when he had a grand mal seizure at home.

His blood levels were drawn, and phenytoin was found to be below therapeutic level. His previous dose was 50 mg with breakfast and dinner and 75 mg at bedtime. Answer the following questions:

1. What could be the reason for the client's breakthrough seizures?
2. Is this client's dose of phenytoin appropriate?
3. Why is the monitoring of blood levels important?
4. Why is the bedtime dose greater than the other two doses?

Exercise 4

A 2-year-old girl visits the nurse practitioner. She is irritable and febrile, and has some nasal congestion. Her parents report that she is rubbing her ears and appears to be very uncomfortable. On the basis of physical examination and history, the nurse practitioner gives a diagnosis of otitis media and prescribes 125 mg of amoxicillin three times daily for 10 days. The amoxicillin suspension is available in 250 mg/5 mL.

1. How much medication should the child receive?
2. How often?
3. The mother asks if she can use household teaspoons. What is your response?
4. The father asks if the child needs to take the medicine for the entire 10 days if she starts to feel better. In two to three sentences, respond to his question.

Exercise 5

You are a home care nurse treating an elderly man who lives alone and whose purified protein derivative test and chest x-ray were positive for tuberculosis. He is being treated with three different antitubercular medications: isoniazid, ethambutol, and streptomycin. He asks why he can't take just one medication.

1. In two or three sentences, explain why multidrug therapy is indicated.
2. He has orders to have his blood drawn in 2 months for liver enzyme levels. Why?
3. After 3 months of therapy, he complains of ringing in his ears. What condition does this indicate and which medication could be responsible?

Exercise 6

A client has a diagnosis of leukemia. He complains of fatigue, shortness of breath, and weakness. The physician believes these symptoms are caused by anemia. The client is ordered to receive erythropoietin subcutaneously. In two to three sentences, describe the action of this medication. In two to three sentences, describe how to give a subcutaneous injection.

Exercise 7

A 52-year-old man is recovering from a heart attack. You are caring for him on a medical-surgical unit. He is ordered to receive digoxin.

1. What nursing precautions are essential during administration of this medication?
2. As a nurse, you are vigilant for signs and symptoms of digoxin toxicity. List several of these signs and symptoms.
3. You are aware that low levels of one electrolyte can potentiate (add to) digoxin toxicity. What is the electrolyte?

Exercise 8

A 16-year-old client with cystic fibrosis is ordered to receive fat-soluble vitamins in a water-soluble form. In two to three sentences, explain the difference between fat- and water-soluble vitamins. In one sentence, explain why this client should not take fat-soluble vitamins.

Exercise 9

A client is ordered to receive sucralfate (Carafate) for treatment of a peptic ulcer. Explain how this medication should be administered in relation to other medications and meals. Provide rationales for your answers.

Exercise 10

A client receives regular insulin at 7 a.m. At 10 a.m. he becomes shaky, irritable, and sweaty. Answer the following questions:

1. What do these symptoms indicate?
2. What characteristic of regular insulin predisposes to this problem?
3. What actions should the nurse take?

Exercise 11

A 22-year-old woman enters the gynecology clinic seeking oral contraception. Answer the following questions:

1. The client asks about the side effects of oral contraception. Summarize these.
2. The client smokes. What would you tell her?
3. The client reports taking St. John's Wort for depression. What would you tell her?

As you can see, **Email Exercises** help students apply classroom principles, use problem-solving skills, and prepare for class. Key to this process is that email exercises are assigned prior to coverage in class. This ensures a level of preparation so that the class can proceed more effectively.

Ideas for Use

- Checking and grading **Email Exercises** can be time consuming and laborious, especially in a larger class. Teaching assistants or graduate students can help with grading.
- Use textbook exercises, **Clinical Decision-Making Exercises,** or **Critical Thinking Exercises** as questions for this strategy.
- Make sure the exercises apply to current classes so students will have to prepare. Some of my students have said they'd prefer to have the **Email Exercises** follow a class discussion. I had to remind them that one purpose of this assignment is to encourage preparation before class.
- **Email Exercises** may be posted to **Online Discussion Groups** or to an electronic bulletin board.

Group Tests

General Description. In this effective strategy, students take a short test as a group. They're directed to answer the questions following a group discussion, in which all members reach a consensus about the correct answers. One of the most valuable parts of this strategy is the analysis of incorrect answers. The instructor leads with the question "Why are the other options incorrect?"

This strategy builds test-taking ability, fosters teamwork, encourages study groups, and helps the instructor assess the knowledge level of the class. Students learn valuable test-taking strategies from each other during group work.[19]

Preparation and Equipment. You will need to develop a group test of five to 15 items, set aside class time, and establish the groups. (See **Group Thought** for some hints on the formation and use of group exercises.) The group at large can discuss the correct answers, you can grade the **Group Tests** and discuss them in class later, or correct answers with rationales may be posted in an **Online Discussion Group.**

Example of the Strategy at Work. This strategy has proved effective in a senior-level seminar course, a portion of which was devoted to NCLEX® preparation. Group tests were well received and gave the students a different way to practice test-taking strategies.

Here are two of my group tests.

Group Test 1 General Nursing Review

1. A nurse is ordered to administer 8,500 units of heparin to a client by IV. The medication comes in 10,000 unit/mL concentration in 10-mL syringes. How many mL should the nurse administer?

   Answer: 0.85 mL

2. A client is crying as she approaches the nurses' station. The client yells at the nurse seated at the desk and says that she needs to see the nurse manager, slamming her fist down on the counter. How would the nurse manage this client correctly?

   a. Setting clear limits on the client's behaviors.
   b. Saying to the client, "You seem upset."
   c. Ignoring the client's behavior.
   d. Referring the client to the nurse manager.

3. A client with diabetes mellitus is admitted to the unit with a history of alternating high and low sugar levels, poor compliance, and

alcohol ingestion. The nurse enters the room, where the client is unconscious but breathing with a strong pulse. What is the first nursing action?

a. Call the physician immediately.
b. Check the client's blood sugar.
c. Administer a STAT dose of insulin.
d. Establish an IV line for dextrose injection.

4. The nurse is changing the dressing on a central venous catheter. Put the following steps in the correct order.

a. Assess the site.
b. Don sterile gloves.
c. Clean the site with antiseptic swabs.
d. Apply the clear transparent dressing.
e. Don clean gloves.
f. Remove the old dressing.
Order: e, f, a, b, c, d

5. A client has a nasogastric (NG) tube for decompression. The nurse irrigates the NG every 4 hours with 20 mL of normal saline solution. When doing the 12-hour shift totals, the nurse empties 260 mL of fluid from the drainage container. Calculate the true NG drainage for the shift.

Answer: 200 mL

Group Test 2   Management of Care and Delegation

1. A registered nurse from the maternity unit is reassigned to the emergency department. Which client would be most appropriate to assign to this registered nurse?

a. A 50-year-old with chest pain, diaphoresis, and an electrocardiogram showing elevated ST segments
b. A 25-year-old who fell from a ladder and has a fractured arm and no other trauma
c. An elderly client in acute respiratory distress for whom the family wants "everything to be done"
d. A 7-year-old with expiratory wheezing, poor air movement, and oxygen saturation of 88%

2. Which client should the day shift registered nurse assess immediately after receiving a report from the night shift?

   a. A 76-year-old man with deep vein thrombosis being converted from intravenous heparin to oral warfarin
   b. A 45-year-old client with type 1 diabetes mellitus with a fasting blood glucose level of 130 who is hungry
   c. A 60-year-old client who had a tracheostomy placed yesterday and has a humidity collar
   d. A 75-year-old who had a transurethral prostatectomy 2 days ago and has a three-lumen catheter

3. A client is to receive a feeding through a nasogastric tube. Which task related to this activity could the registered nurse delegate to the unlicensed assistance personnel?

   a. Checking the placement of the tube
   b. Documenting the feeding
   c. Flushing the tube with water before and after the feeding
   d. Accessing the formula from the nutrition department

4. Which client could the registered nurse safely assign to the licensed practical nurse to care for?

   a. A 70-year-old with a pulmonary embolus
   b. A 69-year-old with Prinzmetal's angina
   c. A 70-year-old who had a total hip replacement 3 days ago
   d. A 78-year-old receiving chemotherapy for breast cancer

5. A registered nurse is assigned to admit a new client to a medical-surgical unit. The registered nurse needs to do which function without delegating the task?

   a. Escorting the client to her room
   b. Orienting the client to the bed and call bell system
   c. Helping the client change into a hospital gown
   d. Interviewing the client about medications

6. A registered nurse from a medical-surgical unit is pulled to the intensive care unit. Which of the following is appropriate to assign to the registered nurse?

   a. A client awaiting transfer to the step-down unit
   b. A client in cardiogenic shock on vasopressors
   c. A client who has a pulmonary capillary wedge pressure monitor
   d. A client who has recently undergone open-heart surgery

7. A registered nurse arrives for work and finds the shift very short-staffed. When the registered nurse receives the client assignment, the nurse feels they have been assigned too many clients to provide safe care for all of them. To whom should the nurse report this problem first?

   a. The nursing supervisor
   b. The charge nurse
   c. The unit clerk
   d. The director of nursing

8. A pediatric client is admitted with a new diagnosis of Wilms tumor. The nurse is teaching the unlicensed assistance personnel key components of the client's care. Which is a critical component of this client's care?

   a. Assess for hematuria
   b. Rate the client's abdominal pain frequently
   c. Monitor urine output
   d. Refrain from palpation of the abdomen

9. A nurse is caring for a client who had major spinal surgery 8 hours ago. The nurse notes that the client has a nasogastric (NG) tube to straight drainage, a peripheral intravenous, and a back dressing that is dry and intact. The belly is distended and the client complains of mild abdominal pain. Which should the nurse do first?

   a. Empty the NG drainage container
   b. Irrigate the NG tube
   c. Assess bowel sounds
   d. Provide an oral feeding

10. A client with ascites is scheduled for a paracentesis. The nurse is preparing the client for the procedure. Which action should be carried out initially?

    a. Scrub the skin
    b. Place the client in a high Fowler's position
    c. Measure the client's abdominal girth
    d. Check that the consent form is signed

11. A client is displaying all of the following lab work. Which warrants the greatest concern?

    a. A BUN of 25
    b. A serum sodium of 140
    c. A hematocrit of 45%
    d. A white blood cell count of 500

12. An unknown relative brings a 6-year-old client to the emergency department. The client appears to need surgery. Which is the first nursing action?

    a. Prepare the client for surgery
    b. Determine who may sign the surgical consent for the child
    c. Teach the client about the operating room procedure
    d. Access insurance information

Ideas for Use

- Using **Group Tests** early in a course allows the students to assess your testing style.
- Provide a **Group Test** as a review before examinations.
- Encourage students to work at a good pace to foster test-taking skills. Even though NCLEX® and many certification examinations aren't strictly timed, they do have a maximum time limit.
- **Group Tests** are a great way to introduce students to some features of NCLEX® alternative items, question formats, blueprints, level of difficulty, and priority setting.
- Make up groups with varying knowledge levels so students can model behavior and learn from each other.
- Use test banks or review books to construct **Group Tests.**
- **Group Tests** may be used in continuing education and in-services. Prizes and incentives make them more fun and increase the competition between groups.
- Administer **Group Tests** to pairs, trios, or larger groups. Encourage students to study together in the same groups.
- **Group Tests** may be constructed for any subject matter. To calculate the time needed for this exercise, allow about 1 minute per question and several minutes for discussion. It takes time to consider all answer options, but the time is well worth it.

Web Assignments

General Description. The internet has opened up a whole new way to access knowledge. We have an unprecedented amount of information at our fingertips. In **Web Assignments,** students are instructed to search the internet for answers to assigned questions. Students discuss their findings informally in class or send their insights as an **Email Exercise** in the LMS assignment function or to an **Online Discussion Group.** Students can also email the URL to the instructor for reference. Although most students and nurses are fully aware of accessing information from the internet, being a critical consumer of information is an important skill.

This strategy promotes awareness of online resources, both for health professionals and for the public. It also develops critiquing skills—students must make sure their information comes from a valid source.

Preparation and Equipment. The only preparation you need for this exercise is to search for internet resources that students will find valuable.

Example of the Strategy at Work. I asked students in a health promotion class to search for smoking cessation websites. Part of the assignment was to print out the exercise or the home page and bring it in for discussion. This paper served as the **Admit Ticket** for the class. I showed a slide from the Centers for Disease Control and Prevention page on smoking cessation strategies. We began by discussing its value as a resource and then covering some of the other sites the students had found.

I've also asked students to use a search engine to determine the number of websites available for selected topics. My students were surprised to find 65,000 websites on diabetes and 33,000 on digoxin. It's important for nurses, especially when providing client education, to appreciate the sheer number of sites available to the public.

Ideas for Use

- Although most students know how to use the internet these days, some are reluctant to enter this realm or are accustomed to personal, not professional, internet use. **Web Assignments** help them practice the skills they need to search for health-related information.

- Devote some discussion time to providing criteria for your students to use in evaluating websites. This guidance will enhance their scholarly writing as well as their nursing practice.

- If your classroom has an internet connection, conduct a sample search in class using different search engines. Compare results and evaluate the selected websites.

- Have students **Think-Pair-Share** about their findings.

- Pose a question and ask students to search for the answer. They'll access an interesting variety of websites and often provide diverse answers. Use this opportunity to discuss the reputability of the internet as an information source.

- For a more extensive class project, have students develop a resource booklet of websites for specific client conditions.

- Use **Web Assignments** to create an in-service that introduces nursing staff to different electronic resources. Teach students to use the intranet within an organization, the agency's internet resources, client education materials, and internet resources approved for client distribution. To provide good education, nurses must know what information is available to clients and how valid the sources are.

- Ask students to critique a website, analyzing the validity of the source. Have them consider the ease of navigating the site. How difficult would it be for someone with less developed computer skills?
- Spend some time discussing the validity of online resources. This is a key skill for nursing professionals.

Student-Led Seminars

General Description. In nursing education, **Student-Led Seminars** are commonly used for clinical, agency, and discussion groups. This strategy provides a forum for practicing presentation and developing organizational skills. It also provides a teaching voice besides that of the instructor.

However, you need to observe some cautions. In its abbreviated, "on-the-run" form, the strategy requires a 10-minute time limit for the presentation. Students must differentiate "need to know" from "nice to know" and focus on information that takes priority. **Student-Led Seminars** could become monotonous if you let them drag on. Besides focusing on priorities, this method encourages creativity and reinforces the premise of this book—that learning can be fun!

Preparation and Equipment. Develop a list of potential presentation topics and provide guidelines. These should include the information to be covered, the time frame, possible use of resources, research, stipulations for internet use, and specific recommendations. For academic settings, make sure that the grading criteria or rubrics include your priorities for the assignment.

Example of the Strategy at Work. During a summer, flipped classroom discussion course, I realized that formal lectures for every class would prove difficult for students and instructors alike. I composed a list of presentation topics equal to the number of students in the class and assigned two **Student-Led Seminars** to each session. All topics began with the phrase "Nursing care of the client with _____." One presentation was given halfway through the class and one at the end. A brief discussion followed each presentation.

I told my students to adhere strictly to the time limit and to focus on nursing priorities and the implications of the condition. I instructed them not to discuss pathophysiology, elaborate laboratory tests or diagnostics, or in-depth management strategies. Instead, I asked them to discuss the disease briefly, nursing assessments, and any care included in the disease management.

Creativity, organization, ability to engage the class, and emphasis on priorities all counted toward the grade. I also asked for a reference list in American Psychological Association (APA) format that included at least three resources, one of which was a nursing research article mentioned in the presentation.

Table 6–2 shows the grading system I use for this assignment in a discussion group.

Students came up with many creative teaching strategies to enhance their classmates' enjoyment of the seminars. One student brought in an older adult relative. Simulating a client education session, the student discussed the client's nursing care and the assigned diagnosis. Another student prepared a presentation on sickle cell disease by baking cookies depicting sickled and nonsickled red blood cells. Another dressed in camouflage to discuss the role of chemotherapy in treating prostatic cancer. A student with computer skills created a newspaper with "articles" about the nursing priorities associated with the assigned condition. Videos, skits, food, costumes, and puzzles were only some of the strategies the class invented.

Table 6–2. Student-Led Seminar Topic

Grading Criteria	Points Available	Points Assigned
Information is comprehensive and based on nursing priorities.	30	
Seminar is organized and adheres to time limits.	30	
Seminar includes creative strategies to engage class participants.	30	
Reference list is appropriate for American Psychiatric Association (APA) format, and nursing research article is appropriate.	10	
Total	100	

Ideas for Use

- As with **In-Class Test Questions,** you can ask students in the audience to develop test questions about the seminar. These may be used in the review session or on actual tests to reinforce attentiveness during the seminars and encourage class attendance.
- If you draw test questions from the seminars, tell students how many questions per seminar they can expect.
- Encourage students to develop a brief handout, like the **Legal Cheat Sheet,** for each of their classmates.
- Allow students a lot of latitude with their creativity to keep the assignment informative and fun.

Self-Learning Mini-Modules

General Description. **Self-Learning Mini-Modules** are a well-documented strategy in nursing education.[20] To adapt them to an "on-the-run" strategy, I've created an abridged form of these modules.

Essentially, the instructor turns one small portion of the class into a **Self-Learning Mini-Module**. In the middle of a lecture, take a moment and pass out this mini-exercise to cover the next topic. The **Self-Learning Mini-Module** replaces the lecture for 5 to 10 minutes, and then the traditional class resumes. The content of the **Self-Learning Mini-Module** is not addressed verbally because the module is enough to convey the information. This strategy may be used in academic and continuing education settings.

Preparation and Equipment. The **Self-Learning Mini-Module** consists of selected readings and questions, both of which you'll need to determine while planning your class. It's usually better to select a less complex topic for the module.

Example of the Strategy at Work. While covering nursing care of the hepatic, biliary, and pancreatic systems, I realized that class time was limited and that the hepatic system could take up most of it. I also noted that the biliary system discussion was largely related to the various terms used for biliary disease and management. I asked the students to bring their text to class and gave them an assignment similar to the one shown in Box 6–7.

Ideas for Use

- This strategy is ideal for an important subject that's a subset of a larger topic. The subject should be simple enough to teach by this method. **Self-Learning Mini-Modules** emphasize the material without taking too much class time.

Box 6–7.
Nursing Care of the Client With a Biliary Disorder

In class, take 5 minutes and read suggested readings in your text. Then define the following terms:

1. Cholelithiasis
2. Cholecystitis
3. Choledochitis
4. Choledocholithiasis
5. Cholecystopathy

Now that you have defined the terms, indicate which of the following disorders in the left column match the assessment or management procedures in the right column.

1. Cholelithiasis	a. Cholecystogram
2. Cholecystitis	b. Choledochoplasty
3. Choledochitis	c. Cholecystectomy
4. Choledocholithiasis	d. Cholelithotripsy
5. Cholecystopathy	e. Choledocholithotomy

Answers: 1 (e), 2 (c), 3 (b), 4 (a), 5 (d)

- Use this assignment as the **Admit Ticket** for the next class.
- Ask students to think of their own mini-modules for class, study, and review sessions.
- Use case studies in your text to construct **Self-Learning Mini-Modules.**
- In academic classes, make sure the material covered in the **Self-Learning Mini-Modules** is represented on tests.
- **Self-Learning Mini-Modules** can coincide with learning of psychomotor skills, such as monitoring of one's own blood glucose, nasogastric intubation, insulin administration, and others.
- For continuing education settings, use this strategy to reinforce concepts and change gears. It can also provide a break for nurses not used to day-long classes or battling the after-lunch "sleepies."

Online Discussion Groups

General Description. The internet provides several ways to communicate with students. The easiest way to conduct **Online Discussion Groups** is to use the school LMS agency server or platform for posting and receiving messages. Instructors post questions, and students participate in the discussion by posting their answers.

Online Discussion Groups stimulate critical thinking, personal problem solving, and universal participation.[21] Harden[22] demonstrated that these online sessions helped students better understand the material being discussed. In addition, they stimulated a positive exchange of ideas and a comfortable forum for sharing thoughts about nursing practice.

Within academic institutions, LMSs usually provide icons that lead participants into a discussion. Clinical agencies may already have, or can develop, a limited-access posting site for staff, new orientees, or unit personnel.

Preparation and Equipment. You'll need to access agency resources to make **Online Discussion Groups** work. Then you'll need to stimulate discussion or provide guidelines for the online groups. Some instructors participate actively; others witness or observe the discussion group. Either way, you can use the electronic platform to evaluate student participation and the quality of responses.

For academic instructors, evaluation and assignment guidelines should be part of the class syllabus. For agency instructors, **Online Discussion Groups** may be voluntary, may provide staff support and access to new policies and information, or may be a professional requirement.

Example of the Strategy at Work. In a large lecture class, stimulating meaningful discussion with all students may be a challenge. Even in smaller classes, total participation is difficult to attain. **Online Discussion Groups** provide an answer to this dilemma. I used this strategy in a winter class of accelerated (all second-degree and some second-career) nursing students. Weather constraints and other commitments made this group responsive to online discussion.

I posted a question to the discussion group each Monday and Thursday. Because the winter session was condensed, the discussion sessions had to take place twice per week. Weekly or biweekly discussions would probably suffice for longer sessions.

I asked my students to respond at least twice to each discussion question, once by answering the question and once by responding to a classmate. After I set this parameter, it was interesting to watch the spirited discussions that followed my questions. Some questions stimulated a higher level of discussion than others, but I always felt rewarded witnessing the level of thinking and passion in the students. Although I did not participate actively in the discussion, I often needed to alert the students to potential test material or provide a closure statement to summarize their observations.

Ideas for Use

- Internet etiquette, or netiquette, should always be respected and maintained. A fellow instructor and I meant well, but we didn't know some of the rules associated with listservs in the early years. We asked students to sign on to a listserv, determine its purpose, view some of the key issues, and follow up with a reflective **Ah-Ha Journal.** We heard from many listserv members that this use was not appropriate because listservs are meant for sharing specific information, not for education. We omitted this assignment, needless to say. It's important to tell your class that listservs are available to support nursing students.

- Social media sites for a specific class, or for nursing students in general, may be another resource. Instructors should clearly delineate their involvement in social media. I was once criticized for having inaccurate information on the class social media site when, in fact, the students themselves had constructed the site.

- Students also may be responsible for initiating **Online Discussion Groups,** establishing "thinking questions," and creating closure at the right time.

- Some internet platforms provide chat rooms for real-time discussion. Chat rooms are a familiar resource for many students. However, students less used to computer chatting or instant messaging may need some orientation. Instructors can sign onto chat rooms at specified times to be available for questions or to set up an instructor-led discussion. They can provide a virtual environment for postconferences in clinical or discussion groups.

- Chat rooms and **Online Discussion Groups** are great tools for assessing students' knowledge level. Students can apply their problem-solving skills and explore class content.

- To make this an "on-the-run" strategy, you can create mini-discussion groups for **Email Exercises** or **Ah-Ha Journals.**

Learning Contracts

General Description. **Learning Contracts** enlist the students' contributions to their own course grade. This practice, especially common in nursing education outside the United States, is being used increasingly in this country. The instructor sets the course parameters and presents options for attaining specific grades, based on the completion of elective assignments. Returning adult and second-career students find **Learning Contracts** a valuable way to determine their own learning goals and to succeed in the course.[23,24]

Most **Learning Contracts** include the number of required assignments as well as the elective ones. Also included is the time frame for completion, instructions for achieving goals, and methods of course evaluation. A key element of the **Learning Contract** is student cooperation. Another is the instructor's explicit articulation of expectations—it's important to make sure everyone understands the contracts. Students agree to complete an anticipated number of assignments, but they may change the contract as they wish during the semester.

Preparation and Equipment. To establish a **Learning Contract,** you need to delineate assignments clearly and explain the credit associated with each one. The class parameters, which allow students to determine their course grade, should be set out in the syllabus and policy statement. Establishing and maintaining **Learning Contracts** can be labor-intensive and difficult. However, when students take responsibility for their own learning investment, the rewards are significant.

Example of the Strategy at Work. Colleagues used a **Learning Contract** in a seminar course for senior nursing students.[21] Five assignments were required: a field trip, practice in standardized testing, weekly class activities, composing a résumé and cover letter, and leading a small-group discussion. Completing all five assignments ensured a grade of C+, four brought a C, and three resulted in a C−. Any student completing fewer than three assignments would fail the class. Each student signed a contract agreeing to these conditions.

In addition to these requirements, students were offered six optional assignments to raise their grades. These assignments included a field trip reaction paper (one-third grade increase), a résumé and cover letter resubmission (one-third increase), an NCLEX® prep option (one-third increase), political meeting attendance (one-third increase), job fair attendance (one-third increase), and a topic reaction paper (two-thirds increase).

Ideas for Use

- **Learning Contracts** give students an effective way to control their grades.
- **Learning Contracts** reflect accomplishment and increase students' investment in their own success.
- **Learning Contracts** may be as elaborate or as simple as needed to meet the course objectives and the needs of the students.
- To make **Learning Contracts** an "on-the-run" strategy, you can let students negotiate contract terms for specific assignments. For example, instructors may provide students with an array of several assignments to meet a course objective. Students may elect to write a paper, carry out a presentation, create patient education material, or another assignment. Key to this contract is to have

students agree to a certain project and follow through, teaching another important lesson about commitment and obligation.

- Several resources document the feasibility of **Learning Contracts** for clinical groups in selected settings, including mental health and community health facilities.

Condensed Portfolios

General Description. **Condensed Portfolios** can enhance a small class. In this strategy, students gather selected assignments and create a personal portfolio of their progress. These portfolios may be maintained on paper or electronically.

This strategy helps students assess their own performance and maintain personal records. They feel more responsible for preserving evidence of their performance and their attainment of course objectives.[25] Portfolios may include completed assignments and papers, clinical evaluation tools, anecdotal notes, reaction papers and journals, evidence of accomplishments, and formative and summative evaluations. They can be used for a single class or an entire curriculum. The ability to collect and save portfolios electronically has changed the way these can be used throughout an individual's career.[26]

Preparation and Equipment. Instructors need to establish clear evaluation policies for the use of portfolios within a course or curriculum. Individual instructors can add **Condensed Portfolio** expectations to their course syllabi. In agencies, orientation personnel can develop standards for nursing orientees to use in recording their professional growth. Agency portfolios might include records of attendance at educational programs, evidence that requirements have been met, certification documents, current résumés, and evaluations. As the literature confirms, the success of this strategy depends on clear guidelines related to expectations and portfolio contents.[25]

Example of the Strategy at Work. In an introductory nursing class, I asked students to create a personal portfolio of their progress through the course. As time went on, I adopted the name **Condensed Portfolios** to make it clear that these portfolios would contain only the information discussed in the course syllabus. By doing so, I eliminated a significant amount of extraneous information.

The course syllabus indicated the following contents of the *Context of Nursing Portfolio*:

- Responses to six **Email Exercises** with instructor comments. (Including these assignments gave students incentive to read my feedback.)

- The instructor-graded copy of the completed Nursing Database.
- The instructor-graded copy of the student's data-analysis project.
- The instructor-graded copy of the student's plan for client care.
- Evidence of a **Web Assignment** answering a class question.
- The instructor-graded copy of the APA formatting exercise.
- Signed documentation of completion of Total Care Test-Out, ensuring competency in basic care skill performance.
- The instructor-graded copy of the Nursing Economics Case Study.
- A final personal growth **Ah-Ha Journal** entry.

This assignment was worth 10 percent of the course grade. Documentation of each assignment was worth 1 point except for the last assignment, which was worth 2 points. The extra point represented the amount of time students should have spent on the final **Ah-Ha Journal** entry, which discussed their personal growth during the semester.

All the portfolio assignments had been required for the class; none were optional. I wanted the students to practice maintaining records, develop an organizational structure for the portfolio, and assume responsibility for completing it. These expectations fit the objective of professionalism that underlies even a beginning-level nursing course.

Ideas for Use

- To establish **Condensed Portfolios** as an "on-the-run" strategy, you can develop assignments or policies aimed at creating an abbreviated portfolio.
- In nursing clinical groups, **Condensed Portfolios** can track individual progress through a rotation. Clinical evaluation tools, lists of skills, and personal evaluation summaries can be included. Schools might establish policies allowing subsequent clinical instructors to assess student skills by reviewing these portfolios. The student's explicit consent would be needed for this use of the portfolio.
- You may want to develop assignments that build on one another and eventually become part of the **Condensed Portfolio.**
- Students can maintain a voluntary portfolio of their educational experience. They can show it to prospective employers or graduate schools, or use it for promotion within an agency.
- Agencies can use **Condensed Portfolios** in annual evaluations, as evidence for promotion or advancement in a clinical ladder, or as documentation for accreditation.

References

1. Cioffi J. Collaborative care: Using 6 hats thinking for decision-making. International Journal of Nursing Practice 23(6): 1, 2017.
2. deBono E. The Six Thinking Hats. Penguin Books, 1985.
3. Gross R. Peak Learning: How to Create Your Own Lifelong Program for Personal Enlightenment and Professional Success. Putnam, 1999.
4. Sweeney J and Moeller L. Decision training—The use of a decision curriculum with an in-basket simulation. Education 104:414–418, 1984.
5. Schroffel A. The use of in-basket exercises. Public Personnel Management 41(1): 151–160, 2012.
6. Maslow AH. The Farther Reaches of Human Nature. Viking, 1971.
7. Breytenbach C, Ham-Baloyi W, and Jordan P. An integrative literature review of evidence-based teaching strategies for nurse educators. Nursing Education Perspective 38(4), 193–197, 2017.
8. Free KW. What Next? www.whatifgame.homestead.com.
9. Paul D and Elder L. Critical Thinking Tools for Taking Charge of Your Professional and Personal Life. Prentice Hall, 2002.
10. Bowles DJ. Active learning strategies . . . not for the birds! International Journal of Nursing Education Scholarship 3(1). 2006 3:Article 22. Epub Sep 22.
11. Ibrahim ER, Richardson N, and Nestel D. Mental imagery and learning. Medical Education 49(9): 888–900, 2015.
12. DeYoung S. Teaching Strategies for Nurse Educators. Prentice Hall, 2014.
13. Rowling JK. Harry Potter and the Sorcerer's Stone. Arthur A. Levine Books, 1999.
14. Aronson E, Blaney C, Stephen C, et al. The Jigsaw Classroom. Sage, 1978.
15. Phillips J and Fusco J. Using Jigsaw technique to teach clinical controversy in clinical skills course. American Journal of Pharmaceutical Education, 79(6): 1–7, 2015.
16. Hunt R. Introduction to Community-based Nursing. Lippincott Williams & Wilkins, 2012.
17. Mosteller F. The "Muddiest Point in the Lecture" as a feedback device. The Journal of the Harvard-Danforth Center 3:10–21, 1989.
18. Aycock M, Sikes ML, and Stevens, G. Physician assistant student perceptions of "muddiest point" classroom assessment technique implementation. Journal of Physician Assistant Education, 29(2): 115–117, 2018.
19. Peck S, Werner JL, and Raleigh DM. Improved class preparation and learning through immediate feedback in group testing for undergraduate nursing students. Nursing Education Perspectives 34(6): 400–404, 2013.
20. Oermann M and Gaberson K. Evaluation and Testing in Nursing Education. Springer, 2016.
21. Osborne DM, Byrne J, Massey D, and Johnson A. Use of online asynchronous discussion boards to engage students, enhance critical thinking, and foster collaboration: A mixed methods study. Nursing Education Today 70: 40–46, 2018.

22. Harden JK. Faculty and student experiences with web-based discussion groups in a large lecture setting. Nurse Educator 28(1):26–30, 2003.
23. Gregory D, Guse L, Dick DD, et al. What clinical learning contracts reveal about nursing education and patient safety. Canadian Nurse 105(8): 20–25, 2009.
24. Watson S. The use of reflection as an assessment of practice. Can you mark learning contracts? Nursing Education in Practice 2:150–159, 2002.
25. McMullen M. Students' perceptions on the use of portfolios in pre-registration nursing education: A questionnaire survey. International Journal of Nursing Studies 43:333–343, 2006.
26. Russell A. Digital portfolios: A method to assess student understanding. Radiologic Technology, 90(2): 183–186, 2018.

Chapter 7

Strategies for Clinical Instruction and Orientation

"I take one minute a few times a day to look at my goals and see what I want to learn . . . . I can teach myself what I want to learn more easily by taking one minute to catch myself doing something right. . . . We are at our best when we teach ourselves what we need to learn."
—S. Johnson and C. Johnson

Challenges

* Clinical education, whether in an academic or an agency setting, is one of the most rewarding venues in which to pass on the craft of nursing. It also provides some of the greatest challenges in nursing education.

* Although the learning needs of new orientees and nursing students are important, the priority in a clinical agency is always safe and effective client care. Instructors struggle to balance client safety with the experiential needs of students. It can be especially difficult to foster learner independence in a clinical area.

* Instructors find it difficult to encourage critical thinking with a large number of students or orientees.

* Experiential learning creates a special kind of tension if some clients' conditions are more acute than others. In such a setting, mistakes and inexperience cannot always be tolerated. This tension increases in environments with intense client needs, as in acute illness or injury. The nurse educator encounters demands in settings with poor staffing, in which nurses are constrained by frustration, or those who don't foster the growth of novice nurses. Clinical site shortages, lack of agency preceptors, and workforce issues exacerbate these problems.

* Instructors must encourage independence in their learners, whether staff employees or nursing students, while maintaining some sense

of organization and control over the learning experience.

- Evaluating student performance, whether for a grade or continued employment, is often difficult to balance with teaching. The question "When does teaching stop and evaluation begin?" can help instructors decide whether learners have met the objectives of the experience.

- The instructor may find it arduous to create a learning environment for multiple students with varying needs and skill levels.

- Preconferences and postconferences and learning debriefings usually take place before or after a hard day at work. It takes planning and effort to give these sessions value for students.

Innovative methods can help you provide a safe and relevant education to novice nurses. In the clinical setting, you'll need strategies that foster learning in a tense environment, safe simulations outside actual client care, and group exercises in which students learn vicariously through each other's experiences. Focus your strategies on critical thinking, priority setting, decision making, and applying theory in the clinical setting. Clinical experience is one of the most valuable tools we have for teaching the nurses of tomorrow and those who already practice.

IDEAS

Scavenger Hunts

General Description. The primary objective of **Scavenger Hunts** is to help students get comfortable within their surroundings so they can work efficiently and effectively. One of the chief difficulties that new employees encounter is not knowing where things are or how to access them quickly. This lack of knowledge may affect their ability to navigate both the physical environment and the virtual world of the computer. **Scavenger Hunts** provide a safe venue for finding, using, and understanding objects employed in daily nursing practice.

Preparation and Equipment. Although it takes a while to make up a **Scavenger Hunt,** the format may be used time and again to orient new students or employees to a clinical area. You can make up a list of five to

Box 7–1.
Clinical Scavenger Hunt

1. Find the tympanic thermometer on the unit. Take the temperature of a partner and record it here: _____.

2. Find a drinking straw and record its location: _____.

3. Access the electronic blood pressure cuff and take your instructor's blood pressure. Record it here: _____.

4. Visit the dietary department and ask to see a low-sodium menu. Consider the lunch choices. Are soup or luncheon meats found on the menu? _____

5. Count the number of Band-aids found at the bedside of a client. Write the number here: _____.

6. Go to an unoccupied bed or crib. Attempt to lower the side rails. Note here whether it is harder or easier than you anticipated: _____

7. Ask the unit clerk to show you how to find clients' lab results. Record one client's most recent complete blood count here:

   _____

   _____

8. Use the computerized telephone directory to find the number for Spiritual Services. Record it here: _____

six things to find or tasks to be completed in order to meet orientation objectives and develop a sense of comfort in the clinical area.

Example of the strategy at Work. Box 7–1 shows the **Scavenger Hunt** I use for clinical orientation.

Ideas for Use

- **Scavenger Hunts** can be used in various ways to orient newcomers to a setting. Asking students to find things in the new environment develops their search-and-explore skills. You can ask them to find a straw, locate probe covers for the electronic thermometer, count the Band-aids at the client's bedside, or hunt for other objects used in daily care.

- You can take **Scavenger Hunts** into the area of skills. Your students can learn to use objects they'll be responsible for in clinical practice. For example, you can ask students to take a tympanic temperature, take an electric blood pressure reading, find an empty crib or bed and raise and lower the side rails, or take their own oxygen saturation reading.

- I find having students working in pairs makes it more enjoyable for them and faster, too.

- You can help your students meet the people associated with the unit function. Ask the unit clerk which phone numbers are used most frequently and where to find the agency directory, how to transfer a call to another phone, or the procedure for printing lab results. Ask the unit pharmacist about the medications prescribed most often on a given unit. Talk with the dietary personnel about their customary times for tray delivery. Talk with a volunteer about his or her role on the unit.

- Some components of the unit may be especially conducive to **Scavenger Hunts.** You can plan searches through the code cart, the medication room, the supply closet, or the utility room. Other searches may be planned throughout the nurses' station.

- You can develop a great learning experience by involving a client's medical record in a **Scavenger Hunt**. Students can practice chart information retrieval by hunting for demographics, historical information, or current data before assuming responsibility for client care. Students should be reminded of the confidentiality of client information before this exercise.

- Enlist the support of your agency in developing **Scavenger Hunts.** Have students or orientees visit the pharmacy to retrieve an insert for a common medication administered on a unit, or stop by central supply to ascertain the cost of selected items. Send students to the medical library for information on a client's condition, to the lab for the latest clinical results, or to the dietary department to retrieve a menu for a specific medical diet. If you go this route, you'll need to spend a little time seeking the assistance of ancillary departments and making sure they won't feel burdened by sudden multiple visits.

- Develop a computer **Scavenger Hunt** based on all the principles I've discussed. Have students sign on to the actual electronic health record or a demonstration unit to access specific client information. Ask them to retrieve lab results, admission dates, birth dates, the number of scheduled and as-needed medications, or the most recent medical orders. You'll be helping the students navigate a computer system and client database that are often unique to each clinical area and specialty. Again, client privacy should be reinforced before students access the client record system, making the training site an optimal option.

- Code, or crash, carts are frequently locked to ensure that they're stocked completely for emergency use. Create a virtual or video tour of the cart, showing each drawer and its contents as part of the presentation. Include a pretest and posttest to measure competency in navigating the drawer.
- Compose a **Scavenger Hunt** that meets the specific needs of your clinical environment.
- It's essential to keep **Scavenger Hunts** both brief and fun. **Scavenger Hunts** that are too long or arduous will frustrate participants. You're simply trying to acquaint them with the environment enough that the next time they need to find something, they'll venture into somewhat familiar surroundings.

Pass the Problem

General Description. I learned this strategy at a nursing education conference and have found it valuable for clinical groups, especially those new to care planning skills. Attributed to S. Kagan,[1] this strategy fosters thinking, teamwork, and planning.

First, I ask my students to take out a clean sheet of paper. At the top, they write their client's age, sex, medical diagnosis, and a brief background description. Next, they write the primary nursing diagnosis to be used for their care plan. Then the fun starts—the paper is passed to each member of the clinical group. Each member is asked to contribute a client goal and a strategy for that nursing diagnosis.

Preparation and Equipment. This strategy needs very little preparation. You can develop a **Pass the Problem** form (Box 7–2) or just have students use blank paper.

Example of the Strategy at Work. I use the strategy as explained here during a clinical postconference early in the rotation. Students are very creative with their ideas, and the exercise often fosters team spirit. Students and orientees learn vicariously about each other's clients because conversation always happens in response to this exercise.

Ideas for Use

- Keep the students to a strict time limit so they can all benefit from each other's contributions. I plan 4 minutes each for an eight-member clinical group, so we are done in about 35 minutes. Usually students can make their comments in that amount of time.
- You can use any problem format you like to teach the **Pass the Problem** concept. Nursing incoming classifications (NICs) and nursing outgoing classifications (NOCs), client problem lists,

Box 7–2.
Pass the Problem

Client: Age: Sex: Medical Diagnosis:
Background Information: _____

_____

Nursing Diagnosis:

Client Goal: _____

Nursing Intervention: _____

_____

Client Goal: _____

Nursing Intervention: _____

_____

Client Goal: _____

Nursing Intervention: _____

_____

Client Goal: _____

Nursing Intervention: _____

_____

Evaluation of client goals; effectiveness of interventions; revisions in care:

medical diagnoses, or patterns of function can also be adapted for use.

- Write **Pass the Problem** at the top of a sheet of paper, or use a form similar to mine, and give each student a copy. This gesture formalizes the strategy and gives it more credibility for some students.

- You may want to review the format for client goals and nursing strategies before this exercise. It's important to make sure that students are clear on these concepts. Client goals are measurable, observable, realistic, and client-centered, with a target date. They should begin with the words "Client will . . ." Nursing strategies are individualized, realistic, understandable, specific, and nurse-oriented and should begin with "Nurse will . . ."

- **Pass the Problem** is great for orientees using simulated clients and for teaching agency care plan formats. It promotes team building; sharing of care plan skills; and assessment of individual knowledge about critical pathways, care plans, standards of care, and other planning formats.

- Students can get their papers back and spend a minute reviewing other members' contributions. Give them time to clarify information with each other.

- If time allows, encourage the students to relate interventions and goals to what they did or witnessed in client care for that shift. They can then evaluate goal attainment and effectiveness of interventions.

- Students and orientees can use **Pass the Problem** to plan care if they're assigned the same clients the next day. Other students may suggest new goals and interventions, enhancing the clinical experience and the client's level of care.

- Postconferences and debriefings are a great time to complete this activity.

- You can use **Pass the Problem** in connection with the **One-Minute Care Plan.**

- A creative conference participant relayed how this strategy was implemented in a clinical group. Students began with copies of the **Pass the Problem** index card and carried it in their pockets throughout clinical. When the students had a free moment, they wrote on the card and passed it to another student, who then gave them their card. They continued this passing throughout the shift until everyone had "visited" each card and then returned it to the originator. This method addressed this great strategy and also the potential for downtime in the clinical area.

Cooperative Strategies

General Description. An important skill for nursing students and new nurses to develop is teamwork. **Cooperative Strategies** build collaboration, not competition. They encourage the group to work together rather than in isolation. They reinforce the knowledge that teamwork is a lifelong skill vital to professionalism in nursing.

Preparation and Equipment. The equipment needed depends on the emphasis of your **Cooperative Strategy.** This task mostly requires a longstanding focus on teamwork and collegiality rather than specific supplies.

The goal is to create a cooperative atmosphere that can translate to more effective and efficient client care.

Example of the Strategy at Work. On the first day of clinical work or orientation, assign pairs of students to take care of clients. Encourage students to assist each other but not to overwhelm the client with their efforts. The students may take turns checking vital signs, cooperate during assessments so they don't duplicate efforts, and share in helping the client with activities of daily living. For the next clinical experience, try assigning the same two students (or you can vary them) to two patients—again they need to learn prioritization and delegation. If the unit and agency allow, try two students with three or four assigned clients.

Reinforce the concepts of delegation and cooperation in this first assignment. As time progresses, make assignments more challenging and independent, always asking students to solicit help as needed. To develop rapport, assign students to neighboring rooms in the early weeks of rotation or orientation. Encourage them to help each other, especially when client assignments are demanding.

Sometimes we praise students who function well independently. It's also crucial to reward teamwork in your evaluation of students and orientees. Recognize the importance of working together to accomplish goals.

Ideas for Use

- Cooperative games marketed for young children can set the stage for team building. There are no winners or losers in these games; the objective is to work together for a common goal.
- Creative strategies described in other chapters of this book are great ways to begin team building in a clinical group, orientation cohort, or any other team in which work may reflect cooperative efforts. **Group Concept Mapping, In-Class Debates,** and **Group Thought** are effective ways to foster cooperation and teamwork.
- Show a film clip demonstrating team building, such as *Remember the Titans*, to corollate with collaborative nursing practice (see **Short Clips** and **Film Clips in Clinical**).
- If you encounter cliques, you may want to assign groups arbitrarily. You can use this tactic to pair more- and less-talented students and help them build on individual strengths. A student with a sound knowledge base but awkward interpersonal skills may complement a gregarious student who's less skilled in technical or analytical components.
- For nursing clinical groups, you can stimulate team spirit with simple statements such as, "We don't leave until everyone is

done," and "We don't eat until everyone is ready." Students who finish an assignment early are encouraged to help the others so all can meet the common goal.

- Many agencies have client lifting and movement policies to prevent back and other injuries. Using **Cooperative Strategies** may help new nurses preserve their health as they develop good team-building habits.
- Using pairs, trios, and groups within the clinical group can foster teamwork and collegiality.
- **Cooperative Strategies** encourage novice nurses to consider clients as partners, reflecting the current model of healthcare. **Grand Rounds, Clinical Quick Writes,** and **Day in the Life of a Client With . . .** may be used to reinforce this partnering message.

Here's a great **Cooperative Strategy** to read to a clinical group, especially one having interpersonal conflicts (see Chapter 5 for another strategy with this story):

His name was Fleming and he was a poor Scottish farmer. One day, while trying to make a living for his family, he heard a cry for help coming from a nearby bog. He dropped his tools and ran to the bog. There, mired to his waist in black muck, was a terrified boy screaming and struggling to free himself. Farmer Fleming saved the lad from what could have been a slow and terrifying death.

The next day a fancy carriage pulled up to the Scotsman's sparse home. An elegantly dressed nobleman stepped out and introduced himself as the father of the boy Farmer Fleming saved.

"I want to repay you," said the nobleman. "You saved my son's life."

"No, I cannot accept your payment for what I did," the Scottish farmer replied, waving off the offer. At that moment, the farmer's own son came to the door of the family hovel.

"Is that your son?" the nobleman asked.

"Yes," the farmer replied proudly.

"I'll make you a deal. Let me provide him with the level of education my own son will enjoy. If the lad is anything like his father, he'll no doubt grow to be a man we both will be proud of." And that he did.

Farmer Fleming's son attended the very best schools, and in time graduated from St. Mary's Hospital Medical School in

London. He went on to become known throughout the world as the noted Sir Alexander Fleming, the discoverer of penicillin.

Years afterward, the same nobleman's son who was saved from the bog was stricken with pneumonia. What saved the man's life? Penicillin.

The name of the nobleman was Lord Randolph Churchill and his son was Sir Winston Churchill. What goes around, comes around.

Messages such as these stimulate thought. Discussion may be directed at developing positive relations among individuals in the group.

Clinical Quick Writes

General Description. In this strategy, students are encouraged to develop and use writing skills to describe their experiences in caring for clients. **Clinical Quick Writes** may be done during conference or as independent assignments. Several different versions of this strategy give students a safe opportunity for reflection.

Preparation and Equipment. No specific preparation or equipment is needed. You should have a plan for the type of writing project to be assigned. Specific objectives and evaluation strategies should appear in the course guidelines.

Example of the Strategy at Work. I have found this strategy especially valuable in postconferences. After a long day of clinical work, students may find the postconference tiring. Allowing time to write and vent some of the day's emotions provides closure and can make students more responsive to your feedback.

The most frequent **Clinical Quick Write** I use is "Write a Letter to Your Client." Students assemble in the conference room and get out a paper and pencil. They spend about 20 minutes composing a letter to one of the clients they took care of during the previous shift. They can also write to a family member about their interaction with the client on that shift. This type of assignment is especially valuable in pediatric and maternity rotations, where family-centered care is very important. A colleague who uses this strategy in the mental health field finds that it stimulates insight and builds empathy regarding psychosocial issues.

Ideas for Use

- You can assign **Clinical Quick Writes** as journal-keeping exercises.
- Ask students to spend a minute or longer writing down what happened during the shift. Obviously, this version is a true

Clinical Quick Write. Students can use a narrative format to write about their day. Another approach is to write down as many words as they can to describe their experiences.

- You can ask students to write a single word or sentence that describes the clinical day. This word or sentence, shared with the group, generates discussion about the day, students' accomplishments, and goals for future clinical experiences. The conciseness of the exercise helps to focus thought and sharpen assessment and prioritization skills.

- The **Clinical Quick Write** strategy is effective for orientation groups, team building, a break in class or a change in atmosphere, and dealing with controversial topics. For example, if a conflict occurs within the group, have all your students write down their thoughts. Let them choose whether or not to share them with the group.

- If a legal or ethical issue arises in the clinical area, students and novice nurses benefit from organizing their own thoughts. Reacting to the issue in writing may offer a chance for you and the group to discuss it. By having students write their personal reactions, you encourage participants to think about their progress and objectives for growth.

- **Clinical Quick Writes** help students explore personal issues about their profession. The strategy promotes a metacognitive approach, in which participants are asked to think about thinking.

- Provide the opportunity for freewriting as part of the **Clinical Quick Write** exercise. Simply instruct the students to write for 5 minutes. It's interesting to see what topics they choose and how they use this time as a chance for catharsis.

- You may use this strategy daily or weekly and keep the writings in the students' electronic or hard-copy folders. Students can review the file at the end of the rotation to appreciate their own growth and new breadth of experience. Assignments may be submitted on paper or electronically.

- Ask the students to answer a written question or **Critical Thinking Exercise** in written format.

- If a troubling event occurred during the clinical shift, use post-conference as a chance for debriefing. Begin this session with private writing time. Conversation will follow from the students' reactions to their own and each other's writing.

- Use **Clinical Questioning** as a subject for **Clinical Quick Writes.**

- Monagle and colleagues[2] relayed the successes in fostering clinical judgment in new graduate nurses through the use of a "clinical anecdote reflection." In this study, new graduates noted better communication, teamwork, ability to respond to the complexities of care, and understanding the role of the nurse following a guided writing experience, much like **Clinical Quick Writes.**
- Use new technologies to allow journaling to be more palatable to students. For some students, emailing is preferable. I have worked with cloud-based journaling sites where students text their journal to the cloud and I have surveillance permission to grade them. For some, texting a journal would be laborious; for others it is a trending way to make journaling happen.
- Keeping a journal is an effective way to focus thinking and investigate thoughts, emotions, and experiences. These may be in writing or digital format.

One-Minute Care Plan

General Description. Many of us remember the elaborate care plans we produced in our nursing education. These long, detailed works drew on a plethora of sources and involved hours of work. Grounded in years of educational practice, this type of care plan provided an excellent learning experience. Because it was specific to the care of one client and required a long preparation with extensive rationales, however, it lacked practicality in today's busy nursing practice.

The **One-Minute Care Plan** streamlines the time and pares down detail. This strategy gives students a useful and realistic means of organizing their thoughts, using the nursing process, and creating an accurate profile of a client.

Preparation and Equipment. You need to decide what client information is essential in clinical rotations. The setting, the objectives of the rotation or orientation phase, and your personal priorities can all influence your decision. You may assign the **One-Minute Care Plan** with explicit instructions or develop a form to be filled in like a worksheet. I've provided an example in Box 7–3, but you can make up your own or adapt this one for your needs.

Example of the Strategy at Work. I developed this form for my clinical groups after reading *The One Minute Teacher*[3] by S. Johnson and C. Johnson. Their book is part of the "One Minute" series, and I recommend it highly. According to the authors, learning arises from the learner, and the teacher provides the framework for learners to teach themselves. The **One-Minute Care Plan** developed from that idea.

Box 7–3.
The One-Minute Care Plan

Client initials: _____ Age: _____ Medical Diagnosis: _____
_____

Brief Background Statement: _____
_____

Nursing Diagnosis: _____
_____
_____

Long-Term Goal: _____
Short-Term Goal: _____
Nursing Strategies:
   1. _____
   2. _____

Short-Term Goal: _____
Nursing Strategies:
   1. _____
   2. _____
Nursing Diagnosis: _____
_____

Long-Term Goal: _____
Short-Term Goal: _____
Nursing Strategies:
   1. _____
   2. _____

Short-Term Goal: _____
Nursing Strategies:
   1. _____
   2. _____

Evaluation of strategies and goal achievement:

Ideas for Use

- Add medication sheets, lab data, and assessment information as needed to make sure the students have a good understanding of the client's condition.
- Use the following guidelines to ensure a comprehensive client profile:
  - Allergies
  - Diet (type and how tolerated)
  - Fluid requirements (based on weight and age or norms)
  - Reason for hospitalization
  - Other medical problems
  - Planned treatments (surgeries, therapies)
  - Current physiological status: vital signs, pain status, oxygen saturation, review of systems
  - Lab and radiological findings
  - Current psychosocial status (fears, stressors, coping)
  - Family involvement (visiting, participation in care)
- Use this form during preconferences to prepare students for the clinical day. You may need to help students choose a nursing diagnosis; they sometimes have trouble anticipating nursing needs on the basis of a medical diagnosis or condition. Confer with them about care priorities, their role in the clinical experience, and their goals for the day for the client.
- Have students take notes on the form during report periods. I'm often surprised that when staff members give a report, students often either write nothing or write selectively. The **One-Minute Care Plan** may help them take down information that will affect care planning for their clients.
- Encourage the students to use the **One-Minute Care Plan** as a worksheet for ongoing assessments, developments in care, and news to be passed on in reports. The strategy helps students decide "things to check," such as turning, medications, and scheduled treatments. This can also be where they take notes throughout their shift (so much preferable to writing vital signs on their hands).
- This strategy also provides the framework for reporting to staff members. Students often just say to the nurses, "We're leaving," without realizing that certain information needs to be passed on.
- The **One-Minute Care Plan** allows students to reflect on the care they've provided and to think about potential revisions. After using the strategy to look back on the day, students can write in

their journals about objectives achieved, potential areas of concern, and personal goals for growth (see **Ah-Ha Journals**).

- Bristol[4] discusses the **One-Minute Care Plan** as part of "prioritization power," wherein students identify the top three: assessments, laboratory and diagnostics tests, interventions, potential and actual complications, client education, and nursing implications. Often, students try to "learn everything" about a topic. Delineating these top priorities ensures that students understand the highest priorities and appropriate nursing actions.

- Establishing a system of organization is one of the biggest challenges for students and orientees. **One-Minute Care Plans** help them organize their day and their client care. These plans can be adapted for individual and agency needs.

- Students caring for multiple clients may want to restrict their care plans to a brief client profile and one nursing diagnosis with goals and interventions.

- Other aspects of paperwork that can be added to the **One-Minute Care Plan** include pending labs, the client's daily/hospital stay/home day schedule, or priorities that need resolution.

- Have students complete their **One-Minute Care Plans** and then develop an SBAR (situation, background, assessment, recommendation) based on this information. Students can be asked to replicate a call to a healthcare provider, a hand-off to the next shift caregiver, or a report to an unlicensed assistive personnel (UAP).

- Use the **One-Minute Care Plan** to develop either a preclinical case study (much like the **Preclass Case Study**) or **Reverse Case Study** (both discussed in Chapter 5). Preclinical case studies allow you to assign students to develop a plan of care for a client who is typical of the unit, their community, or the client population. This assignment helps prepare students prior to the clinical experience and ensures that students consider the nursing priorities when caring for diverse client issues and populations.

- Check agency policies about taking papers from the clinical area. Some sites don't want any papers to leave their area; others allow papers that have been de-identified.

Ah-Ha Journal

General Description. The journal is a common method by which clinical instructors gauge student progress and students' thoughts and emotions. Less often, agency educators use it to assess the progress of new orientees.

The ease and perceived value of journal keeping varies among individuals. For some students, writing even five sentences is a painful experience. For others, page limits may be necessary to rein in their lengthy writing. The value of conventional journal keeping is questionable, especially if journals become chronological records of "things done" rather than "lessons learned." I still remember a five-page student journal that began, "At 6:45 a.m. I hung up my coat and prepared for my observation day in the ICU." Although this journal recounted every event of the day, it gave me no means of assessing critical thinking or any clue to the student's emotional side: hence the **Ah-Ha Journal.** This strategy provides a glimpse of an event, giving some idea of students' thoughts, emotions, and reflections on lessons learned during the clinical experience. This journal technique is based on critical incident theory, in which important events are analyzed based on their context, the writer's reactions to these events, and how to learn from and generalize lessons for the future.[5,6]

Preparation and Equipment. Put **Ah-Ha Journal** guidelines in your class packet or syllabus. Assign a component of the class grade to this assignment, allowing for frequency, estimated page length, and the points assigned to the exercise.

For orientation groups, provide guidelines to validate the use of **Ah-Ha Journals** as a legitimate way to document progress throughout the orientation period. Make sure that you read all journals, comment about students' observations, and demonstrate support of their reflective learning. Students provide more detail and share more readily when they think someone cares and is reading.

Example of the Strategy at Work. Box 7–4 shows the format I use for **Ah-Ha Journals.**

Ideas for Use

- By describing events and thoughts, students can use **Ah-Ha Journals** as learning exercises, which will help them generalize learned lessons to future events.
- By analyzing contributing factors, students learn to appreciate the complexity of and the often-competing priorities and perspectives associated with today's healthcare environment.
- Make sure your students understand the format of the journal—it's not a record of the day or a validation of experience but a reflection on lessons learned.
- Surprisingly, some students go through an entire clinical day and claim, "I had nothing to write in my **Ah-Ha Journal** today." I always find this hard to believe. It's important for students to see **Ah-Ha Journals** as places to write about both positive and negative,

Box 7–4.
The Ah-Ha Journal

1. The Critical Incident (the Episode or Event)
   Note: The incident may be positive or negative.
   A description of the experience including what happened, in sequence
   How and when the event started and ended
   A list and description of the people, things, or content involved in the event

2. Reaction and Analysis
   Your reactions, feelings, desires, and thoughts
   Nonverbal or other physical cues you noticed at the time
   Any associations while these reactions were occurring
   Examination of how you reacted to what happened and why these reactions occurred

3. Generalization
   Application of what was learned to future similar situations
   What you would change about the incident if it occurred again

or even neutral, events. I tell students to think about the day and write about something they found surprising, or something they didn't know or hadn't thought of before the clinical experience.

- Michele Deck[7] describes "whack on the side of the head" experiences as those in which the individual is changed or inspired by an event. Encourage students to find material for **Ah-Ha Journals** in everyday life, and especially in their clinical work.

- For orientees, include **Ah-Ha Journals** as part of weekly debriefings. Share common observations with the orientation group or allow orientees to disclose their own insights.

- **Ah-Ha Journals** give you a great way to observe how students are doing in various sites or on different units. Observational experiences, such as the operating room, emergency department, and intensive care unit, are candidates for these journals.

- **Ah-Ha Journals** let you keep your finger on the pulse of a clinical or orientation group. The process can uncover issues that require aggressive interventions, such as unit conflicts, staffing issues, or management problems. This strategy can help you resolve conflicts sooner rather than later.

- A colleague suggested that students or instructors save the **Ah-Ha Journals** throughout the semester and revisit them to assess trends in behavior, determine personal growth, and see areas of continued effort. This increases the value of the journals and provides even more reflection on progress and personal needs.

Creative Lab Skills

General Description. The nursing laboratory assists students with developing skills in dealing with heightened clinical acuity and more complex psychomotor skills. The number of nursing skills to be learned is always increasing. Nursing and staff development instructors must struggle to find effective teaching strategies that keep pace with students' new level of learning.

Although a comprehensive discussion of teaching laboratory skills is beyond the focus of this book, several strategies can aid in teaching and reinforcing those skills. The emphasis is on learning the steps of a skill, understanding its scientific basis, and demonstrating it safely in the lab or the clinical area. Lab skills focus the sense of accomplishment for a novice nurse—competent completion of these skills gives students more satisfaction than other cognitive achievements do. For this reason, nursing instructors should be sensitive to the stress involved in learning motor skills. **Creative Lab Skills** help students learn them as thoroughly and expeditiously as possible.

Preparation and Equipment. Laboratory experiences take a fair amount of preparation. Depending on which strategy you use, you may need skills checklists, policy or procedure guidelines, and the equipment to practice the skills.

Example of the Strategy at Work. After growing numbers of students overwhelmed our old methods, our program searched for effective and cost-efficient ways to teach lab skills. Each course has certain skills assigned to it. Students attend the simulation resource center for practice and skill evaluation. The lab is staffed by lab coordinators, who foster the learning environment. Several aspects unique to our lab are noted in the Ideas for Use section.

Ideas for Use

- Audiovisual resources help in demonstrating lab skills. Use DVDs with both written content and movie clips. This approach appeals to diverse learning styles and allows you to repeat the demonstration. Be sure to preview commercially available videos and those online to ensure their methods are similar to those taught in the program; drastically different methods may confuse students.

- Each student purchases lab supplies in a duffel bag. The equipment company allows us to choose the supplies, which then belong to the student. The students can practice in the lab while you evaluate their progress. Having their own equipment also lets them try their skills at home. This method is especially valuable for skills that take practice, like sterile gloving.

- Lab coordinators developed learning bins, which sort the equipment needed for different skills. Students can use the contents as an adjunct to their personal equipment.

- Encourage the students to use peer teaching and learning as part of their lab skill training. Rather than demonstrating all the skills yourself, let the students actively coach each other using their skills textbook. Have them open the book at the mannequin's bedside and assist each other through the steps of a skill, providing feedback as needed. This peer teaching is valuable for both learner and coach. It ensures active integration of the skill rather than the passive learning that follows a simple demonstration.

- Laboratory textbooks and checklists of skills are available from multiple publishers. You can either use these or make your own checklists, though doing so can be very time-consuming.

- One faculty member suggested that students wear the school uniform when in the resource simulation lab. Uniforms foster a professional atmosphere in which the students "feel like nurses" and behave accordingly. Uniforms also help them regard the lab as an integral component of the clinical experience.

- Student teaching assistants have made a positive difference in our program. Having senior students assist junior students benefits both parties. More details about this program are found in the literature.[8]

- Actors posing as clients (standardized patients) can be useful in teaching physical assessment skills to prelicensure students and advanced skills at the graduate level. Schools may employ these actors or ask students to cover the cost as part of their course fees. Some schools with theater or other departments collaborate for course credit as students "act" like clients.

- There is increased emphasis on interprofessional simulation as a way to build teamwork and collaboration. Consider working with other departments at your school to foster such alliances.

- Readers are encouraged to delve into the current literature for creative lab strategies. In-class simulation, where entire lab setups are wheeled into the room, are becoming more popular.[9,10]

Instructors use PowerPoint to develop the electronic health record and data; a voice-over lecture allows the client to share her or his story; and the simulation commences with several students as nurses, other healthcare professionals, and family members. The rest of the class members serve as witnesses, taking notes on nursing interventions, appraising lab results as they emerge, and writing individual SBARs. The debriefing discusses the scenario, client responses, nursing judgments, and means to improve.

- Using tabletop activities is another creative option. One school addressed disaster planning by providing disaster patient scenarios, which presented students with patients after a disaster, provided results of appropriate assessments, and required clinical judgment in the management of the patient.[11] Students conducted disaster management from their seats while some students served as disaster logistics officers, liaison officers, and in other roles. This may be a more feasible option than full-scale disaster drills, in which large classes of students are assigned roles and manage a simulated disaster.

- For orientees and nurses new to a specialty, engage more senior clinicians to teach, assist with practice, and evaluate psychomotor skills. In clinical agencies with explicit procedure manuals, ensure that skills are taught and learned according to agency policy (see **Active Reading Conference**).

- Some lab skills or remediation efforts may benefit from station concepts. In these setups, students rotate among separate stations that include psychomotor skills, scenarios requiring clinical decision making, and planning of care. These are great to do at the beginning of the semester when students might be "rusty" or at the end of the semester to reinforce learning and ensure competence.[12]

- The use of simulation mannequins has revolutionized the way nursing skills are taught in both schools and the clinical area. Simulators can be programmed to provide more than just a practice medium for a specific skill. They also can replicate a client's response in a given situation. Numerous resources exist for establishing and maintaining a simulation lab. Educational research has begun to develop an evidence basis for the use of simulators in nursing education across the practice field.

- An innovative colleague developed a very effective and inexpensive lab technique to use in the classroom. This mental health instructor determined that students often do not appreciate the "realness" of client delusions and hallucinations. The instructor sat in the front of the room with one student sitting, facing the instructor. Several other students stood behind the student. The instructor commenced to attempt dietary teaching with the student who was the simulated client. The other students started to speak, simultaneously replicating internal voices. The student felt the frustration of struggling to attend to the content, the temptation to yield to the distraction, and the embarrassment of not attending to a professional. This strategy provides a valuable and expedient means to provide reality-based experiences in the classroom.

Equipment Conference

General Description. This strategy is just what it sounds like. **Equipment Conferences** acquaint students with equipment they'll use in the clinical area. Each agency has its own type of equipment, which may differ from what students used in previous lab work. This strategy reviews the basic workings of a piece of equipment and examines the nuances of a specific machine or set of supplies. Conferences take place away from the active clinical area. Thus, they provide a safe opportunity to discuss the policies and procedures involved in operating and troubleshooting equipment.

Preparation and Equipment. Plan the time and place for the conference and bring the equipment with you. In some cases you'll need other supplies to put the equipment to work and allow students to practice.

Example of the Strategy at Work. Although students practiced clinical skills repeatedly in the lab, they consistently expressed misgivings about their skills. I chose to incorporate tracheostomy care and suctioning into their orientation day. We used several mannequins with simulated tracheostomies and portable suction to allow students to practice the skill in pairs.

The students practiced tracheostomy care according to the agency policy, which was slightly different than what they had learned in lab. They changed tracheostomy ties, did the suctioning procedure, and bagged the mannequin to provide oxygenation between suctioning attempts. They rotated among the stations and practiced each skill. Students were encouraged to teach each other and provide feedback. An earlier tour of the unit had shown them how many clients were ventilated by tracheostomy. Seeing the wide clinical application of this skill helped them appreciate its relevance and immediacy.

Once I taught on an oncology unit, in which many clients had central venous access devices. One of our responsibilities was changing the central line dressings. We used the unit's format for teaching families: venous devices were accessed from staff development and inserted into placemats purchased at a local bargain store. The students brought central line dressing change kits for practicing. First, we all did the procedure together, discussing sterile technique, principles of asepsis, how to change a dressing on a moving client, and troubleshooting line complications. Then each student was able to change the dressing on an individual placemat.

In both examples, students were active during the conference period and reinforced a key skill for the clinical area. They could then be held accountable for that skill when the time came to provide it as part of client care.

Ideas for Use

- Conduct **Equipment Conferences** early in the rotation to ensure competency before your students begin caring for clients. Start with less complex equipment, such as the pulse oximeter. Pass the sensor around the room to have students spot-check themselves. Move on to more complex skills throughout the rotation.

- If you can, obtain the equipment instruction manuals or agency policies to establish the procedures and show the students where they can obtain additional information about the skills.

- Identify the key skills the students will need on the unit: inserting urinary catheters, administering IV medications, using a feeding pump to administer tube feedings, using IV infusion pumps, caring for a client with a ventilator, changing complex dressings, and obtaining and interpreting electrocardiogram strips. These and many other skills can be reviewed in the clinical area if students' motivation is high and agency-specific equipment is available.

- Solicit feedback about what skills the students would like to review in conference time. As the rotation proceeds, poll them to find out what equipment or skills they find puzzling and build an **Equipment Conference** around those needs.

- Conferences may be held before, during, or after clinical or orientation days, or during other clinical meetings.

- **Equipment Conferences** may be instructor-led or student-led according to the needs of the group and the way students are evaluated. The **Equipment Conference** may be assigned to each student as part of the course grade.

- Enlist other professionals at the agency to help with **Equipment Conferences.** Respiratory therapists, dieticians, IV specialists, unit instructors, and staff development personnel can provide a high level of expertise concerning skills and agency-specific procedures.

- Staff development educators may provide frequent **Equipment Conferences** as needed when technology, new designs, and new products become available. Consult manufacturers for their support with training supplies and materials. Combine this strategy with **Learning Carts.**

Active Reading Conference

General Description. I was surprised to find that students often didn't know what resources were available. Then I realized that I, as their clinical instructor, was responsible for showing them these documents. That's how the **Active Reading Conference** was born.

One surprise new nurses and nursing students face is the realization that there's more than one way to do certain procedures. Sometimes different procedures can accomplish the same skill with the same outcome. Another surprise for students and orientees is that clinical agencies have explicit procedures and standards of care, much like the skills texts and care plans used in nursing school.

The **Active Reading Conference** reveals the resources available in a clinical agency and reinforces the importance of those documents for safe practice. This strategy requires both students and instructors to be vigilant for frequently used skills or common nursing problems in the specific clinical area. The instructor assigns each student to seek a procedure or the standard of care for that procedure. Students read this to the group during conference time. **Active Reading** calls for students to condense and summarize the information, making sure to emphasize key points, focus on nursing priorities, and allow for questions and comments.

Preparation and Equipment. Find the agency protocols via the intranet or manuals and show them to the students early in agency orientation. Refer students to those documents frequently to ensure their use during clinical practice. Many agencies have converted their procedures and standards of care to an electronic format, available through the facility's network.

Example of the Strategy at Work. A student needed to insert a nasogastric tube into a client and panicked. The student had learned the skill in the lab and been tested successfully—but now the time had come to really do it. We got out the agency manual, at the time bound in a notebook, read the procedure together, and completed the skill. The student, who marveled at the resource and how much it had helped with the task, wanted to share the experience in postconference. The student copied the procedure and presented key points of the policy to fellow students while discussing the experience of inserting the nasogastric tube.

Ideas for Use

- Have students download and print or copy a policy or protocol and use a highlighter to emphasize key points of the standard of care or procedure before they present it to their peers.
- Tell students the point of the strategy—to emphasize key concepts and focus on nursing priorities. The word *reading* confuses some students, who think they're supposed to report on the document verbatim.
- Pass out company equipment handouts or other materials to help students learn about new equipment.
- Post **Active Reading Conference** information in the restrooms. One participant called this method "Elimination Illumination." Another is "Stall Street Journal."
- This strategy can be incorporated into mandatory skills and orientation to ensure compliance with agency policies.
- The **Active Reading Conference** is especially valuable if the student assigned to read the case will be caring for a client needing this skill or care plan. Encourage the student to enhance the presentation with personal experiences. Students enjoy sharing insights—what it was like to do the procedure, the challenges encountered, and the sense of accomplishment following the task. The discussion can include client responses to the procedure and other nursing interventions, such as teaching, comforting, and client support.
- The **Active Reading Conference** may be effective in a service setting, where seasoned nurses forget the trepidation that skills can arouse in new nurses. Novices can share experiences and learn vicariously from each other.
- An important facet of this strategy is the legal and accrediting aspect of agency procedures and standards of care. Students also need to consider the ramifications of not knowing, not following, or deviating from agency protocols.
- Orientation groups can use this strategy to introduce procedures and standards of care to new employees. **Active Reading Conferences** or debriefings may be used to emphasize key skills and conditions that the new nurse will encounter in the clinical area.
- Many organizations have their policies, procedures, and standards on their intranet, allowing students and orientees to download documents as needed.

Grand Rounds

General Description. Grand Rounds is a common strategy that many of us remember from our days in school. However, some conditions have changed. Clients now expect to be informed about their care; at the same time, they expect that information to remain confidential. We've had to adapt our methods to meet the needs of students and orientees while respecting those of clients.

Grand Rounds requires each student to present cases either at the client's bedside or outside the room. Students are asked to provide a brief description of the client's issues and diagnoses, the course of treatment, and the nursing priorities and implications. An important component of this strategy is to seek the client's and family's permission before undertaking it.

Preparation and Equipment. No equipment is needed. You should preview the clients for whom students will present **Grand Rounds.** Higher acuity levels reflect an increase in the number of clients who may be too sick to qualify for this strategy. Students should understand how to speak about clients in their presence and what information to present. You can give them guidelines, such as a list of needed information: client age, sex, and diagnosis; current course of treatment; nursing issues; and priorities at this time.

Example of the Strategy at Work. **Grand Rounds** is especially valuable when students have gotten comfortable caring for and interacting with clients. Toward the end of the rotation, they generally have the knowledge and poise to undertake the strategy. I let the students decide whether to conduct the **Grand Rounds** at the client's bedside or at the door.

I've also found it important to secure the permission of the nurse manager. Because of Health Insurance Portability and Accountability Act (HIPAA) and confidentiality restrictions, some leaders prefer that we use a conference room for these discussions. In such cases, I assign two or three **Grand Rounds** per clinical day. I ask all the students to introduce themselves to the clients we'll discuss that day, as well as to the clients' families. This tactic gives all the students a visual picture of the client to go along with the presentation. I also reinforce the need to be polite, caring, and respectful during all client interactions.

Ideas for Use

- Questions addressed in the **Clinical Questioning** strategy can become part of the student's presentation in **Grand Rounds.**
- Not only should we ask the client's and family's permission, but we should also ask their perceptions and priorities at this time,

for example: What is troubling you most? What do you expect to get out of this hospitalization? What do you need nursing to assist you with? These questions and others include clients as true partners in care.

- Some instructors find it valuable to include physical and other assessments as part of **Grand Rounds.** This method enlists clients' help in teaching the students or orientees. Again, it takes a special client to agree, and the direction of **Grand Rounds** must change if the client becomes uncomfortable. This is also a great way for you to demonstrate a client assessment on the first day of clinical. You conduct the assessment and the students watch.

- Show the film clip from *Patch Adams* in which Patch so adeptly rehumanizes rounds by asking the client's name. Spend some time discussing that client's reactions to the other physicians and then to Patch as a way to model behaviors.

- **Grand Rounds** are meant to focus on client-specific information. This is not the time for elaborate discussions of pathophysiology or treatment options. For more in-depth discussions, see **One-Minute Class** and **Student-Led Seminars.**

- Students may share their **Ah-Ha Journals,** their nursing priorities in the care of selected clients, and what they would do differently if they cared for the client again. This information must be shared judiciously if the rounds take place at the bedside.

- Use the **One-Minute Care Plan** to guide the structure of **Grand Rounds** if you would like to try a different format.

- As the practice of bedside reporting takes shape in many agencies, use **Grand Rounds** to build on that model and provide for comprehensive reporting along with including the client as a partner in care.

- **Grand Rounds** offers a great opportunity for students and orientees to present with knowledge and a sense of accomplishment. Talking about the client and answering questions gives students a chance to succeed and feel good about their progress. It's important for instructors to take a back seat at this time and allow the students to teach each other.

V-8 Conference

General Description. Students often focus solely on their assigned client or clients. In relation to other unit activities and to the experiences of other students, they sometimes seem to have blinders on. The **V-8 Conference** allows students to share experiences about their clients and to learn from each other.

Essentially, the **V-8 Conference** is a group-experience **Ah-Ha Journal.** Students share information that's newly learned, surprising, never thought about, or not previously known. The strategy gets its name from a familiar vegetable drink.

V-8 Conferences give students an opportunity to discuss their experiences and learn vicariously about clients or clinical issues. Keep a 5-minute time frame but also allow informal discussion to ensure that the entire group participates. The **V-8 Conference** may simply evolve in the direction of the conversation or may have a specific focus selected by the group or the instructor. Students and orientees benefit greatly by hearing about the **Ah-Ha Journals** of every member of the group.

Preparation and Equipment. Little preparation is required with this strategy. In fact, once the conversation is under way, you should provide very little input, allowing the students to lead the discussion. This should be the focus—letting students learn and share while you are a silent observer. You may want to look over your available clinical days and select a focus to provide a direction for each **V-8 Conference.**

Example of the Strategy at Work. As a pediatric nursing instructor, I have two major goals in mind for clinical rotations. I hope that, in addition to learning safe, skilled, and organized clinical care, my students will embrace the concepts of *family-centered care* and *developmental care.* Because these are such high priorities of mine, I use two **V-8 Conferences,** one to address each issue. I present the topic at the beginning. Then the students discuss their personal observations and related client information in terms of their experiences. The assigned focus guides them in asking questions and relating facets of client care.

Ideas for Use

- You can assign a discussion group leader for the **V-8 Conference** or allow the leader to emerge naturally. Discussion leaders can be rotated to ensure equal participation and leadership experiences.
- A few possible topics are:
    - Family-centered care
    - Organizational skills needed to be a nurse
    - End-of-life care
    - Managing the critically ill client
    - Gearing care toward a client's developmental, not chronological, age
    - Clinical research protocols

- Quality Safety Education for Nurses (QSEN)
- NCLEX® Blueprint
- Ethical issues in the clinical area
- Delegation and working with unlicensed assistive personnel
- Staffing and scheduling
- Use **V-8 Conferences** as part of the debriefing process during nursing orientation. Ask students to share their experiences and discuss common issues, frustrations, positive experiences, and areas for growth. Novice nurses may be relieved to learn that others feel the same way or confront similar stressors.
- Use **V-8 Conferences** as times to reinforce teamwork, collaboration, collegiality, mutual support, and learning, and to foster problem solving, decision making, and critical thinking skills. Make sure the **V-8 Conference** doesn't become a complaint session, take on a competitive edge, or become a dreaded part of the clinical day.
- Students should see the **V-8 Conference** as their opportunity to learn and to talk. Intervene only if the conversation is inappropriate or contrary to the objectives of the clinical rotation.
- Conferences may be held before, during, or after clinical or orientation days, or during clinical meetings held at other times.
- Conferences may take place before client care, when students are apprehensive, or after a hard shift, when they're exhausted. Either way, conferences need to be fun, creative, and informative. Encourage students to enjoy this time and see the value of sharing and learning together.
- Provide snacks or have a **V-8 Conference** during a meal to foster a sharing atmosphere.

Documentation Case Study

General Description. The **Documentation Case Study** is one of my favorite clinical strategies. One of the greatest challenges for a nursing student or new employee is to master an agency's unique documentation procedures. Each facility has slightly different forms, expectations, and policies. In addition, different units, groups, or areas may differ subtly in what they mean by "note," "charting by exception," or "keeping up with your charting." Accrediting agencies have certain parameters for safe and legal documentation, but documentation guidelines may be interpreted differently within those constraints.

The **Documentation Case Study** was developed in response to these challenges. The case study is completed during clinical orientation and allows students to practice documentation skills before recording data in an actual medical record.

Preparation and Equipment. The **Documentation Case Study** is one strategy that takes a long time to develop. Once written, though, it can be used again and again. The strategy also makes it much easier to teach and learn agency documentation. First, you need to acquire the flow sheets, documentation policies, and other forms from the agency or you need to become very familiar with the agency electronic health record. Develop a case study and take the client through a care shift. As the shift proceeds, invent little detours that can present a documentation challenges. Develop the case with assessments, clinical information, interventions, and outcomes, all of which need to be documented. For agencies that still use paper charts, this strategy is appropriate. For those with electronic health records, the exercise still may be useful to highlight how to document and what is documented in addition to addressing how charting is done when computers are "down."

You can be as creative as you like. Use this case and appropriate forms to construct an activity best conducted during the orientation phase of learning.

Example of the Strategy at Work. Here is the form I developed. Feel free to adapt it for your personal needs.

Documentation Case Study Exercise

Hello! You and a clinical group member have been assigned a complex case. In this exercise, you'll work together to document the vital data you receive in your assessment. You may work together in any way you like.

You are caring for D. B., a client on the evening shift. He is a 3-year-old admitted for uncontrolled seizures and a history of asthma. On entering the room, you note that he is wearing his ID band and an allergy band indicating an allergy to adhesive tape. The side rails are up, a pulse oximeter is attached with the alarms on, and he is on seizure precautions. His family is at the bedside.

What precautions are indicated in a client at risk for seizure?

_____

_____

You note that his daily weight was not recorded on the day shift. You weigh him during your assessment; he weighs 31 lb. You need to record his weight in kilograms. His admission weight was 12.7 kg; his weight yesterday was 13.1 kg. At 1615 you proceed with the following assessment:

Vital signs: Temperature (axillary): 37.1, Heart rate: 105 bpm, Respirations: 20/min, Blood pressure: 87/56. He is on room air with an oxygen saturation of 89 percent.

Are these findings normal? What would you do?

_____

_____

At 1630 his work of breathing is increased with retractions. His breath sounds are coarse in the upper lobes bilaterally and decreased in the lower lobes, especially the left. He has a productive cough. You provide a prn (as needed) aerosol breathing treatment of 2 mL metaproterenol with 1 mL cromolyn. You suction for a small amount of thin, cloudy drainage. You reassess at 1700 and find he had a positive response to the respiratory treatment.

What would you expect his work of breathing, breath sounds, and oxygen saturation to be after a positive response to the respiratory treatment?

_____

_____

You chart his respiratory response at 1700. Dinner has arrived. He is on a regular diet, eats well, and drinks 240 mL of juice and 180 mL of water.

How would you document his appetite?

_____

At 1730 you move on with your assessment. You find that his color is pink, his skin is warm in all four extremities, he has no edema, and his pulses are strong in each limb. His capillary refill is less than 2 sec in the nailbeds of his fingers and toes.

Is his capillary refill within normal limits?

_____

He is able to follow your commands and assists you with your assessments. He has good muscle strength in his fingers, hips, and legs. His pupils are 4 mm, reacting bilaterally and briskly to lights.

Because of his episode of respiratory distress, he is placed on bed rest with bathroom privileges. He denies any pain. His belly is soft and flat and he has positive bowel sounds in all four quadrants.

At 1800, when you finish your assessment, he asks to use the bathroom. Measuring with a urine hat, you find he voids 75 mL of clear, yellow urine with a specific gravity of 1.030, negative for blood and ketones.

Is that specific gravity within normal limits?

_____

What nursing interventions would you suggest?

_____

At 1900 he has a formed small stool. You estimate it at about 50 mL. A HemaTest is negative for blood. The stool is brown and formed, with a pH of 5. You give the child a complete bed bath.

The client does not have infusing IV fluids but does have an intravenous reservoir, to be flushed every 4 hours with 10 mL normal saline solution. This was done at 1900.

At 2000 he has a grand mal seizure lasting 45 seconds. You record it and the duration on the flow sheet. You document the description in the progress notes.

What behaviors would you expect to describe when documenting a grand mal seizure with full tonoclonic body movements?

_____

_____

After the seizure he vomits 10 mL of thick mucus. He is very sleepy postically. He drinks 60 mL of flat cola at 2030 and voids 120 mL at that time, specific gravity 1.020. You prepare him for bed and assist him with his own oral hygiene. His vital signs at 2100 are:

Temperature (axillary): 36.9, Heart rate: 100 bpm, Respirations: 16/min, Blood pressure: 80/50. His assessment criteria for 2100 is the same as your afternoon assessment. Chart this assessment in the appropriate place.

His mother asks about seizure precautions and you provide teaching at 2130. Chart this in the progress notes.

As you prepare to leave the unit and report to staff, you and your partner sign the flow sheet. Another busy shift!

Ideas for Use

- Use the **Documentation Case Study** early in orientation to teach important documentation skills.
- This exercise is a good way to reinforce the military 24-hour clock often used in clinical agencies.
- Have the students fill out the forms in pairs or trios, allowing for teamwork and team building.
- You may collect this form or allow students to keep it to use as a guide for future documentation.
- This exercise allows students to practice and make mistakes safely.
- The **Documentation Case Study** prevents a common error of new nurses—documenting just as the nurse before them did. Students and new nurses need to see the importance of valid documentation that reflects educated, thorough assessments and interventions.
- For observational experiences such as the operating room, postanesthesia care unit, intensive care unit, and emergency department, obtain documentation forms and flow sheets to discuss with students. These will help to clarify the documentation processes in the different areas.

Clinical Questioning

General Description. Questioning students in the clinical area is a true art. It's not easy to catch up with eight to 12 nursing students or orientees, and it is difficult to assess their progress and preparation for clinical work. **Clinical Questioning** is a valuable tool you can use to determine a new nurse's readiness for increased challenge, safety in the clinical setting, strengths, and areas of future growth. This strategy is designed for the rapid assessment of individual progress. Alfaro-Lefevre[13] discussed the need for students to attend to three concepts in clinical thinking:

1. Thinking ahead (in preparation for the clinical experience)
2. Thinking in action (concurrently with client care)
3. Thinking back (reflecting on care delivered)

These three concepts provide a framework for **Clinical Questioning.**
Preparation and Equipment. Sage nursing instructors in both practice and academic settings can determine quickly when students or nurses are prepared, knowledgeable, and safe in the clinical area. They ask a few basic questions, homing in on clinical decision making, assessment, and critical thinking.

As a clinical instructor, you need several of these questions up your sleeve in today's high-acuity healthcare environments. Select and adapt the questions to the clinical unit or specialty and to your own style. Write them on an index card and carry it with you, tape it to a clipboard, or memorize it. Have the questions available before or during client care. Use these questions readily with students to ensure their eligibility to provide client care. Tell your students that there may be more than one correct answer; this knowledge fosters critical thinking and creative problem solving.

Example of the Strategy at Work. Develop your own questions or adapt these:

> What will you do today to make a difference in the life of this client?
> What will you do to make your client better today?
> What did you, or what will you, spend the most time doing today?
> What equipment will you need to get the day started? As the day goes on?
> What one thing will you do differently the next time you take care of your client?
> Why is *your client* on that medication?
> How will you know the medication or treatment was successful?
> What complications are you worried about with this client?
> What signs and symptoms indicate a deterioration of the client's condition?
> How did you prepare to take care of your client?
> What do you think concerns your client the most?
> What information do you need to get from the client record as soon as you assume his or her care?
> What three things that you heard in report will be priorities for you during your shift?
> What three things will be most important to report to the staff members when we leave?
> What procedures and interventions did you witness that can be done in other ways? What aspect of the procedure would be different?

Ideas for Use

- Students generally find **Clinical Questioning** threatening and can feel judged. If you develop your questions in a nurturing, supportive manner, students will find it easier to express themselves articulately. Try to present **Clinical Questioning** as an opportunity for students to learn and demonstrate their level of knowledge.
- Ensure that students know your expectations for clinical preparation. Be clear about how much they should know regarding the disease process, medications, care plan, and client specifics. Emphasize that preparation for clinical experience is a

professional expectation, not an option, and that it shows the nursing instructor that the student is ready to provide care.

- Make sure students know when to expect **Clinical Questioning** and how it will take place. A colleague of mine announces a set time before which students may solicit information from the client and staff members, consult the medical record, and research questions. After that time, the student should be able to answer the instructor's **Clinical Questions.**

- Provide your **Clinical Questions** in the course materials or syllabus to make students aware of potential questions while they're preparing.

- Use **Clinical Questioning** to assess completion of orientation, achievement of objectives, and safety in the clinical area. Provide students with positive and negative, as well as formative and summative, information. Balancing teaching and evaluation can be one of the great challenges of clinical teaching. **Clinical Questioning** should be part of both processes.

- Use **Clinical Questioning** topics to shape student evaluations. Have students self-evaluate their performance using these questions as the basis for knowledge, preparation, and critical thinking. If you use objective evaluation tools to substantiate clinical performance, the focus stays on clinical course objectives and experiences during rotation.

- Make sure you don't single out any students during **Clinical Questioning.** The tendency is to assess weaker students repeatedly, which can make them feel "picked on." Offer the same amount of feedback to all your students, although its composition can differ drastically from one student to another.

Use the Book in Clinical

General Description. In clinical supervision, it's hard to keep up with what students are learning or have learned in didactic and previous clinical courses. Students sometimes deny experience or knowledge. They may feel overwhelmed, not wish to be held accountable, or truly forget some of the vast amount of information they've learned or heard in nursing school.

Use the Book in Clinical allows instructors, students, and orientees to consider what's learned in class and how it applies to the clinical area. Students bring their texts to the clinical area, look up needed information, and base conferences on their texts and other resources. This strategy also fosters inquiry skills, in which nurses actively research and investigate topics rather than simply learn by rote or authority.

Preparation and Equipment. Instructors who teach both clinical and didactic courses have a head start. Not only do they know what's being taught in class, they can help students apply that information to their clients. Part-time or exclusively clinical instructors often need to pursue such information themselves to know what's going on in the classroom. The same is true for agency staff development instructors embarking on creating a valuable orientation for a new employee.

All instructors should attend to the logic of the curriculum and think about how their courses fit into the total program objectives. Informal conversation with other instructors can clarify what clinical objectives, psychomotor skills, organizational abilities, and assessments students have mastered in previous courses. Course outlines and syllabi are useful. All instructors should have a copy of the textbook that corresponds to each clinical area. The text shows what students have read for class and how they're preparing for clinical rotations.

Example of the Strategy at Work. I use **Use the Book in Clinical** continuously rather than as an isolated event. Clinical preparation is of paramount importance in safe client care. By knowing what's in their textbooks and remembering what has been discussed in their didactic classes, students can be held accountable and encouraged to apply their knowledge clinically. As classroom information grows more complex and students begin to care for high-acuity clients, it's imperative for them to make that connection.

Ideas for Use

- Before their clinical experience, students and orientees can present a client's medical diagnosis and nursing priorities using their textbook preparation. The presentation, which should be kept brief, may be done during preconference time.
- Staff development instructors may find it helpful to consult local nursing programs. They can provide valuable information about their curricula and show how students have learned from clinical experience at their agency.
- During conference, students can discuss what they learned in class about specific conditions, and can apply their knowledge to each other's clients. Your role is to make sure the information is valid and appropriate.
- Students have difficulty with the concepts of multiple diagnoses, comorbidities, and conflicting priorities brought on by

severe health issues. They often expect a client to have only one diagnosis and become flustered with the complexity of the client's actual condition. **Use the Book in Clinical** helps students to unravel information and apply it to individual clients and their needs.

- Have both new and seasoned nurses peruse the textbooks on the unit. This tactic reminds them of lessons learned in nursing school and changes that may have occurred since that time. Reflection on their clinical learning can help them continue to learn and grow. Sharing textbook knowledge and experience can inspire discussion about practice issues, leading to **Research Moments** and **Clinical Area Questioning: Research at Work.**

- Use case studies, critical thinking exercises, and test questions in nursing texts to connect didactic learning with clinical practice.

Field Trips

General Description. We are all familiar with class field trips from our early school years. What we didn't always appreciate is that these trips were carefully planned around our learning needs. Similarly, **Field Trips** are carefully planned facets of nursing clinical instruction. **Field Trips** are useful when additional experience is needed to complement what students customarily learn at clinical agencies.

Preparation and Equipment. **Field Trips** can take a considerable amount of planning or very little. Students may attend alone, in pairs, or in groups.

Example of the Strategy at Work. I experienced this strategy during my own nursing education. My instructor was way before her time: she contended that, to provide holistic nursing care, students needed to be acquainted with the community and the neighborhood around the agency. She had us go to a local restaurant and arranged for us to be given a free portion of a local favorite food, visit the city hall and learn about the town, and window shop through local businesses to get a feel for the community. My students now use this "shoe leather" survey in wellness and community courses to get to know different communities and to learn about the needs of clients outside the agency.

I have used this strategy in a pharmacology class in two ways. Students were asked to take two "field experiences." Here are the guidelines from their syllabus about these **Field Trips.**

Field Experience 1: Pharmacy Visit

For this assignment, you can visit any pharmacy. Select an over-the-counter medication. Take a minute to read the label on the brand-name medication. Find the generic or store-brand medication and read that label carefully.

- Compare the ingredients of both medications.
- Compare the instructions given for both.
- Compare the packaging for both.
- Compare the prices for both.
- What important patient education issues are found on the medication labels?
- Is there a difference between the brand name and the generic or store brand?
- What is the reading level for both sets of instructions?
- Which medication would you purchase? Why?

Field Experience 2: Medicine Cabinet Assessment

Find a medicine cabinet that has at least six over-the-counter or prescription medications in it. Answer the following questions:

- List at least six medications in the cabinet.
- Are any of these medications expired?
- Are prescription medications in the originally labeled bottles?
- What specific precautions are noted for any of the medications?
- Imagine that a client is taking all six medications. What potential interactions should the nurse and the client be aware of?
- What safety issues might be associated with these medications?
- What client education issues can you identify?

Ideas for Use

- Arrange for students to visit and tour large metropolitan medical centers if current clinical sites are limited to community hospitals. Students learn a lot from **Field Trips** to emergency departments with helipads, large intensive care units, and specialty areas. Agencies with significant nursing workforce needs often use these tours for recruitment and marketing.

- Have students complete a community **Scavenger Hunt** as part of a **Field Trip.** As in my nursing school experience, arrange for them to visit local establishments and access local information to understand the community better.
- Pediatric nursing students can visit a toy store to learn about safe toys, developmental guidelines for toy choice, and how children play. If they compare prices, explicitness of directions, age recommendations, and safety aspects, they'll be able to provide anticipatory guidance for parents and caregivers.
- Pharmacology students can visit drugstores to peruse over-the-counter medications. Ask them to compare generic versus brand-name medications. Have them read the directions and determine the reading level of those directions. Ask them to consider the challenges experienced by people with visual impairment, for whom English is a second language, or with poor fine-motor skills. Their assessments can include medication administration instructions, childproof caps, and resources for people with low literacy skills or language disparities.
- Have students visit the local grocery store. Consider the needs of special populations, such as the elderly or those with disabilities, in navigating grocery stores with narrow aisles, carrying groceries inside the store and home, storing food, and preparing foods that come with complex instructions.
- As in the **Scavenger Hunt,** have students take a **Field Trip** within their clinical agency, such as to the medical library, the laboratory complex, or the research areas.
- One nursing instructor used a **Field Trip** to an art gallery to reinforce what the students knew about wellness, illness, and the role of nursing.
- Use shoe leather (walking) or windshield (driving) surveys for students to assess a community. Most community or wellness textbooks have a format for assessing a community's health. These can be adapted for the specific needs of the course and the clinical experience.
- Make sure **Field Trips** are objective driven and a necessary component of clinical education.
- Use **Injection Field Trips** to let your students practice giving immunizations. Contact a school health center, local affiliated healthcare agencies, public health clinics, or local pharmacies for opportunities to give annual influenza injections. Students come away with a great feeling of accomplishment and skill mastery while providing a valuable community service.

To bring home the challenges imposed by living in a wheelchair, one nursing instructor had students navigate the college campus in wheelchairs. Pairs of students, one in the chair and one assisting, experienced wheelchair accessibility or its lack, the reactions of others, and the environmental obstacles related to traffic, crowds, physical strength, and time constraints.

- The ultimate **Field Trip** may be through mission trips, disaster relief efforts, service trips, or study abroad in which students learn the role of nursing in vulnerable settings and focus on clients in grave circumstances, in addition to their own learning needs.
- Use **Ah-Ha Journals** or **Online Discussion Groups** to evaluate the experience and students' levels of learning.

Learning From Each Other: Peer Teaching and Peer Team Leadership

General Description. In one of the quotations used in this book, Johnson and Johnson[2] state, "Everyone is both a student and a teacher." **Learning from Each Other** embraces that philosophy. In this strategy, instructors develop **Peer Teaching** and **Peer Team Leadership** activities in which students may assume the role of teacher. Students are assigned to these experiences on a rotational basis, allowing everyone to gain experience in leading and teaching others.

Preparation and Equipment. Assign students or orientees to both teaching and leadership roles during the clinical or orientation period. Students may be given some instruction on their role, methods of organizing data, and limitations on the role to ensure safe and efficient client care.

Example of the Strategy at Work.

Peer Teaching

The **Peer Teaching** concept has been used a lot in nursing programs. Most programs require that a senior student be assigned to a junior clinical group for 1 to 4 days. During that time, the **Peer Teacher** functions as an assistant nursing instructor, ensuring that tasks are completed, answering questions, and providing an extra pair of eyes and hands for the instructor. Before becoming **Peer Teachers,** senior students must complete the clinical rotation in which they'll be teaching and meet with the instructor to share expectations of the experience.

Students are often more comfortable asking questions of the **Peer Teacher.** In turn, **Peer Teachers** often feel a great sense of accomplishment when they can share what they know and thus realize how much they've learned and grown during their time in nursing school. Nursing students often feel that there's always more to learn. As a result, they may lack a sense of accomplishment about their learning. This strategy gives them insight into how much they know and how far they've come.

Following the **Peer Teacher** strategy, the **Peer Teacher** and the students evaluate the experience and the individual students' levels of performance in both roles. The **Peer Teachers** may also self-evaluate and compare their teaching and leadership styles with those described in the literature.

Peer Team Leadership

The **Peer Team Leadership** concept is similar to **Peer Teaching** except that students from the same orientation or clinical group function as leaders for a specific period. They create patient assignments, assist students with care, monitor task completion, manage changes in the patient load, ensure timely documentation, and seek the assistance of the instructor as needed. This experience helps build organizational skills, models leadership behaviors, and builds rapport within the clinical or orientation group. Again, the evaluation of self and others is an important part of this strategy.

Ideas for Use

- This strategy is helpful for busy nursing instructors in high-acuity areas. It's important to remember that instructors alone are responsible for evaluating students. Also, agencies may have explicit policies about faculty supervision of students giving medications and completing skills.
- Clinical orientees may have a **Peer Teacher** or **Peer Team Leader** who rotates from among the nursing staff, increasing the rapport between staff members and orientees and providing a mentor for clinical work.
- The **Peer Team Leader** may continue as a resource for new nurses who have just come off orientation. This tactic keeps a new nurse from feeling isolated in a newly independent role.
- Make sure that **Learning From Each Other** strategies breed team spirit and foster individual contribution. Students may become competitive in these roles, degrading group collaboration and individual feelings of success.
- Encourage students in the clinical area to **Learn From Each Other** by introducing each other to their clients and engaging in active discussions about client needs and nursing implications. Doing so encourages us to learn from our colleagues throughout our professional career.
- In classroom settings, encourage students to **Learn From Each Other** by setting up study groups, making up test questions

for each other, and tutoring each other after they discover their strengths and areas for growth.

- Creative incentives—course credit, free parking, attendance at educational conferences, award certificates, credit for service learning or volunteer hours—may be given in return for tutoring services.
- Have students and orientees pair up—senior students or those who have cared for complex conditions should assist junior or new students. This method reinforces the teamwork inherent in nursing.
- Use **Pass the Problem, V-8 Conferences,** or the **One-Minute Class** to discuss common client issues, with the **Peer Teacher** or **Peer Team Leader** moderating the conversation.
- Solicit the input of the **Peer Teacher** or the **Peer Team Leader** to enhance student clinical evaluations.

Clinical Puzzle

General Description. I learned this strategy from a class participant. The exercise was developed as a playful activity for clinical groups, with each student responsible for a portion of the project.

First, the group chooses a client with a specific medical diagnosis or condition. Then, before the clinical day, each student is given a puzzle piece with a word or words such as *Nursing Assessments, Lab Data, History, Diagnostics, Medications/Effectiveness, Surgeries/Procedures, Discharge Issues, Family Issues, Developmental Assessment,* and *Psychoemotional Issues.* The number of students in the group will affect what's written on the puzzle pieces and the number of pieces.

Students use downtime in clinical rotations to review the client's chart, consult other resources to investigate the condition, and talk with the client about the assigned aspect of care. Permission must be obtained before the students interact with the client. The instructor should take care to avoid overburdening the client with too many eager students.

During postconference that day or preconference the next day, students put the **Clinical Puzzle** together to create a comprehensive, holistic picture of the client and the medical condition.

Preparation and Equipment. Find a children's puzzle with as many pieces as there are students in the group (see your local bargain store). Writing the individual "assignment" on each puzzle piece is the only other task.

Example of the Strategy at Work. For the first clinical day in a rotation, I generally assign students in pairs. This affords them more time than usual to research a client's condition and care. For the subject of the **Clinical Puzzle,** I select the most common diagnosis on the unit and a client with that condition. I don't assign any student to care for that client; all the students must start this assignment on an equal footing. I've used this strategy to help students understand type 1 diabetes mellitus and leukemia, but it's appropriate for many medical conditions.

Ideas for Use

- You can select the nursing or medical diagnosis most appropriate for the needs of the clinical unit.
- Students can research hypothetical or actual clients to complete the **Clinical Puzzle.**
- Monitor the students' work on this assignment to ensure that clinical work is being attended to. Also, the students' activities must not overwhelm the client or the client's nurse.
- Follow the unit or agency policy for allowing more than one student access to a client's chart or electronic health record.
- Students need to see how each piece of information fits together to make up the client's clinical picture. A missing puzzle piece, just like a missing care component, skews the way we see the client and affects our care planning. To conclude this exercise, it's valuable to discuss how all the different pieces fit together and how each piece of information is needed in providing holistic nursing care.

One-Minute Class

General Description. Like the **One-Minute Care Plan,** the **One-Minute Class** gives students the opportunity to present a client to the group. The presentation must communicate integral information while filtering out anything extraneous. Although the talk may last longer than 1 minute, students are encouraged to condense information to provide a snapshot of the client in a brief period.

One of the greatest skills this exercise develops is the ability to focus. Essentially, students discriminate the "need to know" from the "nice to know." Only the highest priorities are discussed because there's no time for less important details—the student's day, the client's personality, or insignificant aspects of the client's treatment. This strategy differs from **Grand Rounds** in asking students to focus on the nursing care and priorities identified in the **One-Minute Care Plan**.

Preparation and Equipment. Little preparation is required for this exercise. You can develop a format for the assignment or use the **One-Minute Care Plan** to guide the presentation.

Example of the Strategy at Work. Unlike **Grand Rounds,** which is most effective when the students are most knowledgeable, these strategies may be used early. The **One-Minute Class** and the **One-Minute Care Plan** complement each other and provide a means for students to organize their thoughts and their care.

During orientation, I introduce the students to a client on the unit (after getting the client's and family's permission). I assess the client briefly and then leave the room (thanking the client and family again). I then pull the client's chart and show the students where to find the most information: the history and physical examination notes, the nursing database, and the progress notes. These sources give the students a glimpse into the medical record.

I pass out the **One-Minute Care Plan** form and we discuss the client's potential problems and issues. We discuss priorities and select two nursing diagnoses. I then verbally complete the **One-Minute Care Plan** form and demonstrate the **One-Minute Class.** Students are assigned to present their clients in the same way at subsequent conferences. Selecting a variety of clients enriches the experience.

Ideas for Use

- Students can use the **One-Minute Care Plan** or **Pass the Problem** information as the basis for their **One-Minute Class.**
- For deeper pathophysiological perspective on the client's condition, see the **Student-Led Seminar.** For the client's personal experience, see **Grand Rounds.**
- The **One-Minute Class** may take place before the scheduled shift, when students are apprehensive about having to provide care, or after the clinical day, when they're exhausted after a hard shift. Either way, these conferences must be fun, creative, and informative. Encourage students to enjoy this time and see the value of sharing and learning together.
- Conferences may be held at any time and may even take place during clinical meetings.
- Orientees and novice nurses can use the **One-Minute Class** during their orientation period.
- You can use **Clinical Questioning** to form the structure for the **One-Minute Class.**

Film Clips in Clinical

General Description. As in the **Short Clips** strategy, film clips can reinforce concepts during clinical rotations. As we've seen, many films show content relevant to clinical issues. Showing a short clip and talking about it

Box 7–5.
Film Clips in Clinical: Thinking Questions

- How does this clip relate to our clinical experience?
- What is the role of the nurse in this clip?
- In this scene, what are the stated or implied nursing priorities for the clinical area?
- How will this clip affect your clinical care?
- How can you generalize lessons from this clip to future clinical experience?
- What are the nursing implications of this scene?

can generate discussion about issues outside a particular clinical area. If nothing else, **Film Clips in Clinical** provides a diversion from the usual conference format.

For this strategy, it's important to develop thinking questions based on clinical objectives and to reinforce the nursing implications of events shown in the clip. Encourage your students to relate the **Film Clip** concepts to current clients, activities, and experiences. See Box 7–5 for potential thinking questions.

Preparation and Equipment. A laptop computer provides a portable, convenient way to show video footage. Clips saved to a CD or from a DVD may be shown to small clinical groups. Larger groups may need a VCR or DVD player (see **Short Clips** for details). **Film Clips in Clinical** should focus on clinical interactions, care of clients, legal and ethical issues, or other issues not always observable in the clinical area.[14]

Example of the Strategy at Work. Table 7–1 shows some videos you can use to enhance clinical instruction.

Ideas for Use

- Make popcorn and show **Film Clips in Clinical** on the last day of rotations to end the experience on a pleasant note.
- Have students do a **Quick Write, Ah-Ha Journal** entry, or **Online Discussion** to document their reactions to the clip and answer selected thinking questions.
- Show a clip and then have students play **Twosies** as a role-playing response to an interchange between actors. Ask students to rewrite the scene, making it more therapeutic or positive.
- Adhere to copyright and fair use laws while showing **Film Clips in Clinical.**
- YouTube has provided us the ability to show popular movie, television, and streamed clips via computer. Younger learners may

Table 7–1. **Some Films to Use in Clinical Teaching**

Film Title	Clinical Relevance
As Good As It Gets (1990)	Obsessive disorder Myocardial infarction Interaction of sildenafil (Viagra) and nitroglycerine
Awakenings (1990)	Symptoms of extrapyramidal effects Frustrations of chronic illness Concepts of caring Inpatient psychiatric care
A Bag of Knees (2005)	Realities of nursing care Rewards of the nursing profession Survival skills for new nurses
A Beautiful Mind (2002)	Inpatient psychiatric care "Realness" of hallucinations and delusions Family impact of mental health issues Seizure activity Nursing process (separate clips to demonstrate each step)
Clean and Sober (1988)	Substance abuse Cross-addiction Denial of addiction Group counseling
Dead Poets Society (1989)	Teen peer issues Teaching styles Group dynamics Emotional issues of adolescence Suicide and loss
Freaky Friday (2003)	Empathy—living the lives of others Mentoring Conflict resolution
How the Grinch Stole Christmas (2001)	Change theory Loneliness Caring
I Am Sam (2001)	Developmental disabilities Legal and ethical issues The judicial system

Continued

Table 7–1. **Some Films to Use in Clinical Teaching—cont'd**

Film Title	Clinical Relevance
Iris (2001)	Progression of Alzheimer's disease Caregiver issues Disruption of family dynamics Nursing home care
John Q (2002)	Medical jargon Healthcare financing Ethics in healthcare Use of technology in healthcare
Longtime Companion (1990)	AIDS Homosexual relationships Bereavement
Meet the Parents (2001)	Image of nursing Men in nursing Nurse–client interactions
My Flesh and Blood (2003)	Special-needs children Cystic fibrosis Severe burns Developmental disabilities
The Notebook (2005)	Dealing with aging Alzheimer's disease Loss and grief Frustration
October Sky (1999)	Teacher qualities Inspirational learning and goal setting Perseverance
Passion Fish (1992)	Quadriplegia following injury Stresses between client and caregiver
Patch Adams (1999)	What not to do on rounds Humor in healthcare The mind–body connection Inpatient psychiatric care—group session Physical appearance of catatonia
Pearl Harbor (2001)	Depictions of pain and injury Nurses' role in World War II Response to death

Table 7–1. Some Films to Use in Clinical Teaching—cont'd

Film Title	Clinical Relevance
Raging Bull (1980)	Head trauma Chronic traumatic encephalopathy Paranoia Physical symptoms of brain damage
Rain Man (1988)	Autism Developmental disabilities Family dynamics
Remember the Titans (2000)	Diversity Cultural struggles and awareness Team work
Save the Last Dance (2001)	Struggles of teen parenting Diversity Use of nursing theories to interpret issues Adolescence and issues with youth
The Sixth Sense (1999)	Children's perceptions of death Children's response to hospitalization Mental illness Parent interview in suspected child abuse
Steel Magnolias (1989)	Diabetes Chronic renal failure and dialysis Stress of pregnancy Family dynamics
Trainspotting (1996)	Heroin addiction Withdrawal symptoms Effects of addiction on family relationships
Wit (HBO Home Video, 2001)	Dealing with cancer Role of the nurse Interaction with the healthcare community
Young Frankenstein (1974)	Communication techniques Injection techniques (improper) Teaching techniques Research and spirit of inquiry

enjoy clips from situation comedies, television serials, and streaming entertainment shows.

- Have students identify the clips to show in conference; they can develop the thinking questions to meet clinical objectives.
- Make sure students see this strategy as a valuable clinical experience and not a frivolous exercise. Choose your clips and thinking questions carefully, keeping the course objectives in mind.

Let's Be Real in Clinical

General Description. The small size of clinical groups and the intense relationship with instructors often lead to thought-provoking and emotionally charged discussions. **Let's Be Real in Clinical** helps an instructor mold these discussions into positive learning experiences.

Theoretical learning, preconceived notions about nursing, and workplace realities all come together in the clinical area. This part of a nursing student's education can be very stressful. Venting concerns and hearing the advice of a trusted mentor are as valuable as learning cognitive and psychomotor nursing skills. In this strategy, the instructor simply opens a conversation with the words **"Let's Be Real in Clinical."** The discussion that evolves may take many directions and contributes to the socialization aspect of nursing.

Preparation and Equipment. No preparation is needed. You merely set the stage and ground rules for open and honest communication.

Example of the Strategy at Work. I developed this strategy in response to a question I received from a student. During postconference one day, I noticed that the entire group was exhausted. They had worked hard, learned a lot, and had little idle time to reflect on the day's events. In addition, they weren't looking forward to sitting for almost an hour in postconference.

One student stated, "We were all so busy today. There were eight of us and six nurses and everyone was busy. How do the nurses do it when students aren't there to help out?" I suppressed a chuckle and the retort on the tip of my tongue: "Often staff members feel they work harder when students are on the floor than when they're not."

Then I realized this was a great opportunity to discuss some of the realities of staff nursing. We discussed staffing, organizational skills, setting priorities, letting go of "nice to do but not necessary" tasks, and gaining nursing competence through experience. The students discussed these topics in light of the day's experiences, moving on to include their perceptions of reality from both class and clinical work. **Let's Be Real in Clinical** sets a time to voice concerns and discuss the realities of nursing from a personal and a professional perspective.

One question I like to ask involves the role of nursing in the healthcare system. It's often said that nurses have a difficult time defining what we do. To glean students' perceptions, I ask, "If nursing were to disappear tomorrow, what would be missing?" This question stimulates much discussion on the place of nursing in healthcare, the historical development of the nurse's role, and what role nurses will play in the future.

Ideas for Use

- Select questions to open the **Let's Be Real in Clinical** discussion, for examples:
  - How do nursing staff manage multiple client needs?
  - How is the staffing different on off shifts, weekends, and holidays?
  - How do families handle the complex care of clients at home?
  - Will I be able to do this?
  - Is NCLEX® really that hard?
  - What are my job options in nursing?
  - How should I decide where to work after graduation?
  - How do people work and live with that disease?
  - How do I talk with clients about sex and sexuality?
  - What about nursing care is most important to me?
  - What nursing specialty appeals the most to me?
  - What issues affect the smooth management of a nursing unit?
  - How do I care for clients who have value systems different from my own?
  - What characteristics do I value most in a nursing leader?
  - Do I want to pursue a higher level of education in nursing?
  - Why do some nurses leave nursing?
  - What are the pros and cons of 8-, 10-, and 12-hour shifts?
  - What skills do I bring to nursing that guide me toward a certain clinical area or specialty?
  - What qualities do I value in selecting a nursing mentor?
  - Why do they say that nurses eat their young?
  - What are the staff members' perceptions of nursing students in this agency?
  - How has the nursing shortage affected the role of the nurse?
  - How have the costs of healthcare affected the role of the nurse?
  - How do policies and politics affect the role of the nurse?
  - How are clients different now compared to 10 years ago?
  - What legal and ethical challenges does nursing face in the coming years?
  - How will advances in medical technology be reflected in nursing care?
  - Do you prefer the "high-tech" or the "high-touch" components of nursing care—and are they mutually exclusive?

- These questions and a **Let's Be Real in Clinical** discussion give students the opportunity to vent fears, seek information, and share experiences. The strategy enhances team spirit and fosters greater cooperation in the clinical group.
- **Let's Be Real in Clinical** discussions may be adapted for **Online Discussion Groups, Ah-Ha Journal** entries, or **Quick Writes.**
- This strategy is well received at the end of a clinical rotation or orientation period, when trust is high. **Let's Be Real in Clinical** provides a transition to the next clinical experience or to independent nursing.

References

1. Kagan S. Cooperative Learning. Resources for Teachers, 2015.
2. Monagle JL, Lasater K, Stoyles S, et al. New graduate nurse experiences in clinical judgment: What academic and practice educators need to know. Nursing Education Perspectives, 39(4): 201–207, 2018.
3. Johnson S and Johnson, C. The One Minute Teacher: How to Teach Others to Teach Themselves. William Morrow/Quill, 1988.
4. Bristol T. NurseThink, Inc. Waconia, WI, 2019.
5. Butler C. Nurses' experiences of managing patient deterioration: A critical incident analysis. Nursing Education in Practice 28: 96–102, 2018.
6. Vochon B and LeBlanc J. Effectiveness of past and current critical incident analysis on reflective learning and practice change. Medical Education 45: 894–904, 2011.
7. Deck ML. Instant Teaching Tools for the new millennium. Mosby, 2004.
8. Herrman J. Teaching Assistantships in Nursing Education. In Smith MJ, Carpenter R, and Fitzpatrick J. Encyclopedia of Nursing Education. Springer, 2017.
9. Walters B, Potetetz J, and Fedesco H. Simulation in the classroom: An innovative active learning experience. Clinical Simulation in Nursing 13(12): 609–615, 2017.
10. Cole LG, Graves A, and Turner S. Transforming the nursing classroom into a clinical setting. Nursing Education Perspectives 39(1): 46–47, 2018.
11. Evans CA and Schwartz R. Using tabletop exercises as an innovative and practical teaching strategy in response to external disaster scenarios. Nursing Education Perspectives 40(1): 62–64, 2019.
12. Andrea LA and Baxter PM. Incorporating innovative simulation activities into campus lab to enhance skills competence and critical thinking of second-semester associate degree nursing students. Nursing Education Perspectives 40(1): 58–59, 2019.
13. Alfaro-Lefevre R. Critical Thinking, Clinical Reasoning, and Clinical Judgment: A Practical Approach. Saunders, 2015.
14. Herrman J. Using film clips to enhance nursing education. Nurse Educator 31(6): 264–269, 2006.

Chapter 8

Strategies for Discussion Groups

> *"Shared perspectives, shared knowledge, and shared experiences are the key foundational building blocks of creativity."*—Joseph S. C. Simplicio

Challenges

- Discussion groups present challenges similar to those encountered in both large and small classes. Discussion groups are usually smaller than regular classes, with only 10 to 20 participants.

- Smaller groups in academic environments may be graded for participation. The instructor must differentiate valuable contributions from those thrown in merely to gain credit. All participants must have an opportunity to add to the discussion. Sometimes the instructor has to address the problem of students who dominate the conversation.

- Smaller groups can challenge an instructor to maintain a learning pace and keep up interest in the topic. A smaller group may actually be more difficult to teach than a larger one. Such groups are often informal and may lack a concrete agenda.

- The influence of group dynamics may be especially pronounced in small discussion sessions— friendship ties and personal preferences rise to the surface and interfere with group cohesion and functioning. The instructor may have to provide more guidance than usual to ensure a positive learning experience for all members.

- Students who don't understand the material, or who are less gregarious, may find it even harder than usual to participate when the focus is on personal learning and growth.

- New nurses and orientation groups may be reluctant to participate, especially if they are worried about their new jobs, their personal growth needs, or how few people they know. Strategies to enhance comfort and group work are imperative with these smaller groups.

Group learning and innovative strategies can help to deal with these challenges. Discussion groups are a great way to clear up ambiguities, clarify difficult material, and address personal questions. Creative methods may assist in building a team focused on learning and succeeding in both personal and group goals.

IDEAS

In-Class Debate

General Description. This strategy simply asks students to plan and carry out a debate discussing the pros and cons of an issue. The subject of the debate should be relevant to class objectives and may be selected by the students or assigned by the instructor. The instructor specifies the amount of detail in the exercise and how much class time it should take. In an academic setting, the elaborateness of the debate reflects the percentage of course credit given to the assignment.

Preparation and Equipment. The only preparation required for this assignment is the development of a list of debate topics.

Example of the Strategy at Work. I've used **In-Class Debates** mainly in clinical postconferences, although any small classroom setting is appropriate. One of our debate topics was a child in our care who was ventilator-dependent, demonstrated little brain function, had no family support, and was sustained by gastrostomy tube feedings. The child had been born with very little brain structure, had a poor prognosis, and had been cared for by many of the nursing students. The nurses on the unit told the students that there had been much discussion at many levels about withdrawing ventilatory support and enteral feedings. The students expressed concern over the legal and ethical implications of this scenario.

For our postconference, we decided to have a debate rather than the student presentations already scheduled. Six students had not yet presented their seminars and agreed to take part in the debate. With three on each side, the students presented the case, debated the pros and cons of maintaining or withdrawing the medical regimen, and discussed the nursing implications of this type of issue. The experience was extremely valuable for everyone in the group. It felt especially poignant because of the students' intimate contact with the client and their personal investment in the case.

For discussion groups, I've needed to address assisted suicide as part of class content. **In-Class Debate** contributions counted toward the group participation grade. We then used the statements in Box 8–1 to stimulate discussion and spontaneous debate. After a short class on legal and

Box 8–1.
A Right to Assisted Suicide

- Clients have the right to participate in all decisions related to their healthcare.
- Clients have the right to refuse extraordinary treatment.
- Comfort measures should always be provided.
- Clients have the right not to be interfered with in a rational act of suicide.
- Refusing life-sustaining measures is a form of suicide.
- Health professionals should always do their best to sustain a person's life.
- Health professionals have a responsibility to assist in a client's wish for suicide.

ethical decision making, we switched gears to focus on each participant's thoughts about the statements.

As you can imagine, these statements generated a lot of thought and, as the questions became more complex, a significant amount of controversy.

Ideas for Use

- Extemporaneous speeches may be based on class topics. They may be as short as 3 or 4 minutes. Students pick a topic **Out of a Hat** and rapidly compose a debate position speech. Another class member is selected to take the opposing position. Finally, the class discusses both sides of the topic and class participants voice their personal opinions.
- This is a great method for enhancing class participation; quiet students may have a strong opinion about a "hot" topic.
- **In-Class Debates** can occur spontaneously as controversial topics arise in class. Students can take their personal positions on an issue and provide their own arguments for or against it.
- **In-Class Debates** are a great way for new or practicing nurses to begin clarifying their values related to practice issues.
- This exercise has a particularly challenging version: you can ask students to debate the opposite side of their personal beliefs. By taking a stand for the other side, they must stretch their boundaries and carefully consider the pros and cons of the issue. In mounting their case this way, they're required to use true critical thinking.
- Students in discussion groups may be asked to debate each other and be peer graded on how convincing their presentations were. You may assign groups or allow the students to select their own.

- Some real-world topics for debate may be any of the following:
  - Nationalized versus commodity-based or privatized healthcare provision
  - The pros and cons of a practice seen in the clinical area
  - The nurse's role in administering a placebo medication
  - The role of a nurse who discovers that a fellow nurse is abusing substances
  - The use of restraints in a clinical agency
  - Methods of delegation and associated legal issues
  - The pros and cons and the realities associated with cross-training (orienting to multiple specialties within an agency) and pulling (routing staff members to unassigned units to meet staffing needs)
  - The nurse's role when informed consent is lacking
  - The role of a nurse who believes a client has been coerced
  - What is considered professional in nursing uniforms
  - Any other controversial topic with an arguable pro and con
- For students who don't wish to participate in an **In-Class Debate** or when a debate is not feasible, assign a **Clinical Quick Write** or a **Write to Learn** exercise. Other possibilities are an **Email Exercise** or a debate during an **Online Discussion.**
- Clinical and orientation groups may enjoy using the debate format to discuss their previous experiences and the protocols or philosophies of their new agency. Clinical preconferences and postconferences provide a great forum for debates about healthcare financing, ethical issues, professional issues, or evidence-based practices.
- In a practice setting, use the **In-Class Debate** format to guide the development of standards, address organizational policy changes, or discuss the adoption of a controversial practice. This format allows all sides to be heard and ensures that the issue will be deliberated carefully. In the **Six Hats Exercise** strategy, students use the debate template to take on varying roles in a discussion.

Teaching Trios

General Description. This strategy has students form trios. Many of the exercises discussed in this book, such as **Twosies, Think-Pair-Share, Clinical Quick Writes, Skits, Invented Dialogues, Nuts and Bolts, Active Reading Conferences,** and the **One-Minute Class** may be used with trios. All three members of the trio may be active in this exercise.

As an alternative, two participants may take a primary role and the third person act as witness or observer, evaluating the interaction. In both its forms, the strategy helps all three trio members understand what it's like to participate in all three roles. **Teaching Trios** are great for teaching life skills, such as conflict resolution, assertiveness, stress management, decision making, and dealing with difficult people or situations.

Preparation and Equipment. This exercise takes a fair amount of planning to keep it in line with the class objectives. You'll need to create a role for each member of the trio, and enough trios to represent a variety of client issues. You can write each role on an index card. Although it takes time to do this initially, you can use the cards again and again if you remember to collect them at the end of the exercise.

Example of the Strategy at Work. I use **Teaching Trios** to emphasize the role of the nurse as teacher. After the students split into trios, each one gets an index card with a role written on it. These roles are not shared with the other group members. Each student tries to play the role dictated by the card.

After 1 minute, each student passes the card to the next student: whoever had card 1 now has card 2, and so on, for 1 minute. Then they pass again. In those 3 minutes, each student has been both a teacher and a learner with a specific learning challenge. For the final 2 minutes, the students discuss the difficulties they encountered during the exercise, the challenges of the varying tasks, and their responses as they played the different roles. Following are several examples of the trios I've used.

TRIO A

1. You are a nurse teaching a client to give himself insulin injections.
2. You are a 68-year-old client with diabetes, retinopathy, and poor vision.
3. You are the daughter of a client with diabetes. You have three children, a very demanding job, and multiple life stresses.

TRIO B

1. You are a nurse trying to go over a written set of discharge instructions with a client.
2. You are a client who is unable to read and too ashamed to admit it.
3. You are an observer who is aware that the client is unable to read and won't admit it.

TRIO C

1. You are a nurse practitioner teaching safe sexual practices to a young, sexually active male client.
2. You are a 16-year-old who is having a sports physical and admits to having unprotected sex.
3. You are the mother of a 16-year-old boy who, as far as you know, is not sexually active.

TRIO D

1. You are a preoperative care nurse instructing a child who is having surgery in 1 week.
2. You are a 3-year-old child.
3. You are the mother of a 3-year-old and you are very nervous about your child's impending surgery.

TRIO E

1. You are a nurse teaching an Asian client that he must not take certain herbs because of a known interaction with the medicine prescribed by his physician.
2. You are a 55-year-old Asian man who strongly believes in the benefits of Eastern medicine.
3. You are the son of the client, and you believe that Eastern medicine is hogwash and that everyone should follow Western medicine practices.

TRIO F

1. You are a school nurse teaching a 13-year-old and his mother about the use of his inhaler.
2. You are a 13-year-old bilingual boy embarrassed about needing to use an inhaler.
3. You are the mother of a teenager and speak no English.

TRIO G

1. You are a hospice nurse teaching a client and his son about comfort measures for the client, who is dying of cancer.
2. You are an 85-year-old man with very little will to live.
3. You are a 45-year-old man who is unwilling to admit that his father is terminally ill and wants all heroic measures taken to keep him alive.

TRIO H

1. You are teaching a woman the exercises she should do to facilitate recovery after a mastectomy.
2. You are a 42-year-old woman who underwent a radical left mastectomy for breast cancer 4 days ago.
3. You are the husband of a woman who has had a mastectomy. You are appalled by her appearance and are worried that she will notice your reaction.

TRIO I

1. You are an outpatient oncology nurse teaching a client about the side effects of his chemotherapy treatment.
2. You are a man with cancer. You are devoutly religious and believe that "God will heal me, I don't need medicine."
3. You are a wife of a client with cancer and heartily believe in the medical advances that treat the disease.

TRIO J

1. You are a nurse in a Human immunodeficiency virus (HIV) clinic teaching a client about bloodborne exposure and ways to keep sexual partners safe.
2. You are a homosexual client who has just found out that he is HIV positive and doesn't want his partner to know.
3. You are the partner of a gay man and have no idea and you just found out that your partner went to a clinic.

TRIO K

1. You are a staff nurse teaching a student how to complete a technical procedure. You believe in shortcuts to get the job done.
2. You are a nursing student who has never done a certain procedure before.
3. You are a nurse watching a teaching session between a staff member and a student. You disagree with the methods used by the staff nurse.

TRIO L

1. You are a triage nurse in an emergency department teaching a client about injury prevention. The client has been to the

emergency department six times in the last year with various minor injuries.

2. You are a 35-year-old woman whose husband beats her regularly. He always makes sure the injuries are minor and has threatened your children if you tell anyone.

3. You are a 40-year-old man with an 18-year history of alcoholism who believes that what goes on in your house is no one else's business.

Ideas for Use

- For large classes, make up about 10 packs of three cards each. Have the class discuss the various difficulties they encounter in trying to teach clients with differing challenges.

- Ask the students to discuss their challenges and potential nursing interventions related to learning impediments (e.g., language barrier, cultural beliefs, poor vision, developmental issues, illiteracy, lack of motivation, poverty).

- **Teaching Trios** are good practice for dealing with sensitive client issues. Examples of these are death and dying, sexuality, the nurse–student relationship, abusive situations, client advocacy, and conflicts involving spirituality.

- **Teaching Trios** may be used in a clinical group when students encounter a situation they don't know how to deal with or in which they feel uncomfortable.

- Students learn basic critiquing skills by playing the observer and commenting on other students' responses. Because the roles rotate, everyone gets this opportunity. Nurses and nursing students are notoriously "nice" and uncritical of each other. Providing guidelines for peer review is an important lesson for professional practice.

- Like many role-play exercises, **Teaching Trios** provides a safe environment for practicing skills and is well worth the preparation time.

- **Teaching Trios** permit role playing in a comfortable setting because the cards are passed quickly and each member takes a turn at each role.

Same Information

General Description. Empathy and decision making are two of the nursing skills we try to cultivate. These skills are based on the ability to embrace the

context and complexity surrounding an issue. **Same Information** provides two different versions of a case study. Two groups are formed, and each gets one study. Now comes the fun: a key feature of this strategy is that the students don't know there are two different versions of the case study.
Preparation and Equipment. Compose both versions of your story. It's easiest to write the shorter story and then think up the second part, which adds a little twist. This second part may be as short as a single paragraph. Make sure the story is aligned with the objectives of the class.
Example of the Strategy at Work. Split your group in half. Give the first case study to one group, and give the other group the same case study with the information you've added. Then ask the students to read the case and come to some conclusions about the circumstances.

The two versions of the case below (Case One and Case Two) were used to teach a conflict resolution class for staff nurses. I'm sure you can imagine that the two versions stimulated some healthy discussion. As the discussion went on, the students understood that they were dealing with two different versions. **Same Information** demonstrates how unknown details and contextual factors may influence behavior, and how important it is to know the whole story before passing judgment.

Case One

You are a nurse working on a unit. You are making up the schedule for the winter holidays. The custom on the unit is to work every other holiday and to rotate Christmas and New Year's Day in alternate years.

A nurse comes to speak to you about Christmas. She has been working with you for 1.5 years, she worked on New Year's Day last year, and she tells you that she can't work on Christmas for personal reasons. She asks you to schedule her for this New Year's Day and not tell anyone.

Case Two

You are a nurse working on a unit. You are making up the schedule for the winter holidays. The custom on the unit is to work every other holiday and to rotate Christmas and New Year's in alternate years.

A nurse comes to speak to you about Christmas. She has been working with you for 1.5 years, she worked New Year's Day last year, and she tells you that she can't work on Christmas for personal reasons. She asks you to schedule her for this New Year's Day and not tell anyone.

After some discussion, you find out that she is a single parent and that her husband died 3 years ago around Christmastime. Her 9- and 11-year-old children have had a hard time adjusting to the holiday ever since. She is willing to work all the summer holidays. Although she has shared this information with you, she is a private person and asks you to keep it confidential.

You can imagine the colorful discussion about responsibility, taking turns at work, professionalism, empathy, and collegiality. When the information in the last paragraph emerged, the **Ah-Ha Journals** drove home many points about context and knowing the "big picture."

In another class, I was discussing congenital heart defects in children and noted the fact that rheumatic fever is often the sequela of untreated bacterial infections. We examined some reasons why an infection would go untreated: the infection is undetected, children do not receive antibiotics, and others. Several students raised the issue of a family's withholding antibiotics for a streptococcal infection, putting a child at risk for rheumatic heart disease. Following are the two versions of a story that I composed for a subsequent class.

Case One

You are caring for a 6-year-old boy. He is being treated for rheumatic heart disease following a streptococcal infection. He has sustained significant valvular damage that may require corrective surgery. You note in the chart that the client was seen in a doctor's office and that antibiotics were prescribed 5 weeks before this admission. The parents deny filling the prescription and offer no explanation for their refusal to treat the infection.

Case Two

You are caring for a 6-year-old boy. He is being treated for rheumatic heart disease following a streptococcal infection. He has sustained significant valvular damage that may require corrective surgery. You note in the chart that the client was seen in a doctor's office and that antibiotics were prescribed 5 weeks before this admission. The parents deny filling the prescription and offer no explanation for their refusal to treat the infection.

When you enter the room the 6-year-old is surrounded by his family. You learn that the family has eight children and that two grandparents live with them, making a total of 12 people in a three-bedroom home. The father has recently been laid off from his job on the assembly line at an automotive plant. Although his healthcare coverage continues, they no longer have a prescription plan. The parents elected not to fill the prescription because the family is trying to make ends meet. The grandmother has many folk remedies that have served the family well for generations, so the parents have decided to treat the infection in their own way.

These scenarios highlighted the need to ask questions, rather than make assumptions, about situations. We then discussed the need for healthcare personnel to explain why it's important to follow a care plan. In this case, the nurse should use explicit rationales and explain the potential complications of not treating the condition. The family should also receive help in finding appropriate community resources. The strengths of this family must be emphasized while the child receives the best treatment available. This important lesson is difficult to describe without the use of such a story.

Ideas for Use

- Use **Same Information** when students find it hard to understand another point of view or appreciate extenuating circumstances.
- Have students compose their own **Same Information** scenarios with specific objectives in mind.
- Make up a case any time to teach the value of perspective and the need to know the whole story before passing judgment.
- In leadership classes, this strategy is valuable for teaching decision making and helping participants "see the forest despite the trees." If different parties don't have the **Same Information,** or if management bases decisions on unknown factors, new leaders often encounter frustration. This exercise illustrates the need to understand the big picture and respect decision making while adhering to personal principles.
- **Same Information** is an effective approach to topics such as cultural and spiritual diversity, different values, attentive listening, and respect for individual beliefs.

Think-Pair-Share

General Description. **Think-Pair-Share** is most valuable when used with other strategies. Its name describes it well: first, the students **Think** about an issue, then they **Pair** up, and finally they **Share** their thoughts with the rest of the class. Another way to use **Think-Pair-Share** in larger classes is to have students think and pair up in a similar manner but they share their findings with each other. This is a loud but effective strategy when students may not want to participate in a large group.

In this strategy, first described by Lyman,[1] student pairs may share their observations with the larger group or not. Contributing factors are class time, class size, and the intricacy of the material. The key part of this strategy is the opportunity and time to contemplate the exercise and then share it with a partner.[2] Students can pair with a neighbor or pick another partner, or you can assign partners. **Think-Pair-Share** partners may be assigned for a single exercise or for the duration of the class.

Preparation and Equipment. You'll need to decide the partnership terms and create the **Think-Pair-Share** exercises. It's important that the students accept the value of pairing and sharing and that they not use the time for personal conversations or extraneous conversation.

Example of the Strategy at Work. In this strategy, I often ask students to look at a single statement, think about it, and offer comment. These statements resemble those used in **Why Are You in Nursing and Other Mysteries?, Critical Thinking Exercises, Past Experiences With . . ., What's the Big Deal?, What's the Point?, Clinical Decision-Making Exercises,** and **Email Exercises.** Box 8–2 shows examples of some **Think-Pair-Share** statements.

I've also used this strategy as a basis for class exercises. Using pairs in the class gives me a small enough group to work with and ensures active

---

Box 8–2.
Think-Pair-Share

Name the Legal Infraction

- A nurse decides to put a client in restraints so he doesn't have to worry about him at night.
- A nurse is supposed to turn a client every 2 hours but does not.
- A nurse gives a client an extra dose of sedative to keep her quiet all night.
- A nurse removes narcotics from the unit narcotic cabinet and takes them during her work shift.
- A nurse documents that he has assessed the client's IV, but he has not.
- A nurse tells her neighbors about a client who had a therapeutic abortion on her unit.
- A client decides to withdraw from a research study, but healthcare personnel do not allow it.
- A person falsifies records to say that she is an RN, but she is not.
- A nursing student gives medication to the wrong client.

participation from everyone. Students often can get into pairs and begin the activity faster than when larger groups are created, thus encouraging the time spent on task. **Think-Pair-Share** also reinforces the need to think individually and share perceptions. In this way, it differs from **Twosies,** in which students simply pair up and work on a task.

Here are two **Think-Pair-Shares** I use to teach conflict resolution and leadership styles. Effective in both large and small groups, they reinforce material rather than simply present it. The third exercise, a hypoglycemia case study, may be adapted for any diagnosis or client issue.

Conflict Resolution Exercise

You are an assistant nurse manager of a medical-surgical unit. Two nurses you work with on the unit do not get along. They ignore each other when working together, gossip about each other behind each other's back, and do not communicate important client information. One day Nurse A accuses Nurse B of neglecting an important task required for client care. Then Nurse B accuses Nurse A of spying on her and having it in for her. Nurse A says that she is concerned about care; Nurse B feels that Nurse A is being picky.

Each pair is assigned a conflict resolution approach and given the following instructions: Think of a solution to this situation based on the assigned method. What will you do to resolve this conflict? How effective do you believe you will be? What method do you think would be the most effective?

Collaboration: Both sides of the conflict work together toward a solution that does not deny the rights of either. The resolution is fully satisfactory to both sides and is a win-win situation.

Compromise: Both people sacrifice something so they can meet in the middle and agree on a solution. This situation is often described as lose-lose because neither side achieves an optimal solution.

Accommodation: This is a win-lose situation in which one person gives in to the other for the sake of a quick resolution.

Competition: In this approach, both people assert their own needs and deny the other person's desires completely. This is another win-lose situation in which resolution is accomplished to the detriment of one party.

Avoidance: The conflict is denied and swept under the rug. Neither person behaves assertively and the problem is left unresolved.

Alternatively, each student pair can respond in all five styles and then conjecture which style would work best in that situation.

Leadership Exercise

You are an assistant nurse manager delegating work during your assigned shift. You notice that one staff member doesn't seem to be completing tasks, does not interact with clients, and only briefly reports off to staff members. Other staff members have noticed, but no one has attempted to resolve the situation.

Each pair is given a leadership style. Think of one quotation, comment, or technique that represents your assigned leadership style:

Autocratic
Democratic
Charismatic
Laissez-faire
Situational
Transformational

Students then come together to share each leadership style, response, and rationale. First each pair, and then the larger groups, try to reach a consensus about which style would be most effective. Students don't always agree on a style. The difference in their opinions demonstrates the plurality of leadership styles.

Hypoglycemia Case Study

You are caring for an 8-year-old with diabetes. After he returns from physical therapy (PT), he complains of feeling shaky and weak. It is 10 a.m., and you know the dietary department has brought his morning snack. His 7:30 a.m. blood sugar was 458 mg/dL, and his urine was negative for ketones at that time. He is now looking diaphoretic and seems tired and listless.

1. What is the first thing you should do?
    Check his blood sugar.
2. What issues might you need to explore?
    How much insulin was used to correct the 7:30 a.m. hyperglycemia?
    Did he receive insulin glargine (a peakless insulin) last night?
    Did he eat breakfast?
    How did he sleep last night?
    Did he work harder than usual at PT?
3. Should you recheck his ketones?
    No, he is showing signs of hypoglycemia, not hyperglycemia.

4. Should he eat his snack?

If his blood sugar is low, correct with 15 gm of carbohydrates and wait 15 minutes. If his level is still low, he needs another glucose correction.

If his level is normal, he should have a protein and fat snack. Giving him his snack will also depend on its contents and his blood sugar level.

5. What, if anything, could have been done to prevent this episode?

His doses of both a.m. and p.m. insulin should have been lower and he should have eaten more breakfast.

6. What will you do the next day?

Give him a lower dose of a.m. insulin; reschedule PT so it doesn't coincide with the a.m. insulin peak.

Ideas for Use

- **Think-Pair-Share** is also a great icebreaker that encourages students to talk and get to know each other more personally than the average classroom allows. Use the strategy when you sense this need in your classroom.
- **Think-Pair-Share** gives less gregarious students a more private context for sharing their thoughts and insights about an exercise.
- Use **Critical Thinking Exercises, Clinical Decision-Making Exercises,** or **Email Exercises** to provide the structure for **Think-Pair-Share.**
- Ask **Think-Pair-Share** pairs to compose a **Clinical Quick Write** assignment and turn it in for grading. You can also assign a peer evaluation in which pairs trade off assignments.
- **Think-Pair-Share** is a great way to address legal and ethical dilemmas or areas of controversy. This strategy encourages students to think deeply about issues and to share their perceptions in a safe duo.

Admit Ticket

General Description. In this exercise, the assignment is to accomplish a certain task and provide physical evidence that the task has been completed. That evidence is the student's **Admit Ticket** into the classroom (Herrman[3]). The tasks and the **Admit Tickets** may take many forms.

Admission to the class depends on following instructions, completing the task, and remembering to bring the evidence.

Preparation and Equipment. You'll need to set aside a small amount of class time for this strategy. You must compose questions or solicit comments, making sure the assignment is clear. If students show up for class without **Admit Tickets,** policies should be clearly delineated and enforced equally. The syllabus must be clear about both the assignments and the repercussions of not bringing the **Admit Ticket** to class.

For continuing education classes, you can use incentives to reward students who bring their **Admit Tickets.** This method precludes embarrassment and negative feelings for attendees who come without their **Admit Ticket.** It's important to remember that this strategy isn't meant to punish but to reward going the extra mile in the learning environment.

Example of the Strategy at Work. I used **Admit Tickets** in a Friday afternoon class. My colleagues and I were having a hard time getting students to attend because they frequently worked, traveled, or had other activities on Friday. We used the strategy for students who attended class and stayed for the entire session, providing extra credit for each **Admit Ticket** collected. Although the amount of extra credit per assignment was very small, the accumulated points could affect the grade substantially.

Admit Ticket tasks included composing test questions, answering questions based on lecture content, developing a response to a thinking question, and other tasks designed by the course instructors. In continuing education, we routinely require students to bring certain materials to class, especially in critical care, pharmacology, or resuscitation classes. Assigning these materials as **Admit Tickets** reinforces the importance of bringing them to class.

Ideas for Use

- Sometimes we feel that **Admit Tickets** work against us. Some nursing educators are so happy to have students attend class that we don't want to turn anyone away. We worry that students who are unprepared may just decide not to come. One instructor adapted the **Admit Ticket** to create an **Exit Ticket** strategy. The students needed to answer a question or perform some other task before they could leave the class. Especially in continuing education, we want to reinforce rather than discourage class attendance and lifelong learning.

- Combine this strategy with **In-Class Test Questions**. Have students make up test questions about that day's class and hand them in as an **Exit Ticket** or an **Admit Ticket** for the next class.

- **Admit Tickets** encourage attendance even when they aren't due. Students don't want to miss a class in which an **Admit Ticket** might be assigned for the next class.
- **Admit Ticket** may work better in smaller classes. Too many people can create a crowd at the door or make it unwieldy to collect tickets.
- Use **Admit Ticket** in combination with **Muddiest Part.** Ask students to identify the content areas they find the most confusing or complex and to write them on the **Admit Ticket** for the next class. Reviewing the **Admit Tickets** lets you assess the class and provide further instruction about difficult concepts.
- For continuing education programs, ask registrants to bring an **Admit Ticket** related to their objectives for the class (see **Why Are You in Nursing? and Other Mysteries**). Provide incentives such as lunch passes or prizes for those who follow through and bring the **Admit Tickets.**
- Certain **Admit Tickets** are required in some mandatory education classes, such as annual classes and resuscitation renewals. They include certification cards, completed pretests, and competency checklists. These demonstrations of personal responsibility reinforce the privilege of attending class and the professionalism associated with the learner's role.
- Combine this strategy with **Current Events.** Have students bring in news clippings or downloaded copies of articles concerning health and healthcare and use these as **Admit Tickets**.
- This strategy continues the socialization process by emphasizing personal responsibility. It also promotes active involvement in class and preparation for each session.

Write to Learn

General Description. This strategy is based on the premise that writing enhances learning. **Write to Learn** means just that—using writing assignments to help students learn and retain material. These can be as brief or elaborate as time and class objectives warrant. Instructors may assign the **Write to Learn** topic or allow students to write freely.

Preparation and Equipment. For academic settings, you'll determine the written assignment and your method of evaluating it. The syllabus should specify whether the writing exercise is to be graded or is simply a classroom teaching strategy. You may also decide to incorporate the **Write to Learn** assignment in the class participation grade; assignments handed in during class also provide an attendance record. For continuing education, **Write to Learn** is a valuable way to keep the class active and involved. Even if you don't evaluate the assignments, you can use them to assess understanding and attentiveness. Prizes can provide incentive to participate in **Write to Learn** activities.

Example of the Strategy at Work. **Write to Learn** is effective when several topics are discussed in a single session and time is at a premium. When teaching a class about eye disorders, I found that the students were puzzled by the differences between retinal detachment, glaucoma, and cataracts. They were especially confused by the differences between closed-angle and open-angle glaucoma. The **Write to Learn** I assigned was a 1-minute paper defining each condition or differentiating open- and closed-angle glaucoma. (A 1-minute paper is a quick writing assignment with a specific focus. The students actually had 3 minutes to complete the exercise.) Another few minutes were spent discussing students' answers. I did not collect or grade the assignments, but I assured the class that those concepts would appear on the examination.

I assigned another **Write to Learn** as part of a lecture on the nursing care of clients with neuromuscular diseases. Students typically have a tough time differentiating myasthenia gravis, Guillain-Barré syndrome, amyotrophic lateral sclerosis, multiple sclerosis, muscular dystrophy, and Parkinson's disease. These complex diseases, all involving neurological, muscular, and orthopedic sequelae, are confusing and difficult to remember. Key knowledge for nursing students, however, is that the nursing priorities for these conditions are very similar.

Another idea for **Write to Learn** has students integrate and synthesize a class or presentation key points by asking students to identify the "Five Main Points." In this exercise, students spend 2 or 3 minutes listing the five most salient points discussed during a class. By condensing class material to five main points, participants engage in priority setting and critical thinking about class material.

In another application, after a fair amount of class time spent on the different diseases, etiologies, assessments, and diagnostic procedures, I assigned a 2-minute **Write to Learn** on the common nursing care priorities and interventions. As in **What's the Point?** or **What's the Big Deal?**, students wrote about issues in nursing care for such illnesses. These issues included airway comfort, elimination, dealing with immobility, avoiding injury (e.g., aspiration, skin breakdown, falls), and emotional issues. I encouraged students to list their ideas and think of as many issues as possible in the time allowed. We then discussed the commonalities and differences among the nursing priorities. The students benefited from the subsequent discussion, which explored the depression, frustration, loneliness, and anger that can accompany these conditions.

The assignments were handed in and included in the class participation grade. They also gave me an opportunity to assess the knowledge level of the class. Because students get caught up in the need to memorize facts about pathophysiology, they sometimes need a reminder to focus on the nursing care common to many different conditions.

The last **Write to Learn** example comes from an elective course on adolescent health. We were discussing adolescent sexual activity and the pros and cons of abstinence-only versus comprehensive sex education for teens. The class started to evolve into an unplanned debate. Because I had a few very quiet students, I assigned everyone an individual **Write to Learn.** I asked them to spend 5 minutes writing down their thoughts on the topic and to substantiate them with personal experience or information. We then had a verbal **In-Class Debate** with a high level of participation. The **Write to Learn** strategy allowed all the students to solidify their thoughts on the issue.

Ideas for Use

- See **Clinical Quick Writes** for the use of writing assignments in the clinical area. Writing a letter to your client, describing the clinical day or class in one sentence or word, or writing freely can also work in a classroom or discussion group.

- Writing in the classroom gives you an effective way to assess learning and comprehension. If you hit a **Muddiest Part,** you may want to take a few moments for a **Write to Learn.** It can help you determine whether you'll need to revisit the **Muddiest Part** in subsequent classes.

- **Write to Learn** exercises can be incorporated into **Learning Contracts.** Use the written assignments to gauge each student's performance against the standard work requirements.

- Discussion group participants can use **Write to Learn** to lay the groundwork for an **In-Class Debate.** Students can write their thoughts about a controversial issue and then share in a debate format. The written precursor ensures that each student has thought about the issue and may have reached some conclusions.

- Continuing education students may not embrace the idea of **Writing to Learn** during a presentation. Keep written exercises short and fun. If you provide handouts, include a **Write to Learn** space so the exercise looks like a formal teaching strategy and not just a whim of the instructor.

- In general, include the **Write to Learn** question or topic in your handouts or audiovisuals to formalize the assignment and add credibility to your request.
- Use peer critique and grading on a set rubric. This tactic gives the students experience and eliminates the need for you to evaluate all the assignments.
- Have students **Think-Pair-Share** about each other's compositions.
- Ask students to summarize the main point of the class discussion in one sentence. For an easy **Write to Learn,** each student may complete the sentence "Today's class was about . . ."
- Provide a dataset about a client or condition. Ask students to analyze it and think of client issues and nursing interventions. Use this with **Pass the Problem** to encourage students to share insights.
- For graded assignments, use a scale of 0 to 2, with 0 is not acceptable or not done; 1 is acceptable but incomplete; 2 is acceptable and comprehensive.
- Here is a good exercise for beginning nursing students:
  - You are caring for a client in the clinical area. He refuses a bath for the third day in a row. What rationale could the client have for his refusal?
  - What would you do?
  - What are the consequences of your actions?

Group Concept Mapping

General Description. Concept mapping is a well-documented strategy in nursing education. Sources indicate that concept mapping promotes critical thinking.[4] Concept maps are two-dimensional diagrams of a process, illness, concept, or construct. **Group Concept Mapping** is a slightly different version of this strategy: students in a discussion or clinical group work together to map an assigned or selected topic. The relationships between boxes or circles are established with connecting arrows (see Figure 8–1 for an example). These relationships illustrate the complexity and the interrelation of conditions that students will encounter in practice. Many software packages provide the designs of concept maps with major elements and connections, allowing students to focus on the thinking components of the maps.

Preparation and Equipment. Little preparation is necessary for this strategy. You'll need to think of a study topic that relates to class objectives. For materials, you'll need large writing surfaces, large paper, and markers or

Fig. 8–1. Group concept map. Solid arrows show the interaction of risk factors. Dotted arrows show the nurse's conclusion based on assessment of these factors.

BUN = blood urea nitrogen; GT = gastrostomy; I&O = intake and output; LOC = level of consciousness; NG = nasogastric.

pens. As an alternative, you may have students use their laptops or tablets to produce concept maps. This strategy can take some time, so students need to be clear about the time limit. Assigning the topic in advance gives them an idea of the main concepts to be mapped. If the assignment is being graded for an academic class, the details and evaluation rubric should be set out in the syllabus.

Example of the Strategy at Work. I used **Group Concept Maps** as a postconference for a clinical group. The pediatric nursing instructors had agreed that students should assess each client's hydration status carefully and calculate maintenance fluid requirements according to their clients' weight. Students were puzzled about the priority given to fluid status, which is an area of emphasis in pediatric nursing.

We discussed the developmental and physiological characteristics that predispose pediatric clients, especially infants, to dehydration. I asked the students to research fluid status in children and be ready to do a project in the next postconference. The **Group Concept Map** they developed is shown in Figure 8–1. In this map, fluid input and output and physiological function all influence the client's dehydration potential. Clearly, vigilant assessments can prevent future episodes of dehydration.

Ideas for Use

- **Group Concept Mapping** requires a significant level of cooperation within the group. It's a good way to develop or to refine team-building qualities.
- Develop concept maps for complex conditions seen in clinical settings, such as burns, congestive heart failure (CHF), chronic obstructive pulmonary disease (COPD), and diabetes.
- Concept maps can include physical signs and symptoms, precipitating factors, nursing diagnoses, discharge planning, risk factors, stages of illness, lab and diagnostic studies, medical and surgical treatments, and medications. The lines between components are important because they represent the establishment of relationships, a form of critical thinking.
- **Group Concept Mapping** provides a valuable review of conditions discussed in class but not encountered in the clinical area.
- Any medical or nursing diagnosis or client need may be developed into a **Group Concept Mapping** exercise.
- Include a **Group Concept Mapping** assignment in your final evaluations of learning. Students will have to meet on their own time to complete the task and hand it in for grading.
- As in all group work, students must share responsibilities, delegate appropriately, and ensure total group participation. These lessons in themselves are valuable components of **Group Concept Mapping.**
- In continuing education classes, use this strategy to teach complex algorithms and unfamiliar diseases or specialties.
- Everyone's idea of a concept map is different. With **Group Concept Mapping,** negotiation is a key element.
- Software is now available to create concept maps or mind maps. Standard word processing packages can also be used to develop them. Students generally hand in creative and attractive concept maps that reflect thought and hard work.
- See **Research Concept Maps** for details about using concept maps in research classes.
- The literature is replete with the use of individual concept mapping in nursing education.

War Stories and Clinical Anecdotes

General Description. We all have stories from our past. We tell them to relate experiences or illustrate important lessons we've learned. We also remember stories we were told that drove home a point or made an impression. Humans learn well via stories, especially auditory learners, who develop an internal "tape" of information they've heard.

War Stories and Clinical Anecdotes is based on these ideas. The strategy has become a common mode of teaching in the healthcare field. The work of nurses and other health professionals, filled with human drama, real-life application, intrigue, and mystery, provides a fertile field in which to root our stories. People outside healthcare are often fascinated by the life-and-death nature of our work, our view of people's intimate sides, and the miracles we perform regularly.

New students and nurses are just as enthralled by our stories. Because of the interest we stimulate and the memories we create, **War Stories and Clinical Anecdotes** is a stalwart of many nurse educators' portfolios. This strategy comes with some caveats, however. It's important to make sure that your stories enhance retention and don't detract from learning or from other strategies. The key lessons should be clearly evident; this is not a time for hidden messages or covert lessons.

Preparation and Equipment. **War Stories and Clinical Anecdotes** may seem spontaneous and unplanned to students. In reality, personal stories should be well planned and should coincide with class content. Stories that stray from course objectives may mislead students and throw you off focus. They also take up precious time, limiting your ability to keep the class on schedule.

When you prepare your lecture on content, consider which **War Stories and Clinical Anecdotes** relate directly to the class. Which ones do you think of when you revisit the information? Write a few notes about the story in the margins of your lecture guide. Add two to three key words you'd like to use in retelling it.

It may also help to decide how much time you can devote to the story. One to two minutes will let you make a concise point without dwelling too long on a single incident. I've learned the importance of preplanning to make sure I include only the most relevant information and maintain the focus of the class. Marginal notes give me prompts for the components of the story I want to relay to the class.

Example of the Strategy at Work. Nursing instructors use **War Stories and Clinical Anecdotes** across the learning spectrum. Many of us remember stories from our education that have stuck with us for years. I've found that relaying stories from my childhood, education, early nursing practice, parenting experiences, and current life can trigger memories for students.

One story I've found useful comes from my early practice as a nurse. I was caring for a child who had sustained significant trauma in a motor vehicle accident. The child had been cleared of internal injuries and was stable. On the night shift, we were assessing his vital signs with neurological checks every 2 hours. The child rested comfortably between my visits, with his mother at the bedside. He was voiding in his diaper and his assessments remained unchanged throughout the night—except for his heart rate, which increased throughout the shift.

I began checking his heart rate every hour. Worried that I was missing signs of pain, I carefully checked behavioral and physiological signs to assess his comfort level. I noted early in the morning that his heart rate was markedly above baseline despite no other change in vital signs or assessments. My gut feeling was that something was wrong. I called the resident and reported the finding. The physician examined the child. We tested his hemoglobin and hematocrit and found them remarkably low. Despite no physical signs, this child was bleeding. He was taken to surgery soon after, all because of a subtle sign and regular assessments.

I use that story to drive home the importance of the gut feeling and of vigilant assessments for postoperative, posttrauma, or ill clients. That story reinforces the need for high-quality nursing care far better than a simple statement. It also reflects the independence of nursing assessments, especially on the off shifts.

Ideas for Use

- Establish a repertoire of stories for content you teach often. Ensure that the stories meet course objectives and are kept brief.
- Use caution when sharing stories about previous students, especially if a story is derogatory. Students may begin to feel like potential fodder for your stories and may resent hearing about others' weaknesses or mistakes. Even "I heard of a student who" stories may be offensive. Stories should have a learning focus, not a judging one.
- Gauge audience members for their ability to tolerate graphic detail. Nurses are notorious for gory, detailed work stories, even at the dinner table. Use your discretion to make sure your **War Stories and Clinical Anecdotes** don't horrify the students.
- Carefully weave the story into class content and objectives so students see the connection. It should be clearly evident and memorable.

- Make sure students comprehend that the story is only an example or prototype of the study topic. Novice students may generalize facts about your story to everyone with the same condition. They may have a difficult time transferring knowledge to the wide and varying array of human illness and trauma.
- Ask students, new nurses, and experienced nurses to share their **War Stories and Clinical Anecdotes.** As the class moderator, keep the stories on track. Make sure the sharing doesn't become a gripe session or a "Can you top this?" conversation.
- Use PowerPoint slides to provide visual prompts for the stories.
- Have students do a **Clinical Quick Write, Write to Learn,** or **Ah-Ha Journal** entry in which they reflect on and derive personal lessons from your story.

Nuts and Bolts

General Description. **Nuts and Bolts** parallels the typical case study approach, with an added emphasis on fun and creativity. The difference between this strategy and a case study is what's missing: participants provide words to complete a story, focusing on the **Nuts and Bolts** of a situation. The format, shown in Box 8–3, recalls a familiar childhood travel game.

Preparation and Equipment. No preparation is needed for this exercise, although you may wish to show the format as a slide. You can interject **Nuts and Bolts** into any class to generate discussion about a condition and the related nursing priorities.

Example of the Strategy at Work. I've used this strategy in a class to differentiate the issues associated with left- and right-sided CHF. Students often have a difficult time understanding the similarities and differences between these conditions. See Boxes 8–4 and 8–5 for the two **Nuts and Bolts** stories I use to clarify, respectively, left- and right-sided CHF.

Box 8–3.
Nuts and Bolts Format

Once upon a time there was a(n) _____ who had _____ and was _____ . The nurse assessed the client, determined that ____ had _____ , and began to _____ . As a result of the nurse's actions, the client _____ .

Box 8–4.
Nuts and Bolts Exercise

Left Congestive Heart Failure (CHF)

Once upon a time there was a *63-year-old man* who had *a history of chronic left ventricular CHF* and was *admitted to the unit with shortness of breath.* The nurse assessed the client; determined that *he had significant dyspnea, orthopnea, and an O_2 saturation of 83%*; and began to *elevate the head of the bed, provide oxygen by nasal cannula, and auscultate breath sounds.* The nurse called the physician and received *an order for IV furosemide.* As a result of the nurse's actions the client *experienced diuresis and decreased work of breathing and had an O_2 saturation of 93%.*

Box 8–5.
Nuts and Bolts Exercise

Right Congestive Heart Failure (CHF)

Once upon a time there was a *78-year-old woman* who had *chronic right ventricular heart failure* and was *brought to the emergency department for treatment by her 85-year-old husband.* The nurse assessed the client and determined that *she had hepatomegaly, a pedal edema score at +4, related pain in the extremities, hypertension (BP 160/106 mm Hg), jugular vein distention, and a weight gain of 4 kg in the last 2 weeks.* The nurse began to *arrange the client in the position of comfort.* The nurse called the physician, who examined the client and ordered *IV furosemide.* As a result of the nurse's actions, the client *experienced diuresis, the pedal edema decreased to +2, and her weight decreased 1 kg.*

As students become knowledgeable and get the gist of the strategy, the underlined areas of each case may be left blank. Students can fill in the blanks by asking questions such as the following:

- What signs and symptoms would a client with this illness demonstrate?
- What are the initial nursing priorities?
- What is the medical treatment?
- How would you evaluate the effectiveness of the nursing or medical treatment?

The same exercise is used to differentiate hyperglycemia and hypoglycemia in Boxes 8–6 and 8–7, respectively. This distinction is a common

Box 8–6.
Nuts and Bolts Exercise

Hyperglycemia

Once upon a time there was *an 8-year-old boy* who had *type 1 diabetes mellitus* and was brought to the pediatric emergency department for evaluation and treatment. The nurse assessed the client and determined that *he had dry skin and fruity-smelling breath, was thirsty, complained of frequently needing to pee, was disoriented, and felt nauseated. The client voided, and the nurse found large ketones in his urine. The nurse assessed the blood sugar, found it to be 450 mg/dL, and began to set up an IV for hydration and prepare to administer ordered insulin.* As a result of the nurse's actions, the client *became more lucid, his urine tested for small ketones, his blood sugar decreased to 300 mg/dL, and he stated that he felt better.*

Box 8–7.
Nuts and Bolts Exercise

Hypoglycemia

Once upon a time there was *an 8-year-old boy* who had *type 1 diabetes mellitus* and was *brought to the pediatric emergency department for evaluation and treatment.* The nurse assessed the client and determined that *he had a decreased level of consciousness and visual disturbances and was sweaty. The client complained of hunger, a headache, and "shakiness." The nurse checked his blood sugar level, found it to be 45 mg/dL, and gave the client 4 oz of juice (15 gm carbohydrate). After 15 minutes, the nurse rechecked the blood sugar and found it to be 55 mg/dL. The 15 gm of glucose was repeated.* As a result of the nurse's action, *15 minutes later, the client's blood sugar was 95 mg/dL. The nurse provided a snack with fat and protein.*

subject of NCLEX® questions. Test participants analyze symptoms to determine high or low blood sugar levels and then decide the appropriate nursing interventions.

Ideas for Use

- Use this exercise as the subject of a **Clinical Quick Write** or an **Email Exercise.** You can give out the forms and let the students pick the scenarios, or you can have them complete the assignment on a client you've selected.

- Ask students to compose the initial sentence for a **Nuts and Bolts** exercise and then switch papers in class so they can complete a classmate's story.
- Use **Think-Pair-Share** to encourage discussion.
- **Nuts and Bolts** is especially valuable for discriminating between difficult concepts. This strategy requires critical thinking skills: identifying the first nursing action and the highest nursing priority, and understanding the gravity of the client's signs and symptoms.
- This is a good strategy for helping students differentiate the subtle differences between two similar conditions. It works for mental health disorders (e.g., borderline personality and bipolar disorders) and medical-surgical conditions (e.g., arterial and venous peripheral vascular disorders). You can use it to differentiate conditions within specialties (e.g., bacterial versus viral meningitis, abruptio placentae versus placenta previa, bone conduction versus nerve conduction hearing loss).
- Have students split into groups and reach a consensus on how to fill in the blanks in the **Nuts and Bolts** exercise(s).

Teaching Tools

General Description. The main premise of this strategy is that we often undervalue the teaching tools we use to educate clients. These tools can be easily adapted for teaching both students and new or experienced nurses. **Teaching Tools** also reminds nurses to see clients as knowledgeable healthcare partners and to remain current about what clients need to know.

Preparation and Equipment. You'll need to consider your own methods of educating clients about disease, treatment, diagnostic testing, medications, symptom management, and activities of daily living. Look in books and other resources on client education, general nursing, community health, and self-care; your class may well find them useful. Use diagnosis- or condition-appropriate teaching resources and clarify the level of information a client should receive. Students are often shocked at the amount and technical nature of client education materials. The role of the nurse in client education takes on new meaning for them.

Example of the Strategy at Work. I used **Assessing the Learner** in a lesson on client education. It not only emphasizes the importance of assessing the client's learning style but it also reminds students to assess their own as well. **Assessing the Learner** is inspired by a learner assessment recommended by Hunt.[5] This kind of **Teaching Tool** also works as an icebreaker and as a way to assess learning styles in your class.

Assessing the Learner

Brain Dominance

1. Likes words, numbers, letters, parts, sequential order, linear thought, language; is detail-oriented and organized (left-brained, analytical learner)
2. Likes images, patterns, entirety, simultaneous actions, music; is nonverbal, creative, intuitive, spontaneous, and graphics-oriented (right-brained, global learner)

Learning Modalities

1. Prefers verbal instruction; remembers names, not faces; is distracted by noise; enjoys music; likes answering machines (auditory learner)
2. Remembers faces, not names; has a vivid imagination; thinks in pictures; uses colors; likes postcards (visual learner)
3. Learns by doing and touching; remembers what was done; is impulsive; loves games (kinesthetic learner)

Favorite Learning Activities

Visual: Television, reading, videos, handouts, flip charts, signs, writing

Auditory: Books on tape, tapes, music, radio, conversation, listening to steps

Kinesthetic: Games, simulations, group activities, role playing, demonstration

Ideas for Use

- Lead a class discussion on the reading level and comprehensibility of client education material. Ask students to brainstorm obstacles and solutions (see Box 8–8).
- Reinforce in every class the complexity of material that nurses need to learn. Ask students to consider the impact of that complexity on the average client and family.
- Many nursing textbooks include client education materials. Students, and nurses new to a condition or treatment, can use those **Teaching Tools** to educate themselves as well as clients.

Box 8–8.
Brainstorming Session

What do you do when a client:
- doesn't read?
- reads at a third-grade level?
- doesn't speak or read English?
- is visually impaired?

- Ask students to develop short client education materials based on a reading level. Computer programs, books, and word-processing software can be helpful in calculating reading levels.
- In an elective class on diabetes, I was able to acquire the education packet for newly diagnosed clients with type 1 diabetes. This became the primary textbook for the course. It provided an excellent resource for both the material itself and the information that a client with this condition would need.
- Do an online search for patient education tools that may prove invaluable for nursing students and nurse orientees. Again, assist new nurses in the development of critiquing skills to ensure sound, evidence-based information.
- Experienced nurses can review client education materials provided by agencies. Ask them to evaluate the materials for their currency and usefulness in nursing orientation. This technique teaches both content and the policies and procedures of the agency.
- Sign on to Web-based listservs within the specialty and encourage the sharing of education materials. Use these materials in the clinical area to teach the value of sharing in this capacity.
- Assign students or orientees to research client education materials for a specific illness or client need. Have students present these to each other in a **Student-Led Seminar.**

Day in the Life of a Client With . . .

General Description. This is a great strategy that was suggested to me by a class participant. Each student selects a disease, condition, or lifestyle and spends one day "living the life" of a client in that situation. The students research the illness, consider its impact on the client throughout the day, and then plan how to live that life in conjunction with daily routines. Then comes the hard part: they actually simulate living with the illness. The students then compose a journal, much like an **Ah-Ha Journal,** to summarize their experiences and reflect on the lessons learned.

Preparation and Equipment. In an academic setting, you need to assign disease, condition, or lifestyle for students to simulate. You also need to design the assignment and evaluation methods. In the practice setting, use **Day in the Life of a Client With . . .** during orientation to teach new employees about predominant diagnoses or client conditions.

Example of the Strategy at Work. I used this strategy in a didactic class discussing vulnerable populations. Students selected from a list of such cohorts, such as people who are homeless, have significant mobility issues such as paraplegia, are incarcerated, are part of a religious sect, are immigrants, are victims of interpersonal violence, are in recovery from substance abuse, and others. Students described the issue using data about prevalence, relayed the potentially typical day for that individual, and developed nursing interventions to meet the client's needs. Another instructor assigned each member of the clinical group to a different illness. In this exercise, students explored and experienced diagnoses such as type 1 diabetes mellitus, heart block with a pacemaker, COPD on oxygen therapy, end-stage renal disease on dialysis, liver failure requiring a paracentesis, inoperable cataracts with significant visual impairment, cystic fibrosis requiring chest percussion and postural drainage, cerebrovascular accident sequelae with aphasia, breast cancer postmastectomy and on chemotherapy, spinal cord injury with paralysis, and CHF with significant activity intolerance.

Students considered the equipment needed, the dietary restrictions, the symptoms and limitation imposed by the illness, and activities of daily living. Then they worked out how to survive with the limitations and accomplish the instrumental activities of daily living (e.g., shopping, home maintenance and cleaning, banking).

Ideas for Use

- Students may do this exercise in pairs. One participant "lives the disease"; the other records challenges and issues and provides assistance as needed.
- **Day in the Life of a Client With . . .** is a great empathy-building exercise. It may be carried out as elaborately or as simply as class objectives require.
- In practice settings, this strategy can be more cognitive. Novice nurses or nurses new to a setting can conjecture what it would be like to live a **Day in the Life of a Client With . . .**
- This strategy may be very helpful in community nursing classes so that students understand the needs of clients in their home, the needs of a population, or the concepts of public health nursing. Shoe leather (walking) and windshield (driving) surveys may assist students in gathering data and anticipating client needs.
- Many nursing diagnoses may be adapted to this strategy.
- Ask students to keep a log of activities throughout the day, including meals eaten, obstacles encountered, and experiences with symptoms such as shortness of breath or fatigue.
- Each assigned condition should have a significant physical limitation. The student should experience inconvenience, potential pain, diet and activity restrictions, or a change in daily routine.

- This strategy introduces students to the different skills and equipment needed to care for their diagnosis. Skills may include principles of oxygen therapy, insulin administration, chest therapy, and others.
- Have students **Write to Learn** by doing a reaction paper based on preliminary research and personal experience.
- **Day in the Life of a Client With . . .** may be done in discussion groups, small classes, orientation groups, and clinical groups.
- Students can report their findings to other students in **One-Minute Classes** or **Grand Rounds.**
- Students can use **Ah-Ha Journals** to document their experience.
- A quick rendition of this exercise has students or new nurses navigate the campus or agency in a wheelchair. This experience offers poignant insights. Students encounter firsthand the challenges of wheelchair dependence and of accommodations that are theoretically wheelchair appropriate yet remain an obstacle for many clients.

Invented Dialogues

General Description. Nursing students and novice nurses must master the challenge of communicating and interacting outside their comfort zone. Nurses have the privilege of quick entry into their clients' private lives, often being privy to intimate details. New nurses may not be equipped to deal with such candor, nor do they have the tools to respond therapeutically.

In this strategy, students respond to statements designed by the instructor. The responses should be appropriate, feasible, and comfortable for both participants in the conversation. **Invented Dialogues** are based on the class objectives and may be used in a variety of ways.

Preparation and Equipment. Clinical practice provides you with the potential statements to begin forming this exercise. Think about times when clients have confessed personal facts to you and you were either at a loss for words or needed to formulate an appropriate response quickly. These are the types of statements that make great conversation starters for **Invented Dialogues.** Think about times in the clinical area when students appeared to be stymied by a client's comment or question and how they should, or could, have responded.

Example of the Strategy at Work. I've used this strategy in a class on sex and sexuality. The idea of responding to clients' comments about sexuality made the students uncomfortable; **Invented Dialogues** gave them a chance to practice. Because this topic was so sensitive for some participants, I showed the statements on the screen, read each aloud, and paused to let the students consider their personal responses. Then I asked each student to formulate one response and send it to me as an **Email Exercise.** Here are some of the statements and questions used in that class:

- "I told the doctor I don't take Viagra but I really do."
- "I'm afraid my husband doesn't love me since my mastectomy."
- "I'd like to take you out to dinner once I get out of the hospital."
- "Will the diabetes prevent me from having an erection?"
- "I don't take my medicine because I heard it causes impotence."
- "I don't want to wear condoms when I have sex."
- "I'm a homosexual, but I don't want anyone at the hospital to know."

You can use **Invented Dialogues** in class discussion, with class members suggesting responses. I also used this strategy, with statements from students instead of clients, to teach nurse educators about creative teaching strategies. Here are the statements from students that I used to stimulate responses during our class discussion:

- "I had to cheat on the assignment; I ran out of time."
- "I didn't have time to give the bath because I needed to look up my medications today in clinical. I didn't look up all my meds last night because I didn't have time."
- "My client says he doesn't want to get out of bed and the MD wants him to walk three times a day."
- "The nurse yesterday said meds can be 1-hour late. The nurse today said only one-half hour. Who do I believe?"
- "Just tell me what's on the test."
- " Why do I have to participate? I'd rather just listen."
- "I can't come to class; I have to work."
- "I don't like to write things on a calendar."
- "I have to text my friend during clinical; it's important."

Ideas for Use

- In a large classroom, you can show the statements as a PowerPoint slide and ask for immediate responses.
- This strategy can be used as a **Think-Pair-Share.** Student pairs develop responses to the statements and discuss how the client might react. This method highlights the circular nature of communication and the impact of a nurse's answer on a client's attitude and behavior.

- **Invented Dialogues** are generally more comfortable than more elaborate role-play exercises. Its brevity keeps the discussion from becoming more detailed and perhaps uncomfortable.
- Another application of **Invented Dialogues** is to have instructors role-play in front of the classroom and then have students develop next lines or responses to their role play. Instructor role play in the classroom, though labor-intensive, provides role modeling for students and allows instructors to design the script tightly to meet class objectives. Then students can play an active role in the portrayal of the scenario and engage in deep thinking about responses to the instructor statements.
- For larger classes or to provide anonymity, you can combine this strategy with **Clinical Quick Writes, Email Exercises, Online Discussion Groups, Guided Discussion Groups,** and **Admit Tickets.**
- Use class objectives to develop statements, especially for sensitive subjects such as spirituality, sexuality, high-risk behaviors, and legal or ethical conflicts. It may also be helpful as students learn to deal with inappropriate questions from clients.
- **Invented Dialogues** are great for practicing responses in clinical situations. Comments from clients may include:
  - "I don't want to take a bath today."
  - "I don't want a student nurse."
  - "I haven't had any pain meds since yesterday. I'm sorry the nurse told you I did, but I haven't had any."
  - "I don't want to quit smoking; why should I?"
  - "I don't know how to read."
  - "I don't understand the surgery I'm having today."
  - "I don't take my medicine because it's too expensive."
  - "I take herbs with my medicine, but I haven't told my doctor."
  - "I don't want to be in this research study anymore."
  - "I feel like I have no reason for living."
  - "My dad hit me really hard last night and I'm not allowed to tell anyone."
  - This last statement touches on the topic of the nurse's role in an abusive situation and how it may depend on the age of the client.
- The following situation can help to clarify a nurse's role when a fellow nurse is impaired: A nurse colleague says to you, "I need to sign out some narcotics, so don't ask any questions."
- The following example may be used in teaching isolation precautions: Ask the class for their response if a nurse says, "You don't need to use all these isolation procedures. I've been a nurse a long time and I've never caught anything."

Guided Discussion Groups

General Description. Discussion groups can be difficult to maintain. They're especially vulnerable at the beginning or end of the semester, at other busy times, in summer, and near holidays. At these times, instructors need strategies that are objective-driven and valuable but also fun and a change of pace from the normal classroom routine. A **Guided Discussion Group** can help. When traditional teaching methods become too mundane, the instructor can entertain the group with creative exercises that also reflect their learning needs.

Preparation and Equipment. This strategy may take a little more work than usual. It's actually a combination of several creative strategies woven into a single learning session.

Example of the Strategy at Work. **Guided Discussion Groups** have been effective in teaching concepts such as wellness and the nurse's role in stress management. Used in both academic and clinical settings, the following exercises focus on nurses' need to manage their own stress while fostering stress management strategies in their clients.

Are You Stress Resistant?

We begin with the following assessment to set the stage for continued discussion.

I. This is a quick measure of your ability to resist stress! Score 0 if the statement is not true for you, 1 if it's usually not true, 2 if it's somewhat true, and 3 if it definitely is true.

1. _____ When I work hard, it makes a difference.
2. _____ Getting out of bed in the morning is easy for me.
3. _____ I have the freedom I want and need.
4. _____ I have sometimes sacrificed for an exciting opportunity.
5. _____ Sticking to my routine is not important to me.
6. _____ I vote because I think it makes a difference.
7. _____ I make my own lucky breaks.
8. _____ I agree with the goals of my boss, company, school, or family.
9. _____ I've been lucky in love because I try to be a loving person.
10. _____ I believe I get what I give but I don't keep score.
11. _____ It is important for me to try new things.
12. _____ Free time is a gift I really enjoy.
13. _____ I work hard and I'm paid fairly.
14. _____ My family is a great pleasure to me.
15. _____ I speak up for what I believe in.

SCORING

Add your scores for questions 1, 6, 7, 9, and 13. This is your stress management score. The higher it is, the more control you feel you have over your own life and the better able you are to manage your own stress.

TOTAL: _____

Add your scores for questions 2, 3, 8, 10, and 14. This is your commitment score. The higher it is, the more committed you are to enhancing and enjoying your life.

TOTAL: _____

Add your scores for questions 4, 5, 11, 12, and 15. This is your risk score. The higher it is, the more willing you are to take risks.

TOTAL: _____

Add the three scores together:

OVERALL TOTAL: _____

This is your overall stress resistance score If you score 35 or more, congratulations, you are very resistant to stress and your attitudes help you.

If you score 27–34, you are somewhat stress resistant but could be more so. Look at each item and choose a few to work on.

If you score 18–27, you need to look at your habits and attitudes and improve your resistance to stress. Select one area to improve each month.

If your score is less than 18, you could be in trouble if stress gets serious—take time now to change your habits and attitudes.

Happy stress resisting!

II. Following the assessment, we discuss common stressors in a lecture-discussion format in which I write down the stressors on a flip chart or blackboard.

III. After this activity, students are asked to discuss the following questions in a **Guided Discussion Group.**

QUESTIONS TO THINK ABOUT

1. How do you know when you're stressed? What physical and emotional signals let you know that you're stressed?
2. How do you generally manage your stress? Do those strategies work?
3. What interventions would you like to employ to deal with stress more effectively?
4. What lifestyle habits keep you from being stress resistant? What lifestyle habits enhance your stress resistance?
5. What is the role of the nurse in assisting clients to recognize stress and become stress resistant?

IV. The final activity has students frame stress management in terms of the nurse's role. Students write a **One-Minute Care Plan** for a partner based on a brief **Think-Pair-Share** about stress assessment and management. Each student is asked to use the nursing diagnosis of *Ineffective individual coping related to* _____ *as evidenced by* _____. Each student develops one long-term goal, two short-term goals, and two interventions for each short-term goal. These **One-Minute Care Plans** should be individualized for the client using the data collected in previous conversations as discussed in this book.

Ideas for Use

- Use a **Guided Discussion Group** when addressing controversial or difficult issues. Nursing ethics, values clarification, assertiveness skills, professional issues, and therapeutic client relationships may all require more than lecture and discussion. As I've shown, this strategy combines several different strategies in a concerted learning package. This approach may prove more effective and enjoyable than one strategy used alone.
- One of the greatest assets of **Guided Discussion Groups** is the repetition of material in several formats. Repetition is a form of mental aerobics in which the mind practices material and exercises the brain.
- Combine several strategies with **Guided Discussion Groups** to yield the best results: **Think-Pair-Share, Admit Ticket, Same Information, Critical Thinking Exercises,** and others can augment the learning and the fun.
- The final **One-Minute Care Plan** may be handed in at the end of class, written and handed in later, or submitted electronically as an **Email Exercise.**

- **Guided Discussion Groups** may be adapted to any course content. You'll meet class objectives simply by collecting several exercises and strategies and developing a schedule for their use.

Out of the Hat

General Description. In this strategy, the instructor creates a pool of topics to be discussed or evaluated. Students then select one or more topics **Out of the Hat** and are asked to demonstrate understanding and competency in those areas. This is a common testing strategy when a lot of material must be assessed in a limited amount of time; examples include physical assessment and basic nursing skills. Alternatively, students can create a **One-Minute Class, Student-Led Seminar,** or **Ah-Ha Journal** based on the selected topic.

Preparation and Equipment. The equipment you'll need depends on the skills to be tested. You will need to write down the testable items so that they may be selected. Smartphone apps exist to allow this level of randomization. You can use this strategy to test psychomotor skills. Ask students to assemble the supplies needed for the task they've just pulled **Out of the Hat.**

Example of the Strategy at Work. This strategy has traditionally been used to assess psychomotor competency. Health assessment courses teach skills sequentially. You can use **Out of the Hat** to test assessment of neurological, respiratory, cardiac, integumentary, gastrointestinal, and other systems. Students come prepared to be tested on any system. They don't know which one they'll be tested on until they pick it **Out of the Hat.**

Out of the Hat also works for testing fundamental skills. We thought of a Total Care Test to test basic skills. Students practiced hygiene, body mechanics, assessing vital signs, making beds, moving clients, and various other basic skills throughout the semester.

In the Total Care Test, pairs of students demonstrated hand washing, vital signs, giving a bed bath, brushing a client's teeth, and making an occupied bed. Then they picked two other skills **Out of the Hat.** These included putting a client on a bedpan, applying wrist restraints, teaching walker or crutch walking, stretcher transfer, and shaving. They also selected a position (supine, prone, Fowler's, Sims', lateral) **Out of the Hat.** This strategy cut down on the time needed to test each student while ensuring that each one had prepared every skill.

Ideas for Use

- **Out of the Hat** allows you to evaluate competency in any psychomotor skill.
- This strategy is appropriate for discussion groups, clinical groups, or small groups in classes with a psychomotor component.

- **Out of the Hat** allows students to demonstrate their knowledge of a topic orally. Evaluate content mastery by having students pick a class concept or topic **Out of the Hat** and explain it to classmates.

- Let students pick one of the topics for that day's class. Each **Out of the Hat** topic is then discussed at length. Students may also pick discussion questions and potential issues related to a class topic. You're available to clarify issues, but the students lead the discussion.

- For orientation groups and nurses accomplishing mandatory requirements, **Out of the Hat** makes a good alternative to written posttests. Each nurse picks a topic **Out of the Hat** and answers orally or does a **Clinical Quick Write.** Staff development instructors can use checklists to document these demonstrations.

- **Out of the Hat** may be used for part or all of a class session. It can add flavor to another exercise: students pick the topic for an **In-Class Debate,** a partner for an icebreaker or **Think-Pair-Share,** or a role in a **Teaching Trio.**

- Students may pick topics for oral presentations **Out of the Hat.**

Legal Cheat Sheets

General Description. Cheating is a funny thing. If students spent as much time studying as they did preparing eloquent cheat sheets, their test performance would excel. **Legal Cheat Sheets** let students select priority points in any class and develop them into study sheets with the instructor's help. These **Legal Cheat Sheets** become flash cards for studying material, focusing on most important content, and setting priorities among key issues.

Legal Cheat Sheets work well with material that's often memorized, such as lab values, norms, difficult concepts, and numerical data. This strategy moves such information from one category to another: "need to remember" becomes "need to know where to find it." Students find more freedom to think critically and develop prioritization and decision-making skills. Less encumbered with the need to memorize, they can look beyond the facts to the potential contexts that surround those facts and influence nursing practice.

Preparation and Equipment. Your only preparation for this strategy is to guide students in developing personal **Legal Cheat Sheets** for later use. You can help by suggesting a format for the sheets. In addition, you can create a classroom environment in which **Legal Cheat Sheets** are an accepted aid to learning, studying, and evaluation.

Example of the Strategy at Work. Students are encouraged to use **Legal Cheat Sheets** as study guides for test preparation. Often they spend a significant amount of time selecting which material should go on the sheet. This prioritization process encourages students to select and study material that's integral to the test or the course. After the initial reading and class preparation, students revisit the material while selecting integral information, formatting the cheat sheet, writing information in the cheat sheet, reviewing, and finally while studying for the test. This is a good example of the mental aerobics—the repetition—so important in learning. This strategy works regardless of learning style.

Ideas for Use

- Allow students to bring **Legal Cheat Sheets** to examinations. They'll feel more at liberty to use critical thinking and decision-making skills rather than focusing only on memorization. This method replicates many clinical practice settings in which memorization is no longer emphasized. Standard practice emphasizes the ability to find accurate information quickly, especially in emergency situations.
- Use this strategy as a means to study and review for final examinations. A semester's worth of **Legal Cheat Sheets** provides a compendium of review materials. Keeping up with **Legal Cheat Sheets** throughout the semester or the course creates a study guide for comprehensive final examinations.
- Have students recopy and reformat the sheet as much as they would like to ensure that they learn and cement the information in their understanding.
- Encourage students to work in pairs, trios, or groups to enhance their **Legal Cheat Sheets.**
- **Quizzes, Student-Led Seminars, Gaming,** and **Email Exercises** may all be combined with **Legal Cheat Sheets** to add to their educational value.
- Students may be encouraged to share their **Legal Cheat Sheets** through **Online Discussion Groups** or in **Group Thought.** Students can rotate responsibility for compiling **Legal Cheat Sheets** in different subjects.
- Students can help each other by sharing their **Legal Cheat Sheets** during study groups and review sessions.
- Use **Legal Cheat Sheets** to summarize and reinforce key material from slides and class notes.

Mock Trials

General Description. **Mock Trials** serve two purposes. They address the legal and ethical conflicts inherent in nursing and healthcare, and they provide practice in organizing and delivering a presentation. This presentation mimics a courtroom trial.

Preparation and Equipment. Because this strategy requires a lot of work from students, it's probably most effective in the academic setting. You will need to determine the evaluation method or rubric for the assignment.

Example of the Strategy at Work. In a continuing education program, an attorney was asked to present the legal aspects of nursing documentation. Knowing that this could be a dry issue, she created a **Mock Trial** about the hazards of poor documentation. Volunteers from the audience were solicited in advance to take roles and were given mini-scripts to follow.

The attorney then created a courtroom vignette. A nurse on the witness stand was asked to relate events of several years ago that had ended in a client's death. The nurse was provided with the documentation surrounding the incident. Her testimony exposed major lapses such as illegibility, documenting infrequently, undocumented care, spelling errors, electronic health record discrepancies, and other poor practices. The speaker masterfully met all the class objectives in 1 hour and had the rapt attention of the class the entire time.

Ideas for Use

- A **Mock Trial** may be incorporated into a continuing education program as an entertaining way to address a legal issue or conflict.
- **Mock Trials** can reinforce the need for careful documentation at all levels of nursing.
- Agency ethical rounds can use a **Mock Trial** as a platform to discuss the needs and roles of the multidisciplinary team in ethically difficult circumstances.
- Have students select a legal issue and act as a group to establish roles and scripts. Group members may serve as defendants, lawyers, plaintiffs, a judge, witnesses, and jury members.
- Plan a discussion group in which the **Mock Trial** is an impromptu event, allowing students to take roles and wade their way through the dialogue.
- In a more formal **Mock Trial,** you can assign roles and have brief scripts written out on index cards. Students may be encouraged to ad lib as necessary.
- **Mock Trials** may be used in a research class to help teach the rights of human subjects. These rights include autonomy, informed consent, the risk-to-benefit ratio, and beneficence. You develop a case representing an infringement of these rights, the **Mock Trial** follows, and the class discusses the issue. Other

concepts may include failure to disclose risks, participation under duress or coercion, or unethical research practices.

- Use a **Mock Trial** to approach several legal issues, such as negligence, malpractice, false imprisonment, and fraud.
- Use case law to develop a realistic subject for the **Mock Trial.**
- As in a debate, students should be evaluated on their level of research, knowledge of the topic, ability to present their case within their role, and contribution to the group.
- A small group may present the **Mock Trial** for extra credit. Other students may write their reactions as an **Email Exercise** or a variant on the **Clinical Quick Write.**
- The **Mock Trial** can be a component of teaching about the electronic health record using an agency training site or using a marketed digital health record product.
- Students may witness the **Mock Trial** and then be asked to apply their knowledge by answering questions related to a different case study.
- Encourage groups to share the preparation and dialogue evenly. Students can share roles and assist each other in presenting extensive material.
- Have an attorney visit the class to discuss major legal concepts and then use them in a **Mock Trial.**
- Use the **Mock Trial** as a way to reinforce documentation skills in the clinical area. After students complete the **Documentation Case Study,** create a **Mock Trial** scenario. Ask students to go back and look at the care they "delivered" in the case and use their documentation to reconstruct that care. Discuss gaps or discrepancies that could be misinterpreted or are difficult to evaluate. Emphasize that it's this type of documentation issue that creates legal conflicts. This is a great way to reinforce accurate and comprehensive documentation.

Learning Carts

General Description. This strategy works the way it sounds: you place your educational materials on a cart and take it to your students. This cart conveys the message "I am here to teach you" and signals that learning is the order of the day. **Learning Carts** allow instructors to bring in all the necessary equipment and to move the learning location as needed.

Preparation and Equipment. Of course, this strategy requires a cart—or a box, carrying case, or whatever allows you to transport teaching materials easily. The size depends on what you plan to transport. Some **Learning Carts** include a laptop computer with Wi-Fi capacity and a projector. A blank light-colored wall on which to project images eliminates the need for a screen. Other equipment depends on the skills or material being taught and on the needs of the instructor. You could bring handouts, games, puzzles, prizes, models, pretests and posttests, audiovisual equipment, supplies for skills, other materials, and snacks and beverages (which always attract learners).

Example of the Strategy at Work. **Learning Carts** are most effective in staff development and agency settings, where unit-to-unit education meets the needs of busy staff nurses. This strategy communicates your desire to teach and your appreciation of the factors that often keep nurses from participating in educational programs. **Learning Carts** also keep you ready for repeated teaching sessions. You just take the cart and go! Agencies have used this strategy to teach staff members about a new piece of equipment or a hospital-wide policy change, to help them meet mandatory requirements, to prepare for an accreditation survey, and to assess the competency of nurses in or just ending their orientation.

In academic settings, in which lab or hospital space is at a premium, **Learning Carts** can bring the setting to the students rather than the students to the setting. Sometimes labs become so crowded that it's difficult for every student to see a demonstration. A colleague of mine wheels a hospital bed into a traditional classroom to teach moving the client in bed and positioning. She packs a **Learning Cart** with needed supplies, a DVD demonstrating the skills, a short pretest and posttest, and supplies (e.g., draw sheets, pillows, towels). The entire class sees the demonstration at once, and each student has a clear view of the procedure. Students then go to the lab to practice the skills on their own.

Ideas for Use

- Invent your own **Learning Cart** contents and use them consistently for every class you teach.
- Have students or orientees develop a seminar or presentation and set up their own **Learning Cart.** Role-model the use of a **Learning Cart** during orientation.
- Keep **Learning Cart** teaching sessions short and to the point. Leave handouts or graded posttests to reinforce the sessions.
- Allow students to work in pairs, trios, or groups to create a **Learning Cart.**
- Do a procedure review by having clinical groups work in pairs and develop a **Learning Cart.** Encourage them to set up an

Active Reading Conference to review the procedural protocol and the necessary equipment and supplies needed for the procedure. Have them use active teaching strategies to involve the entire group. Let students pick the skill to be discussed **Out of the Hat.** Students may research the skill and use **Clinical Area Questioning** or **Bring on the Evidence** to determine the evidence base for the skill or procedure.

- Make sure you hand out prizes or small gifts as a way to thank learners and student teachers for their time.
- Use a variety of **Case Studies** along with equipment from the **Learning Cart** to address a learning topic.
- Provide URLs for YouTube videos so learners can watch videos before and after the learning session.
- When the teaching materials allow, use bins or boxes to carry class supplies from one area to another. Let the bin be the signal that learning is about to occur during units, satellite clinics, or a clinical rotation.

Pass the Stick

General Description. This quick strategy helps to control a discussion group. Simply, the stick is passed around the group, and whoever has the stick has the floor.

Preparation and Equipment. You guessed it—you need a stick! You'll also need to set ground rules for its use. Parameters may include timing, which way to pass it, the need to observe the rules, and other details specific to the exercise.

Example of the Strategy at Work. I learned this strategy from a colleague who has taught first grade for a long time. Simple though it is, it meets two important goals. Discussion groups always have some participants who rarely contribute and others who monopolize the conversation. The stick ensures that those who don't generally talk are given that opportunity and those who talk excessively have some limits on their participation. The stick provides parameters for all group members—it allows all members to participate. Only those with the stick may talk and you don't talk unless you have it.

Ideas for Use

- You can use a toy magic wand instead of a stick. You could also use a baton.
- This strategy is an effective way to get everyone in a group to talk. In a discussion of conflicts or sensitive issues, some group

members may not disclose their thoughts readily. **Pass the Stick** requires that they participate at least to some small extent.

- **Pass the Stick** may be used with **Imagine** or **Remember When, Reality Check, Mock Trials, In-Class Debates,** or **Case Studies** to ensure contributions and equal sharing.
- In a clinical group, **Pass the Stick** may be used to facilitate **Grand Rounds, V-8 Conferences, Learning From Each Other,** and other postconference topics.
- **Pass the Stick** may be used to assess or test the class. You can **Pass the Stick** around the group to ask questions, pose issues, or test skills.

Put It All Together

General Description. **Put It All Together** gives students an opportunity to synthesize material. Students pick a condition or a diagnosis (medical or nursing) that interests them. As an alternative, they may pick a client they've cared for in clinical rotation. Then they augment their past experience or clinical knowledge with continued research in the chosen area. This strategy thoroughly investigates many aspects of nursing or of a particular client. **Put It All Together** is a good summative assignment for a clinical or senior-level course. Pared down and used at the end of an agency orientation, it can reinforce knowledge of conditions seen frequently in that facility.

Preparation and Equipment. You'll need to think of the criteria for this strategy. When the exercise involves a particular client, the following topics should be addressed:

- Description of the medical or nursing diagnosis
- Client demographics
- Pathophysiology of the condition
- Physical signs and symptoms
- Assessments
- Diagnostic, lab, and medical imaging data
- Client history and risk factors
- Nursing care—specific to the condition (may include client goals and nursing strategies)
- Nursing care—general (may include client goals and nursing strategies)
- Nutrition and diet therapy
- Medical treatment: medications, hydration, treatments, procedures, surgeries
- Potential complications—both rare and common ones and associated nursing monitoring

- Appropriate precautions (e.g., bleeding, aspiration, seizure, neutropenia, fall)
- Client teaching, discharge, family teaching
- Psychoemotional issues

In certain conditions, other topics may need to be addressed.

Once you decide which information needs to be included, you can choose a variety of formats for this exercise. Possibilities include a conference or seminar, a poster or chart, a report, a nursing care plan, a client profile, and a discussion group. These are only some of the ways your students can show their ability to **Put It All Together.**

Example of the Strategy at Work. This strategy allows students in discussion groups to develop a capstone assignment at the end of a course. Using the information previously listed, each of my students created a database, developed and handed out a one-page nursing care plan, and presented a 10-minute seminar in class. It's critical to tell the class that this assignment is meant to **Put It All Together.** After sifting through a wealth of information, students must establish priorities before they can condense it all into a 10-minute presentation.

In this exercise, I place a lot of emphasis on laboratory diagnostics. Although students understand the lab abnormalities associated with a diagnosis, they don't always grasp their dynamic nature. A change in lab values means a change in the client's status, and the nurse has a vital role in monitoring these values.

My students have presented topics such as pancreatitis, hepatitis, spinal cord injury, different types of cancer, COPD, asthma, diabetes, epilepsy, and head injury. These presentations often lead to interesting discussions about which aspects of care are common and which differ according to condition.

Ideas for Use

- Students may select a client who interests them or one they cared for in a clinical rotation. You can also assign a client whose condition ties in with class objectives.
- You can establish guidelines at your discretion. For example, you can gear the assignment toward clinical specialty, course needs, student level, available time, and percentage of the course grade.
- In orientation groups, each participant can present a client and a brief care plan for that client. A new nurse can present a selected client, cared for during orientation, whose condition is commonly encountered on the nursing unit.
- Combine this strategy with **Grand Rounds** or **Learning From Each Other.** Students can present the highlights of a case to the group and hand in the comprehensive report.

- Ask students to consider **What's the Big Deal?** and the **Muddiest Part** when selecting information to present to their colleagues.
- Allow students some creativity with this assignment. **Group Concept Mapping, Dress-Up or Skits,** and other creative exercises can enhance their presentation.
- Use a **One-Minute Care Plan** to establish nursing priorities and allow students to focus on nursing care.
- **Put It All Together** cultivates presentation skills and assertiveness in addition to building students' knowledge base and appreciation of their role in client care (Herrman[2]).
- **Put It All Together** can form the structure for an entire course. Students use readings and course objectives to prepare for class. Rotating presentations feature different prototype conditions at each class session. Finally, the instructor rounds out the information in a summary discussion. In this form, **Put It All Together** develops priority-setting skills and confers many of the same benefits as **Learning From Each Other.**

FYI—Classroom Questioning

General Description. Here, **Classroom Questioning** is the strategy; for your information (**FYI**) is the purpose. It's important to note that the word *your* refers to both instructors and students at any educational level.

FYI—Classroom Questioning is an effective way for learners to assess their own level of knowledge, find out if they're on track, assist in reflective practice, determine whether their knowledge base can meet course objectives, or clarify areas of confusion.[6] Instructors can find many uses for **Classroom Questioning** (see Box 8–9). Use of audience response systems may contribute to **Classroom Questioning**[7] (see **In-Class Test Questions**).

Box 8–9.
FYI—Classroom Questioning

Learn About Your Students
- What do they know?
- Are they well prepared for class?
- Are they ready for the next topic?
- Do they need a pep talk to get them going?
- Do you need to revisit a topic?
- Should you change any assignments or due dates?

Preparation and Equipment. Little preparation is required. **FYI—Classroom Questioning** is more a teaching philosophy than a distinct strategy. You may find yourself using it in every class to assess your students and create a reciprocal atmosphere. You should consider potential questions while preparing your class.

Example of the Strategy at Work. Classroom questioning can be tough. Students may come unprepared or busy themselves with note taking or other activities. They'll ask you to repeat your content, spell a word, or clarify a simple concept. This type of questioning is not what **FYI—Classroom Questioning** refers to. In this strategy, students and instructors ask and answer questions that demonstrate, provoke, and encourage critical thinking.

Both instructors and students must learn to ask "good" questions. This type of questioning is usually on the application or evaluation level. Classroom and staff development instructors should consider reviewing and adapting objective multiple-choice questions before class. When I give a test on venous thrombosis and anticoagulants, I might include the following question:

1. A client you are caring for has thrombophlebitis and is receiving heparin. You are providing client teaching and the nurse instructs the client that which of the following is the action of heparin?

   a. Prolongs the clotting time
   b. Decreases the clotting time
   c. Dissolves the blood clot
   d. Inhibits the bleeding time

This question may be adapted to "What is the action of heparin?" This question and the resulting discussion are at the retention level. We then use the next question to generate continued discussion:

2. A client with a chronic deep vein thrombosis is ordered to receive Coumadin (warfarin) at bedtime every night. The client complains of indigestion and is given an antacid with meals and at bedtime. Which client statement indicates a need for more teaching?

   a. "I take the medications together at night with a snack."
   b. "I need to stop the Coumadin 2 weeks before I go to the dentist."
   c. "I take the Coumadin every day and the antacid as needed."
   d. "I need to take my medications with water."

The resulting discussion may include issues such as bleeding precautions, discharge instructions for a client on anticoagulant therapy, and interactions with other medications. This classroom discussion has reached the application level. To take it a step further, you can ask students to apply information about the disorder to teaching, evaluation for complications, nursing implications, and other issues that foster critical thinking. You might ask some of the following questions:

- Your client complains of significant mouth bleeding. What do you do?
- Your client needs to have dental work. What are your recommendations?
- Your client is switched to warfarin after heparin and tells you he eats spinach every day. What recommendations do you have for this client?
- Your client notices dark red blood in his stool. What could this be? What actions are appropriate at this time?
- Anticoagulant therapy is ordered for your client after a cerebrovascular accident. He tells you that he doesn't take any medications and doesn't want to start now. How do you respond?

The key to this strategy is to stimulate thinking. The answers should be longer than the questions; fewer words are needed for the question than are needed to develop a complex and complete answer.

Ideas for Use

- You don't need to use written questions in this strategy. Just remember to pause every so often to question and be questioned by the class.
- Be supportive of questions in the classroom. Make sure students who ask questions receive positive reinforcement, such as "That's a great question," or "I meant to cover that; thanks for the reminder."
- While preparing the lecture or presentation, consider what questions you'll ask and where you'll place them. **Use the Star** in your notes and to reinforce key pieces of information from the lecture.
- Oermann[8] suggests the One-Minute Question and Answer. Difficult areas of content are examined through a short questioning period. Both instructors and students form pairs or groups to consider potential answers, and a class discussion follows.
- **Classroom Questioning** should be reflected in tests. **Use the Star** to signify a study topic for students and a question area for the instructor.
- Watch for those quizzical looks in class. They're a sure sign that you've reached the **Muddiest Part** and that some points need clarification. Things are also getting muddy when students start

shaking their writing hand or ask you to repeat something two or three times, or when you hear a murmur go through the crowd. Be alert to signals that the students are off track and help them get back on. Trudging ahead only leads to frustration and an increased sense of being lost.

- See **Clinical Questioning** to adapt questions for the more intimate setting of the clinical environment.
- Use **Pass the Stick** to encourage questions that both stimulate the questioner and set off a discourse within the class.
- Try to stimulate students who don't participate by asking, "Are there any questions from someone I don't often hear from?" Follow that with eye contact to give the quieter students license to participate in class.
- Pose questions whether or not you plan to discuss them during class time. Ask students to provide answers through **Email Exercises, Clinical Quick Writes,** or **Online Discussion Groups.** This method generates discussion and rewards class attendance. Give extra credit for the correct answers relating to that day's content.
- Go around the room and ask questions of each student. Class participation and the level of preparation will certainly increase. However, this technique can discourage class attendance, so it should be used carefully. Never use it to embarrass students who can't answer a questions.
- Respond positively when a student asks or answers a question. It rewards students to hear, "Good question, let me see if I can answer that for you," or "As we discussed, your question brings up . . ." Responses such as "We already talked about that" or "That questions is off track from this class" discourage participation on a regular basis. Students who answer questions need the same respect. Rather than saying, "No, that's wrong," try "That is an interesting point, but let me clarify by saying . . ." or "Sometimes what you say may be true, but more often . . ." Of course, if a student's conclusions are truly wrong, he or she needs to be corrected. Again, framing that correction in a polite way invites the student to participate in class again.
- Use **Gaming** to stimulate questioning. In a variant of the 20 Questions game, students ask 20 questions to try to identify an illness or condition. Twenty questions may include:
  - Do both men and women get the illness?
  - Is it contagious?
  - Is it painful?

- Can it be treated with antibiotics?
- Does it happen with mostly older clients?
- Does it change the complete blood count?
- Is it visible?
- Is it treated with surgery?
- Does it affect the lungs? Gastrointestinal tract? Nervous system?
- Does it require involved nursing care?

- Question–Question explores a case scenario by having each student pose a question. Each question is answered with another question. Students rotate throughout the room, asking questions that answer the previous question, being careful not to repeat questions or to speak in statements. These questions uncover increasing levels of complexity about an illness or condition and foster discussion of nursing priorities. *Jeopardy* and other game shows can model ways to structure questions and foster questioning skills.

- Make sure you leave enough time for students to either answer or ask questions. Nursing instructors often feel pressured to fit lessons into the allotted time frame and may not feel free to allow a **Classroom Questioning** period. When we ask a question, we often pause for 1 or 2 seconds and then answer our own question. You should allow 30 seconds for students to construct an answer. Although that seems like an eternity, it's important to impress on the students that you truly want their answers and will wait patiently for them to assemble their thoughts.

- Use **FYI—Classroom Questioning** to create healthy competition among students in **Gaming** or just within class discussion. Encourage questioning through **Prizes.**

- Have students ask their questions as part of the **Admit Ticket** or **Exit Ticket**.

References

1. Lyman F. Think Pair Share: An expanding teaching technique. MAA-CIE Cooperative News 1: 1–2, 1987.
2. Fitzgerald D. Employing think pair share in an associate degree curriculum. Teaching & Learning in Nursing 8(3): 88–90, 2013.
3. Herrman J. The 60-second nurse educator: Creative strategies to inspire learning. Nursing Education Perspectives 23(5): 222–227, 2002.
4. Garwood J, Ahmed A, and McComb S. The effect of concept maps on undergraduate nursing students' critical thinking. Nursing Education Perspectives 39(4): 208–214, 2018.
5. Hunt R. Introduction to community-based nursing. Lippincott Williams & Wilkins, 2012.

6. Mahon P, Lyng C, Crotty Y, and Farren M. Transforming classroom questioning using emerging technology, British Journal of Nursing, 27(7): 389–394, 2018.
7. Farrell T and Mom V. Exploring teacher questions through reflective practice, Reflective Practice, 16(6): 849–866, 2015.
8. Oermann MH. Using active learning in lecture: Best of "both worlds." International Journal of Nursing Education Scholarship l (1):1–9, 2004.

Chapter 9

Strategies for Teaching Research

> *"Education is not the filling of a pail, but the lighting of a fire."*
> —William Butler Yeats

> *"The highest result of education is tolerance."*—Helen Keller

Challenges

- Students express fear and anxiety about learning concepts important to nursing research and evidence-based practice.
- Nursing research may be taught in basic nursing curricula as a stand-alone course or integrated into content.
- Students and nurses don't see the clinical application of nursing research concepts.
- Students and nurses don't generally like to learn about nursing research, although some may enjoy learning about research in general and its concepts.
- Nursing research and evidence-based practice are integral concepts for practicing nurses and agency accrediting organizations.
- Students busy with clinical courses see nursing research as a fluff course rather than as a tool for improving nursing care and client outcomes. There may be a perception that research is not tested via NCLEX®, providing direction for informing students about the value of evidence-based practices and quality improvement efforts.
- Content tends to be abstract and difficult to understand. Terminology may be totally new to both students and practicing nurses. Complex statistics and data analysis procedures often

present roadblocks for nurses trying to grasp research concepts.
- Nursing research concepts usually differ greatly from other nursing clinical content.
- Educators vary widely in their knowledge of quantitative and qualitative research methods.
- Practicing nurses may take the attitude that nursing research is a subject they *had* to learn in school, or they may claim they're old enough to have missed it.

Our evidence-based teaching and practice should include nursing research. The challenge is to make it understandable, useful, clinically relevant, and interesting.

IDEAS

Market Research—Cookies, Candy, and the Research Process

General Description. Comparison study in the classroom leads students through the steps of the research process.[1,2] This strategy may also be used to illustrate specific research concepts.

Preparation and Equipment. Put two objects in a ziplock plastic bag for each student in the class. These objects must be comparable at some level.

Example of the Strategy at Work. To teach the research process, I distribute cookies or candy and caution the students not to eat until they're directed to do so. On the screen or board, I show the research process step by step (see Box 9–1).

I've found it interesting to compare two kinds of chocolate chip cookies because so many comparisons are possible (number of chips per cookie, taste, size, price, texture). As a class we discuss each step and raise interesting questions:

- What is the problem we are trying to research?
- How would we design the study?
- What key words would we include in the literature review?
- What does the literature have to say about market research and this study?
- What is the sample?
- How many sample members do we need for the sample?

Box 9–1.
Cookie Research

1. State the research question.
2. Define the purpose.
3. Review the literature.
4. Formulate a hypothesis; define variables.
5. Select the research design.
6. Select the population, sample, and setting.
7. Conduct a pilot study.
8. Collect the data.
9. Analyze the data.
10. Communicate conclusions and implications.

Eventually we move into a more complex discussion:

- Is this class (sample) representative of the target population?
- If I coerced you into participating in this study, what rights would I violate and what threats would I expose you to?
- What are the threats to internal and external validity?
- Why do businesses perform market research?

The last question leads to a discussion of the needs that motivate nursing research.

Ideas for Use

- Students enjoy food. You can use candy, cookies, crackers, or any food small enough to carry around. In large classes, consider your time and expense.
- You can ask students to develop hypotheses or research questions based on this strategy.
- After the exercise, you can open a discussion about sampling, sample sizes, or random sampling versus random assignment.
- Use **Market Research** for an entire class; as a group, trio, or pair exercise; or as a story incorporated into lecture content.
- Student groups can report their results to the rest of the class.

How Do You Pick Your Shampoo?

General Description. In a large or small group, students can be asked about the decision-making process used to select a brand of any product. Using the steps of the research process, students correlate research, decision making, and the nursing process.

Preparation and Equipment. No special equipment is required. Bringing pictures of the product will stimulate your students to think creatively.

Example of the Strategy at Work. I show a slide of a model with gorgeous hair and ask the students what criteria they use to select their personal shampoo. We discuss variables such as cost, recommendations by friends, availability in the shower, desire for certain hair qualities, store displays, custom, exposure to advertising and marketing, recommendations from authority figures, previous experience, supermarket versus hair salon accessibility, expert advice from a hair stylist, and more (Box 9–2). These considerations echo the "ways of knowing" that often guide nursing practice.

When we've exhausted those ideas, we turn toward a discussion of evidence-based practice. The research process, like the nursing process, is one of the tools we use to help us make decisions and solve problems. Then I expand the research discussion with a hypothetical case: "What happens if you purchase a shampoo and your hair turns green after shampooing with it?"

This is a good time to reinforce the steps of both the nursing process and the research process. "Hair turning green" is an important piece of data. Even if the shampoo was recommended by an authority figure (a parent, perhaps), the data would lead the buyer to question its use. You can extend this situation to the authority figure in the clinical area (nurse educator or experienced nurse) who recommends a nursing intervention.

Box 9–2.
Shampoo Research

What influenced your purchase decision?
- It's cheap.
- My friend likes it.
- I can hang the bottle in the shower.
- It makes my hair silky.
- It looked so pretty in the store.
- I've always used it.
- I kept seeing the ads on TV.
- My neighbor used to work as a beautician, and she says it's great.
- I can pick it up at the supermarket.
- My hair stylist likes his own special kind.

Nursing research can determine the effectiveness of an intervention without relying on customs and beliefs about nursing practice. Discussing the need for continued nursing research, tight research designs, and replication studies is an effective way to relate nursing research and nursing practice.

Ideas for Use

- Ask students to consider the influence of the internet, television, radio, and print media on different types of decision making.
- You can ask students about any product they choose to purchase and use that item to describe the decision-making process. Personalize your teaching by using an object someone brought to class—a smartphone, laptop, or tablet, for example.
- Begin the discussion with the ways of knowing. Compare literature, customs, policies, peers, instructors, intuition, family members, or other experts with the research process as a way to validate knowledge.
- **How Do You Pick Your Shampoo?** is a playful way to open a research discussion with both students and practicing nurses.

Issues in Measurement

General Description. This strategy uses practical methods to teach measurement concepts, including reliability (consistency) and validity (accuracy). The exercises demonstrate the differences between these concepts and their relevance to the research process. See Froman and Owen[3] (an old but great resource) for examples in addition to those presented here and for details about each exercise.

Preparation and Equipment. In the measuring exercise, each group of four students needs one 6- or 12-inch ruler, a 3-foot piece of string, a 1-foot piece of elastic, a pencil, and a tape measure. You may want to hand out data sheets to each student. See Table 9–1 for an example.

Table 9–1. Head Measurement Data Sheet

	Head A	Head B	Head C
Tape measure			
Ruler			
String			
Elastic			

Example of the Strategy at Work. I've used **Issues in Measurement** with both staff development and nursing student classes. I split the class into groups of four. After I distributed the equipment and gave instructions, each student measured the circumferences of the three other heads in the groups using the supplies I'd given out. No other directions were provided.

When all the measurements were completed, group members discussed the validity of each method used to obtain a head circumference. They related each method to the types of measurement used in the clinical area. The group also identified the difficulties of using a straight ruler to measure head circumference, the inaccuracies of measuring with elastic, and the interference caused by different hair styles and types of hair.

Ideas for Use

- This active, entertaining strategy gets students out of their chairs and involved in exercises.
- You can use both metric and standard measurement rulers and then discuss the discrepancies that result from using different units of measurement.

Reliability and Validity Darts

General Description. This is a general strategy that helps students differentiate between reliability and validity. The reader is also referred to Froman and Owen[3] for additional details. **Reliability and Validity Darts** depicts the differences between validity (accuracy) and reliability (consistency).

Preparation and Equipment. Prepare a slide or sign that resembles Figure 9–1. Use it during class discussion to explain the concepts of reliability and validity.

Example of the Strategy at Work. You can let your slide work for you to illustrate how reliability and validity work. The darts are self-explanatory within the context of measurement issues.

Ideas for Use

- Include the diagram on a test. Students can indicate in pictures whether they understand the concepts of reliability and validity. As an alternative, they can discuss these concepts in an essay question or a short, written assignment.
- Ask students to create their own diagrams depicting the concepts of reliability and validity.

- Froman and Owen[3] demonstrate a great way to describe reliability called "Steve's Scale." In this story, they relate that Steve weighs himself on a scale and he is 130 pounds on Monday, 225 on Tuesday, 178 on Wednesday, and so on. This scale is neither reliable nor valid. A replacement scale yielded 140 pounds each morning. It is noted that the scale is reliable (consistent) but that Steve was not apparently this size so the scale is not valid. Another scale reads an accurate weight of 190 pounds that is both valid and reliable.

RELIABILITY AND VALIDITY DARTS

No Reliability
No Validity

Reliable,
Not Valid

Reliable and Valid

Fig. 9–1. Reliability and validity diagram.

Mock Studies

General Description. Students plan and carry out studies that reinforce concepts used in research. These include protection of human subjects, data collection, analysis and interpretation, and nursing implications. The **Mock Study** and its conclusions illustrate the value of nursing research and evidence-based practice.

Preparation and Equipment. You'll need a blackboard, dry erase board, or flip chart to gather ideas. You may bring in computers, classroom screens, and internet access to demonstrate accessing databases, search tools, and data organization methods. Keiffer discussed teaching students about informatics and the technology associated with the research process to link research with improving patient outcomes.[4] Other authors discuss the use of livestream, interprofessional simulation activities to teach research and evidence-based concepts; these activities require extensive equipment and preparation.[5]

Example of the Strategy at Work. One group of students I taught couldn't seem to appreciate the need for nursing research. We were talking about issues that bug us in clinical practice. One student brought up her concerns about performing chest percussion on postoperative clients. She wondered whether the risks (pain inflicted) were outweighed by the benefits (mobilization of secretions) in these clients. Her question turned on a light bulb for me. Suddenly I saw how to create a study that would interest these students.

I let the class decide on the problem and the research question. Then I split them into groups of three or four and gave each group a different assignment. These assignments included designing the study, developing a sampling plan, discussing the literature review, anticipating issues with human subjects and data collection, considering methods of data analysis, understanding the conclusions, and tracking the dissemination of the results. The class quickly learned the interconnections of each step of the research process and understood the need for regular communication between groups.

Ideas for Use

- Ask your students to identify an area of conflict or questionable practice in the clinical area. Use this assignment as preparation for a future class.
- Have students do the assignment individually as an **Ah-Ha Journal** or **Email Exercise.**

- Extend the assignment by asking students to identify a clinical issue, conduct a review of the literature, and propose research designs.
- Whalen[6] discusses the importance of teaching systematic searching to students as part of the literature review. The students completed a worksheet outlining the systematic review process along with reflective questions. The students compiled research logs of search terms, databases, keywords, and other search-related information. These search skills provide the foundation for research projects.

Group Research Critique

General Description. In this strategy, the instructor divides the class into pairs, trios, or small groups. These groups then select and critique a research article. They may use a specific format, found in nursing research texts, or simply discuss the positive and negative aspects of the article. This strategy is also valuable for highlighting current science during coverage of a clinical content topic.

Preparation and Equipment. A critiquing format is essential to this exercise. Most research texts include one. Make sure you use a format that meets the needs of the group and the level of detail needed for this assignment.

Although many different formats exist, most are fundamentally similar, asking the reader to appraise the study and evaluate its validity. Class content can also reinforce critiquing skills.

Example of the Strategy at Work. **Group Research Critique** works well if students are given a critiquing format. Sometimes I let students pick their own article, which increases their level of interest in the assignment, and sometimes I assign one. Having the entire class critique the same one or two articles ensures that you, the instructor, are well versed in the articles' assets and weaknesses. If students pick their own, I ask to approve it to make sure it is a nursing research article. If you do this, you may generate a discussion around the question, "What is nursing research?"

I've also used one article through the entire course or program. We refer to it as the class learns different research steps: design, data collection, analysis, interpretation, and so on. Students prepare for class by critiquing a certain element or the entire work; class discussion can then reinforce concepts. Even some basic concepts, such as "Is the study qualitative or quantitative?," may be unclear during this process. Class discussion provides an opportunity to clarify concepts and reinforce lecture material.

Ideas for Use

- **Group Research Critique** can help you teach the different aspects of a research article.
- You can use the article critique as the final examination.
- In hospital education, nurses can critique articles individually and then discuss them in group meetings or journal clubs.
- In agency education, **Group Research Critique** can enhance a class on research consumerism and application.
- Staff nurses can select articles appropriate to conditions they see often in their client population. Results of several articles or meta-analyses may be referred to agency practice or standard committees.
- Participants can discuss the value of research application. How might their personal nursing practice change as a result of their reading and critiquing nursing research? Their practice may not change immediately. However, it's valuable to examine the influence of research on the ways in which nurses practice and gain knowledge.
- Another potential strategy is an abstract critique. Have students read several abstracts and critique the understandability, readability, and validity of each. They should also critique for inclusion of all components essential to the prescribed abstract format.
- Another author suggests a research scavenger hunt. Students search through assigned studies and look for selected components in a scavenger hunt style.[7]

Clinical Application of Findings to Case Studies

General Description. The instructor asks students to find a nursing research article that applies to their personal nursing practice. A general case study leads them through evaluating the merit of the article. Emphasis may be on the critique of the research and on the ability to use the results in clinical nursing practice.

Preparation and Equipment. Use the case study and questions that follow or develop your own. Ask the students to bring a nursing research article to the class or program.

Example of the Strategy at Work. I asked my students to bring an article of interest and to read it through once before class. In class, I distributed the following case study and questions. The students were asked to consider the questions individually for 15 minutes; then we discussed them as a group.

Answering Questions Through Research

You are a practicing nurse with a strong foundation in evidence-based practice. You have a question about a nursing intervention common on your unit and decide to research the science behind that intervention. Use the information in your article to answer the following questions:

1. After one reading of the article, what nursing problem or practice do you think the study addresses?
2. After one reading of the article, what changes would you make in your personal nursing practice?
3. Now look more closely at your article. What information supports a change in practices, policies, or procedures?
4. Now review your article for weaknesses. Focus on the population, sample, sample size, methods, data collection, data-analysis techniques, or conclusions. How does this information affect the potential changes you would make in your personal nursing practice?
5. What does this exercise teach you about critiquing nursing research and evidence-based practice?

Ideas for Use

- You may need to reinforce the importance of nursing research and its components. This lesson is important in itself.
- You can use **Clinical Application of Findings** after a critiquing exercise. This approach reinforces the need to appraise research before using its results to change nursing practice.
- Liven up the case study by adapting it for application to specific nursing specialties.
- Use a case study to illustrate the ethical issues that surround the research process and the role of the nurse as client advocate in research studies. You can present the following case to generate discussion about the ethical and legal aspects of research in regard to clients. Discussing these issues provides an interesting angle for both students and practicing nurses.

Deceiving the Client: Legal and Ethical Issues in Research

Immediately after a diagnosis of ovarian cancer, a client is offered chemotherapy with an experimental drug. In this research protocol, neither the effectiveness nor the side effects of the drug are known. The client was given a written description of the drug's action and effects before her nurse and physician asked her to sign the consent form. The client did not ask questions about the chemotherapy and felt obligated to accept this treatment because the physician offered no other choices. During 6 months of treatment, she weakened dramatically and at times seemed incoherent. The chemotherapy was continued despite the deterioration in the client's physical and mental condition.

Use this case to illustrate the nurse's role as client advocate and as a proponent of research. It's a great way to generate a discussion on research, advances in medical science, and associated ethical dilemmas.

Research Moments in Every Class

General Description. This strategy reflects the principle that nursing research should be introduced into every area of content. For clinical and nonclinical information, the instructor briefly shares current research with the students. A focus on nursing implications highlights the need for evidence-based practice.

Preparation and Equipment. Before class, take a moment to search an electronic full-text database quickly. Use "research" as one of your keywords to ensure that you access a study about a content area.

Example of the Strategy at Work. I've found **Research Moments** especially effective for relating research findings to current practice. An active search for each class topic reinforces the value of research and evidence-based practice.

I've used this method in many classes, including a class on cystic fibrosis (see Box 9–3). A quick literature review yielded several articles related to current research. I summarized their content briefly on a slide, which led to a short discussion.

Box 9–3.
Research Moment

Examples of Current Research About Cystic Fibrosis (CF)

- Avoidance of summer camps for groups of children with CF (to prevent cross-infection).
- Screening of carriers and affected individuals to assist with early diagnosis and treatment. implications for genetic counseling.
- Success of heart or lung transplants/quality of life for patients with CF.
- Genetic manipulation to enhance diagnosis and treatment.

Ideas for Use

- In continuing education programs, **Research Moments** helps to relate findings to current, local practices.
- You can encourage attentiveness in your students by telling them they'll be tested on research results. Then include a question about the research in a comprehensive examination.
- Ask your students to research topics related to daily class content. If the class is small enough, they can share their results with the group. When their peers become research information finders, other students discover the incentive to apply research to their own practice.

Research Corners—Electronic or Bulletin Board

General Description. **Research Corners** resembles the **Research Moments** strategy. The difference is that abstracts and interesting findings are posted either on cork boards or electronically. Like **Research Moments,** this strategy doesn't take much time.

Preparation and Equipment. You'll need a bulletin board if you plan to post research results on paper. For electronic postings, use a Web-based platform that allows attachments to a page that the class can view.

Example of the Strategy at Work. **Research Corners** enhances knowledge of a content area while reinforcing the need for nursing research. For physical postings, I either type a brief summary of an article or cut the abstract out of a journal. Interesting clip art and colors add to the visual appeal of the board. Citations are kept brief and are limited to interesting findings at the students' level. For electronic postings, I attach summaries or abstracts to the class page for viewing.

Ideas for Use

- Allow students to provide research ideas, abstracts, or summaries for posting.
- Use **Research Corners** as either a required assignment or for extra credit.
- Use bulletin boards to promote research in break rooms or common nursing areas.
- Use **Online Discussion Groups** to discuss current research findings.
- Provide incentives to encourage staff members or students to develop visual displays about a particular topic. Encourage them to change these displays frequently. Students can receive extra credit for assignments. Staff nurses can be given clinical ladder credit, agency "freebies," or books to reward their participation.
- Brief, eye-catching messages are important for busy nurses and students.
- A colleague posts **Research Corners** on her door, making a statement about nursing research and providing reading material for visitors.

Film Clips in Nursing Research

General Description. The instructor shows clips of current films to stimulate discussion of research concepts. These film clips should delineate a problem or issue in current research or healthcare.

Preparation and Equipment. You'll need a supply of video or DVD clips, cued to specific scenes. Before class, you'll need to establish objectives for the exercise, consider the questions you'll ask, and speculate on areas for future investigation. YouTube provides many opportunities for use of video clips to clarify research topics.

Example of the Strategy at Work. Many popular films raise issues that nursing research can and should address (for guidelines, see the **Short Clips** section of Chapter 3). After showing a short clip, I ask the class to formulate a research question or develop a research design addressing the topic. I've used clips to illustrate the steps of the research process, to stimulate research ideas, and to make research "real" from a movie perspective.

Ideas for Use

- Potential film topics include specific illnesses, clients dealing with symptoms, legal and ethical dilemmas, and social science content.

- Ask the class how nursing research might have changed the outcome of the film clip.
- Have students develop a **Mock Study** based on the research questions derived from a film clip.
- After showing a clip, use **Email Exercises** or **Ah-Ha Journals** to brainstorm ideas for research design.
- Discuss with students the importance of replication studies and the cautions associated with practice changes. Reinforce the idea that one or two studies do not warrant changing practice, but they may inform potential future study into evidence-based practices.

Clinical Area Questioning—Research at Work

General Description. Clinical instructors are attuned to the value of research. In this strategy, the instructor investigates the literature to determine what is known about a topic and then presents the findings to the class. Clinical and practice issues present an opportunity for **Clinical Area Questioning.**

Preparation and Equipment. To begin, you need an inquiring mind in the clinical area. The clinical question or issue determines the need to research the literature and find out what is known about the topic.

Example of the Strategy at Work. Students and staff nurses were asking questions about a clinical problem. A client had been admitted with a diagnosis of aspiration pneumonia. This client had been receiving nasogastric tube feedings at home.

I saw this situation as a great opportunity to demonstrate the value of nursing research. A literature review discovered studies that addressed ways of checking nasogastric tube placement. Auscultation of air injected into a tube, aspiration of gastric contents, pH of gastric contents, and chest x-ray were compared for feasibility, effectiveness, and other criteria. Our summary of the findings generated much discussion about local practice and the procedures recommended by nursing textbooks.

Ideas for Use

- Ask unit instructors, senior clinical ladder nurses, or student leaders to do literature searches and disseminate information.
- Information may be posted on electronic bulletin boards or cork boards.
- Like **Research Moments in Every Class, Clinical Area Questioning** should be inherent in every clinical experience.

- Keep a log of questions asked in day-to-day clinical practice so you can research problems later on.
- Ask students to determine their own clinical problems or issues to be researched and examined.
- Colleagues used this strategy to share "Nursing Research Myth Busters" with fellow nurses. Clinical questions from the group listserv were used to stimulate research, gather evidence, and come to practice-based conclusions. By using the questions and issues from active bedside practice, participants not only received information valuable to enhancing patient care but also saw the value of investigation to solve clinical problems and the potential for research to improve patient outcomes.

Paper Towel Ideas

General Description. In this strategy, a common roll of paper towels can inspire creative thinking. Students list their ideas, one per sheet, unrolling the towels as their ideas evolve.

Preparation and Equipment. You'll need one roll of paper towels for each individual, pair, trio, or group. Each roll needs a marker for writing down ideas. For added incentive, you can bring in prizes to reward the greatest number of ideas. **Paper Towel Ideas** is a relatively inexpensive strategy.

Example of the Strategy at Work. A colleague asks students to use their paper towels by listing researchable ideas, one to a sheet. Other instructors have used this strategy in research groups to list other concepts, such as types of sampling criteria and methods of data collection.

Ideas for Use

- You can give prizes to the individuals or groups who think of the greatest number of ideas, measured in the number of paper towels they unroll.
- The competitive atmosphere stimulates different, creative ideas.
- You can use **Paper Towel Ideas** any time you want to brainstorm new ideas.
- Some faculty use toilet paper to create lists. Others reject this variation on the strategy, attaching a negative connotation to the use of toilet paper.
- You can use **Paper Towel Ideas** at the beginning and end of a course or program to demonstrate how far the students' thinking has evolved.

Faculty Research Sharing

General Description. Instructors share personal nursing research experience to demonstrate that professionals participate in and are invested in research. Unlike **War Stories and Clinical Anecdotes,** this strategy focuses on research concepts rather than day-to-day clinical experience. **Faculty Research Sharing** works well in any class.

Preparation and Equipment. You may want to use slides or overhead transparencies to describe research findings.

Example of the Strategy at Work. **Faculty Research Sharing** illustrates important concepts and highlights the challenges and rewards of research. In my experience, it's better for students to hear brief discussions without elaborate discourses on design and implementation. For example, when differentiating quantitative and qualitative data, I avoided a theoretical discussion and stuck to examples from personal research.

Ideas for Use

- Maintain a focus on research concepts and keep **Faculty Research Sharing** brief and relevant to class content.
- As you share your research, make sure to keep the presentation at the knowledge level of the students.
- Have other speakers or instructors share their research experiences with the class.
- You can take as little as 10 minutes to share research findings. Presented in the middle of a class, they can reinforce the importance of research in any clinical area.
- Clinical experts can share a policy or practice that was developed or changed on the basis of clinical research.
- When discussing in-depth data analysis procedures or complex theoretical frameworks, take care not to discourage the students.
- Ask instructors or guest speakers to discuss a single step of the research process—consent of human subjects, data collection, and so on—to keep the focus on class objectives.
- This may be expanded to a research mentor program where instructors lead students through mentored experiences in review of literature, data collection, data entry, and other roles related to the research process.[8]

Poster Sessions

General Description. Student groups create a poster based on a research article or a review of several articles. The research must reflect a practice issue. Because the posters are based on specific criteria and resemble those displayed at professional meetings, they prepare both students and nurses for scholarly presentation.

Preparation and Equipment. You should develop a specific grading rubric or evaluation criterion for submissions. The students contribute poster boards, illustrations, information, and the effort of making the poster.

Example of the Strategy at Work. Colleagues have used **Poster Sessions** in research and continuing education classes to promote active participation and research evaluation. One colleague split a class into groups of five. Each group picked its own topic and found an article or review. Students used the assignment criteria to critique the study and used the posters to display their analysis. Afterward, the instructor graded the posters.

Some of my colleagues have organized a poster display day. Student posters are graded, and the best ones win a small prize or award. Students also work individually with instructors on literature reviews, **Mock Studies,** or pilot studies and present their results in a **Poster Session.**[8]

Ideas for Use

- Invite your colleagues to the poster displays. They can help you evaluate posters and assist in disseminating the students' research findings.
- In the clinical area, assign units to complete a quality improvement activity, a literature review, or a pilot study. Then have them develop posters. Display the posters during nurses' week or in conjunction with an educational program. Provide rewards and recognition for participants.
- Encourage students and nurses attending conferences to view and evaluate research posters created by other nurses.
- Encourage students to submit posters to local conferences that foster student involvement in research.

Research Concept Maps

General Description. Visual maps of research concepts and methods are used to reinforce the research process or to critique individual studies. See Rooda[9] (another old but good resource) for the use of mind mapping in a research course.

Preparation and Equipment. For individual assignments, you'll need drawing supplies or software that can generate concept maps. For class or group concept mapping, you can use a blackboard, dry-erase board, overhead projector, or flip chart. If an entire class or large group is working on one poster, spread a large sheet of paper over a desk or table so they can all contribute to the concept map.

Example of the Strategy at Work. I've had students map out the research process on the blackboard. As with any concept map exercise, lines can be drawn to show connections between concepts reflected in circles or squares. Colors, shapes, and placement on the map can represent categories, steps, or differences in concepts. Concepts may be as elaborate or as simple as desired. See Rooda[9] for examples of research concept maps.

Ideas for Use

- You can use **Research Concept Maps** with pairs, trios, or groups.
- Try using the strategy as a test question: ask students to draw the research process.
- Design a homework project in which students critique an article using a concept map.
- Another strategy, similar to the concept map, is the research puzzle. Each step of the research process is written on a puzzle piece. Each student is given a puzzle piece and asked to dissect a research study for the assigned step. The group convenes to discuss and analyze the study based on each research component. Students then discuss the integral nature of each step and how every step interrelates to produce a sound study design.

Campus or Unit Research and Nurse Interviews

General Description. Students survey peers and other students to learn the elements of tool development, field research, observational research, and data analysis. Practicing nurses can live the experience of data collection by polling each other on selected information. During their clinical rotations, students interview staff nurses about the use of nursing research in the clinical area. Practicing nurses ask colleagues similar questions. These interviews can be either formal or informal.

Preparation and Equipment. No equipment is needed. Students or nurses may conduct interviews before a scheduled class discussion. Interviewers should agree on topics to make sure that all interviews are on similar subjects. You may want to consider topics ahead of time to help your students brainstorm ideas for interviews.

Example of the Strategy at Work. I've used this strategy early in a course or program to determine the research climate in which nurses work and the local attitudes toward evidence-based practice. Students can generate questions and then discuss their interviews in subsequent sessions.

Effective questions are, "Do you use research to guide your nursing practice?" and "Do you use evidence to guide your practice." I've also expanded this question to include areas such as level of research education, participation in policy and procedure development, reading of nursing journals, and involvement in research studies. I've asked students and nurses to conduct informal studies of their peers. For student peer interviews, I sometimes pick a topic before class and instruct the students to ask others about that topic. They can use sample questions or develop their own.

For nursing students, topics should reflect daily life. I've instructed students to ask as many people as possible if they shower in the morning, in the evening, or at some other time. Early in the spring semester, I've asked students to poll peers about their plans for spring break. For practicing nurses, demographic surveys may be valuable.

My students conduct interviews either alone or in pairs. We tabulate the results in a subsequent class. This method allows us to explore the data collection and analysis phases of research.

Ideas for Use

- **Campus or Unit Research** can be combined with **Mock Studies** to simulate study design and implementation.
- This strategy can generate enthusiastic interest in nursing research at the unit or group level.
- On a unit, you may want to include nurse managers, physicians, and clinical specialists in the interviews.
- According to the local research climate, this method may highlight the need for increased evidence-based practice in clinical settings.
- Work with community agencies to develop mutually beneficial research projects. School nurses, unit educators, small health agencies, and research staff at clinical sites may assist in identifying one or more populations, interventions, comparisons, and outcomes (PICOs) for meaningful research collaborations.
- Survey the class for selected information (demographics, satisfaction questions, opinions) and show students how to collect, analyze, and interpret data as descriptive statistics.
- Nurses may claim that they don't use research in daily practice. You can guide a student's line of questioning with queries such as "How does your agency develop policies and procedures?," "How does your unit conduct quality assurance?," and "How do standards of care change a client's course of stay in the

hospital?" These questions may uncover a deeper appreciation of evidence-based practice for both the student interviewer and the practicing nurse.

- **Campus or Unit Research** makes a good icebreaker. Ask students to poll their peers on a topic and then use their findings to stimulate a discussion.
- You can use this strategy to explain different types of data and the methods used to organize them.
- Descriptive statistics, such as mean, mode, and median, can be calculated and discussed as data descriptors.

In the Know

General Description. The tabloids in the grocery store have taught us that human nature reacts to the different, exceptional, and outrageous. Although not all nursing research findings meet these criteria, research sometimes uncovers surprising results that warrant further study and exploration. These are the facts that will catch your students' attention in class. **In the Know** requires the instructor to be in tune with these data and to be able to summarize them simply.

Presenting a potential medical or nursing advance, much like those announced on the evening news, provides an opportunity for discussion and a point of interest. Of course, validity and reliability should be weighed before the data are accepted as fact. This critical process is educational in itself.

Preparation and Equipment. Follow the introduction of research information to the lay public, peruse research journals, or do your own quick study of current research. Any of these methods can provide insights that will engage your students' thinking. You must include the source and validity of that information to avoid misconceptions or misunderstandings.

Example of the Strategy at Work. I used this strategy with a research group to assess the current data and evidence related to multi-tasking. We examined the research in the lay and scientific literature and discussed the implications for studying, personal habits, and nursing practice. In this way, **Current Events** can be combined with **In the Know** to generate class discussion.

Newspapers and online news sites frequently publish information about current scientific research. Issues such as stem cell research, medical advances, and development of new medications are part of everyday news. Busy nurses and nursing students are sometimes so absorbed with work and study that they are insulated from the news.

Current events that affect nursing practice or exemplify nursing research are especially useful. Recent exposés of widespread errors in medication administration have created a public outcry and call for a change in healthcare practices. Clearly, changes are needed to ensure cautious and careful medication administration and eliminate inferior standards of care. Being **In the Know** about such findings is an important way to validate good practice. Discussing these studies and their nursing implications underlines to students the importance of prudent nursing practice.

Ideas for Use

- **In the Know** may be used to discuss both sound and unsound research. Encourage your students to analyze any method or interpretation they find questionable.
- This strategy is a great way to reinforce the fascinating nature of research and scientific inquiry.
- Use **In the Know** to discuss the need for replication of nursing studies. In addition, replication with varying samples is necessary to ensure that results can be generalized. It's important to emphasize that changes in practice should occur only after findings are validated and the literature has been reviewed thoroughly.
- Students can search media to find **In the Know** topics. These topics can be collected as an **Admit Ticket,** written about in a short assignment, or used to guide class discussion.
- Assign groups to review the media portrayal of current advances in disease treatment. Thanks to the internet, we can view archival news clips to learn what the lay public has been told about a medical issue. These clips are often generated from large-scale studies in reputable nursing and medical journals. Students can compare the public information with the scientific study to determine the accuracy of the portrayal, the implications for nursing practice, and the need for further study.

Bring on the Evidence

General Description. Nurses and nursing students at every level are hearing about the importance of evidence-based practice. Novices often have trouble understanding what data count as evidence and how to assess their validity. Sometimes information is accepted as truth because the messenger has a convincing manner, not because the information has been appraised accurately. **Bring on the Evidence** allows students to function as "research sleuths" on a clinical or nursing issue.

Students select or are assigned a clinical problem or research dilemma. They develop the research question, essentially conducting a literature review. The difference is that the students are uncovering and collecting research evidence in a "private investigator" style.

Preparation and Equipment. You may want to use **Bring on the Evidence** as a final project for a research class. You need to develop the assignment, determine how many grade points you'll award for different aspects of the work, and develop a list of potential clinical issues or problems.

Example of the Strategy at Work. This strategy is especially valuable for smaller classes or clinical groups. The assignment may be done alone or as a group activity; I've found that groups work especially well.

First, students select a clinical problem or issue. During the first class session, we discuss and define this topic, and the class brainstorms potential keywords to use in a search. The brainstorming session and choice of keywords are essential, especially for novice researchers. I like to organize a field trip to the library or at least to a computer that allows access to library databases. This type of practice provides a certain level of comfort with the research process.

I encourage my students to download articles and print or bring electronic copies to class to allow for ongoing review. Students are encouraged to highlight hard copy or annotate a PDF article. Students can list their evidence and bring the list to class. Subsequent classes review the evidence and discuss implications for further research and nursing practice.

Ideas for Use

- Students can present their evidence as a **Poster Session** accompanied by a short discussion of their conclusions.
- In a clinical setting, students can use the policies and procedures of the unit to generate their clinical issue. They can then **Bring on the Evidence** to inform the unit staff about their findings and to recommend further inquiry to the agency procedure committees.
- Students may frame their evidence as an **In-Class Debate,** presenting their research findings versus a traditional or institutional practice. Ask them to analyze the evidence and to decide whether it's time to recommend a change in practice.
- Award prizes to students who find the most definitive evidence.
- This strategy may be combined with a **Mock Trial** to continue the "sleuth" theme.

Author Guidelines

General Description. Once students appreciate the value of nursing research, they discover an incentive to become research consumers themselves. The **Author Guidelines** strategy simulates the experience of developing a manuscript for publication. This strategy is meant to be coupled with other projects to teach the next step in the research process—dissemination.

Students use an original research idea or some other project to explore the publication process. The project can be a **Campus or Unit Research Interview, Mock Study,** or any other strategy that replicates the research process.

Author Guidelines takes that strategy a step further. Students review current journals that would potentially publish their idea and bring the author guidelines for that journal to class. As an alternative, the instructor can download or obtain author guidelines to be distributed in class.

Preparation and Equipment. Preparation begins with another assignment related to the research process. You can use one of the other research strategies described in this chapter.

Example of the Strategy at Work. **Campus or Unit Research** and **Mock Studies** are the best foundation for preparing a simulated manuscript. After designing and completing the first step of the process, students then use their **Author Guidelines** to complete a short assignment. They can write the abstract, lay out the sections of the article, or develop an outline of the potential manuscript. Encourage your students to review the guidelines for specific requirements, such as formatting, length, and audience. Many editors suggest reviewing other articles in the journal to learn its literary style.

I've used **Author Guidelines** to discuss the difference between writing school papers and writing for journals (a challenge for many of us). I also emphasize the importance of meeting the needs of the audience. This is a good time to discuss the peer-review process, acceptance rates, the challenges of writing for publication, and opportunities to begin a career in writing. Letters to the editor, any type of commentary, smaller community and local nursing publications, and professional organizations all provide good opportunities for the beginning writer.

Ideas for Use

- This assignment can be adapted for a group activity, a single homework assignment, or a class writing exercise.
- Students can compare the author guidelines of different journals to discover the particular priorities of each publication.

- Classes can peruse issues of a journal to get a feeling for its target audience. Encourage discussion questions such as "Who is this journal designed for?," "How does the audience determine the writing style?," and "How much research is published in this journal?" Discussion questions can be reviewed in pairs and trios to encourage participation.

- Advanced students can use **Author Guidelines** to develop concept papers for publication or assist faculty members with research, leading to a joint publication.

- Have students view and complete components of an institutional review board (IRB) application, including criteria associated with expedited, exempt, and full review applications.

- Provide an exercise on how to set up a research project budget, including expenses such as incentives for participants, data collection, data analysis, and other costs.

- Have your students draft a query letter for a particular journal using the **Author Guidelines** or journal rules.

References

1. Hagle ME and Millenbruch JL. Retooling the Great American Cookie experiment for nursing grand rounds. Clinical Nurse Specialist 25(5): 220–223, 2011.

2. McCurry MK. The Great American Cookie experiment updated for the millennial learner. Journal of Nursing Education 53(3): 180, 2014.

3. Froman RD and Owen SV. Teaching reliability and validity: Fun with classroom application. Journal of Continuing Education in Nursing 22: 88–94, 1991.

4. Keiffer MR. Engaging nursing students: Integrating evidence-based inquiry, informatics, and clinical practice. Nursing Education Perspectives, 39(4): 247–249, 2018.

5. Lanier Y, Bryant K., Budin W., et al. Interprofessional development of a livestream simulation activity to enhance an undergraduate nursing research course. Nursing Education Perspectives, 40(1): 50–52, 2019.

6. Whalen K and Zentz SE. Teaching systematic searching in a baccalaureate nursing research course. Workviews on Evidence-Based Nursing, 12(4): 246–248, 2015.

7. Phillips RM. Creative classroom strategies for teaching research. Nursing Education 39(4): 199–201, 2014.

8. Wheeler E, Hardie T, Schell K, and Plowfield L. Symbiosis: Undergraduate research mentoring and faculty scholarship in nursing. Nursing Outlook 56(1): 9–15, 2008.

9. Rooda LA. Effects of mind mapping on student achievement in a nursing research course. Nurse Educator 19: 25–27, 1994.

Chapter 10

Creative Teaching Strategies to Enhance Clinical Decision Making and Test Taking

"A good teacher can inspire hope, ignite the imagination, and instill the love of learning."—Brad Henry

Challenges

- Even though graduation from a school or program of nursing signals a great milestone, there is one more hurdle to becoming a professional nurse—passing NCLEX®.

- Across the spectrum of nursing educational levels and programs, nursing students find the NCLEX® examinations stressful!

- Although nurse educators do not want to teach to the test, we are responsible for teaching students about the examination and to ensure that the curricula include information about the NCLEX®-identified domains of nursing practice and how these domains coincide with professional nursing practice.

- There are no tricks to test taking—nothing replaces knowing the material. But using strategies that assist students to further develop test-taking skills, and knowledge of the NCLEX® Blueprint and integrated processes provide students with the tools to succeed on the examination.

- Patient safety is a critical priority of nursing education. The Quality Safety Education for Nurses (QSEN) initiative is a landmark work that identifies integral components of safe patient care, teaching strategies, and content.

- As noted in previous chapters, Next Generation NCLEX®, with a focus on clinical judgment, reinforces the need for active learning and opportunities for students to practice and build skills in clinical decision making and critical thinking.[1,2]

Creative teaching strategies may be interlaced with lecture and other strategies to ensure effective student learning of test-taking strategies, the NCLEX® Blueprint and Integrated Processes, the QSEN initiative, and Next Generation NCLEX®. This chapter presents novel strategies and cross-references to methods mentioned in previous chapters to provide new and exciting information to nurse educators across experience levels, specialties, and practice settings.

STRATEGIES TO BUILD TEST-TAKING SKILLS

Test taking is often one of the most stressful parts of education—for students and instructors. Instructors may provide valuable information to allow students to enhance their skills and prepare for the NCLEX® examination.

IDEAS

Assess Your Own Learning Style

General Description. Important skills for students are analyzing their personal learning style, trying different methods of studying and learning, and developing study and testing skills that are successful for them. As discussed in earlier chapters, instructors may evaluate their students' styles. These learning styles are related to generational skills and priorities, attention spans, sensory experiences, brain hemisphere dominance, and other factors. Just as educators need to analyze these factors, students will also find it valuable to assess their own learning skills. We often study what we are good at and what we know—personal assessments allow students to identify areas that need extra study time and emphasis (see **Teaching Tools**).

Example of Strategy at Work. I provide this to students as a **Think-Pair-Share** exercise. Students discuss their personal style and share with the class. Strategies specific to test taking, class content, or the NCLEX® examination then may be discussed.

Assessing the Learner

Brain Dominance

1. Likes words, numbers, letters, parts, sequential order, linear thought, language; is detail oriented, organized (left-brained, analytical learner)
2. Likes images, patterns, entirety, simultaneous actions, music; is nonverbal, creative, intuitive, spontaneous, graphics oriented (right-brained, global learner)

Learning Modalities

1. Prefers verbal instruction; remembers names, not faces; is distracted by noise; enjoys music; likes answering machines (auditory learner)
2. Remembers faces, not names; has a vivid imagination; thinks in pictures and uses colors; likes postcards (visual learner)
3. Learns by doing and touching; remembers what was done; is impulsive; loves games (kinesthetic learner)

Favorite Learning Activities

Visual: Television, reading, videos, handouts, flip charts, signs, writing, handouts, pictures, graphics, charts/tables

Auditory: Books on tape, tapes, music, radio, conversation, listening to steps, lecture, recorded lectures

Kinesthetic: Games, computer and live simulations, group activities, role playing, props and toys, demonstration, practice, and return demonstration.

Write Your Own Test Questions

General Description. Studies reveal that practicing writing test questions is an effective way to enhance test-taking skills. The act of developing a scenario, composing a stem, writing credible distractors, and isolating a correct response allows students to build their skills. This strategy also helps students learn about application and analysis level questions to ensure that they are ready for NCLEX®-style questions. Using this as a homework assignment, an **Admit Ticket**, an in-class activity, or **Quizzes That Count** or **Quickie Quizzes** allows students not only to learn the skills of test construction but also to appreciate the difficulty associated with item writing!

Example of the Strategy at Work. When I notice the students' attention is waning or when I have a few extra moments in class, I have students write a test question about the previously discussed content. I encourage students to think of viable distractor options and reinforce the need to have a "best" answer to represent the correct response. I also recommend that students make the test question application and analysis level questions to ensure that the question conforms to testing guidelines. Students are given 5 minutes to compose their questions and then switch with a neighbor. Make sure the students do not indicate the correct answer to the question. Students discuss the correct answer and collaborate with their peers on the question and answers. As time allows, students can switch with other students around them, further spreading the learning. These questions may be scrutinized for use as **In-Class Test Questions**, for future test items, or for study guides for student use. Another variation is to have students develop remembering or understanding level questions. Students are then asked to revise the questions for higher levels, including applying and analyzing to demonstrate the increasing complexity of items.

Alternate-Item Practice

General Description. The NCLEX® examination includes alternate-format items for the registered nurse (RN) and practical nurse (PN) exams. Many believe that these alternate-format questions better discriminate between critical thinking and decision making than traditional multiple-choice items do. These items may be constructed in a variety of formats, including select all that apply, hot spot, drag and drop, fill in the blank, chart exhibits, graphic interaction, auditory interaction, and video interaction. These last three categories of items ask students to make decisions about pictures, audio recordings, and video clips. Readers are encouraged to refer to the National Council of State Boards of Nursing (NCSBN) website (www.ncsbn.org) for further details about alternate-format questions and practice quizzes for student use. Many standardized testing packages now include alternate-format questions for student practice. These items may offer an additional challenge for students, may take additional time, and should never be a surprise to students when they sit down to the examination! As Next Generation Items continue to evolve to clinically based, technologically sophisticated, and unfolding questions, student exposure to clinical judgment exercises and independent and group work will be even more critical.[3] For further information, check the NCSBN website (www.ncsbn.org/next-generation-nclex.htm). You may want to sign up for email notifications and review the resources closely to ensure that you and your students are well informed.

Example of the Strategy at Work. I provide PowerPoint slides and handouts of five to eight examples of alternate-format questions. You may also use the assignment function of your local learning management system. These questions may be used as homework, an in-class activity, or a **Quiz That Counts**.

Take-Home Quiz on NCSBN Website

General Description. Take-home quizzes are a valuable way to save time in class, to ensure that students are prepared for class, and to reinforce complex topics. One of the most valuable strategies to assist students in preparing for NCLEX® is to review the NCSBN© website. Sending students home to explore the website is a valuable introduction to the site's features. The **Take-Home Quiz** may also be used for many topics and is especially effective when the students' comprehension and mastery of class content would be enhanced by their preparation and preclass work.

Example of the Strategy at Work. I provide this assignment in the students' senior year, when NCLEX® begins to loom over their heads. The assignment asks them to search the website and consider their own learning needs. This may also be used as a **Quiz That Counts** or a **Write to Learn**.

1. If you had to take the NCLEX® examination today, what would be your greatest personal challenges?
2. View the NCSBN website. Last week we discussed the alternate-format questions on NCLEX®. Why does NCSBN use alternate-format questions in addition to traditional items on the NCLEX® examination?
3. Using the NCSBN Test Plan that we discussed in class and that is discussed in the blueprint on the NCSBN website, on which areas do you believe you will need to focus your study efforts?
4. How does NCSBN use the practice analysis to develop the blueprint?
5. From the NCSBN website, what types of topics are included in the Management of Client Care section? Why are these important?
6. Why is the topic of priority setting so important on the NCLEX® examination?

These may also be used as **Email Assignments.** Here are mine.

Assignment 1

1. How much have you prepared for the NCLEX®? What materials have you used in this preparation? Do you have a review book or other resources?
2. If you had to take the exam today, what would be your greatest personal challenges? Why?
3. View the NCSBN website. What is an alternative item? Why does NCSBN use alternative items in addition to traditional items on the NCLEX® exam? Look at the frequently asked questions (FAQs)—what surprises you about this information?
4. Find a scholarly article in the literature that discusses the use of alternative items on the NCLEX® exam. How do alternative items relate to nursing clinical decision making?
5. How has your previous experience with studying, study skills, test taking, computerized testing, and multiple-choice exams prepared you for NCLEX®? Discuss two or three aspects of this preparation.

Assignment 2

1. On the NCSBN website, what types of topics are included in the Management of Client Care section? Why are these important?
2. Why are decision making and delegation so important on the NCLEX® exam? Why are they important in nursing practice?
3. Find a scholarly article in the literature that discusses priority setting in nursing practice. Why is this area emphasized on NCLEX®? How do priority-setting skills relate to clinical nursing practice?
4. When do you perceive you will be taking the exam? What time of day and what day do you prefer? What other things are happening to influence your scheduling the exam?
5. How do you plan to prepare for the NCLEX®? Be specific with time frames, areas, resources, supports, and so on.

Assignment 3

1. How are NCLEX® items established? What processes and variables are attended to when writing items and placing them in the NCLEX® test bank? Address how bias is handled on NCLEX® items.

2. How is the NCSBN NCLEX® blueprint established? Describe the complex process that goes into the establishment of the blueprint.

3. Why does NCSBN change the percentages of the test every three years? On what criteria are these changes based?

4. Find a scholarly article in the literature that discusses the NCLEX® blueprint. How does the blueprint relate to clinical nursing practice?

5. What area of the blueprint do you think may offer the highest level of difficulty? Why?

Assignment 4

1. Ask people in your clinical (or another nursing) setting about NCLEX®. What are the perceptions of those in your current clinical setting (or another nursing setting) related to the NCLEX®? If your clinical setting does not yield rich information, ask other sources or search the internet about perceptions of NCLEX®.

2. Using the NCSBN Test Plan, on which areas do you believe you will need to focus your study efforts? How will you do that? Why is this extra focus needed in these areas? Develop your practice PASSPOINT exam based on these priorities and list these priorities in your CANVAS assignment (see below).

3. What application materials have you received and how have you attended to the application procedure? What types of materials do you need to complete the application? What websites are used to apply? How much will the application cost?

4. How is "NCLEX® World" different from and how is it similar to "real-world" nursing practice? Ask a practicing nurse about her or his thoughts on "NCLEX® World."

5. Find a scholarly article in the literature that discusses how NCLEX® does or does not replicate nursing practice.

Progressive Quizzes

General Description. **Progressive Quizzes,** like **Quickie Quizzes** or **Quizzes That Count**, provide a mechanism to assess student learning, identify **Muddiest Parts**, take attendance, and provide graded items that contribute to the course grade. This strategy is novel because it allows the teacher to ask questions periodically throughout the course of the class. This may be of assistance if you have problems with students coming to class and leaving after the quiz, coming to class late, or not paying attention.

Example of the Strategy at Work. I use this mechanism quite a bit. Quizzes that I have used include a quiz on the syllabus (given the second day of class to ensure that students really read the syllabus), a quiz on the last day of class, or just in the middle of the semester to offer some variation to the course. I make the questions reflect a variety of modes, including **Write to Learn** (short essays), multiple-choice, fill-in-the-blank, and personal reflection items. Students really seem to enjoy this reason to stay attentive, and it reinforces class attendance *and* focusing on content. I find, as many other educators might, that students often do not read the syllabus or that they ask questions that pertain to the content of the syllabus. A participant in one of my presentations suggested a quiz on the syllabus, and I found it very effective. It may be taken with the syllabus in hand or not. Because I do not expect the students to memorize the syllabus, the open-book method allows them to look up answers and to retrieve information later.

- I found this a great strategy as the last class of the semester when the students, and I, are tired. Every 10 minutes I show a slide that has a question. By the end of the 75-minute class, there are eight questions and the quiz is completed.
- Try to ask reflective questions so that students will have thoughtful, personal answers. This will discourage copying from others. Students hand in their answers at the end of the class, keeping them interested and attentive, especially when I remind them that quiz questions may assist in studying for the exam.

Other strategies from the book that may be used related to this content:

- **In-Class Applications:** When discussing topics, ask students to start thinking immediately about content priorities, important application to patient cases, and potential test questions. Critical information about content that should be represented on the examination may be difficult to delineate for novice students.

Guiding this discussion as part of class time prepares students for the class examination and for future testing situations.

- **Student-Led Seminars/NCLEX® Questions:** Seminars about professionalism, patients, or components of care are often part of class expectations. These seminars may be enhanced by having students compose and deliver NCLEX®-style questions to the entire class that relate to the content in the seminar. These questions may be from books or test banks, or they may be developed by the students. Both the students presenting the seminar and the class participants benefit from the practice offered in completing these questions.
- **Write to Learn:** Write about why priority setting is important. Analyze study habits that worked in the past and what areas to improve.
- **Common and Different:** Have students ask each other about personal study habits and concerns about NCLEX®.
- **Group Tests:** This is an especially valuable strategy. Make up a short test (six to 10 items). Have the students work in groups of four to six. Group tests are unique because students identify correct responses to questions, and they also discuss why the incorrect answers are wrong. This discourages guessing and reinforces critical thinking, and students report that it is really fun! These **Group Tests**, with their instant feedback and group interactions, also enhance learning, increase student preparation for class, and are positively evaluated by students.[4] I believe these **Group Tests** are critical during the senior year when taking the NCLEX® examination is imminent for many students and continued development of test-taking and clinical decision-making skills is critical.

STRATEGIES FOR THE NCLEX® RN AND PN EXAMINATIONS

The NCLEX® is designed to assess students' levels of knowledge, thinking, and decision making and provides a measure to differentiate candidates who can practice safety as entry-level nurses. Because nursing is multidimensional, the examinations have evolved from their focus on knowledge to one of application and clinical problem solving. The examinations are divided into eight major areas that represent client needs (see Box 10–1). The blueprint percentages are revised every 3 years based on a practice analysis of staff nurses who are surveyed about their daily work and other parameters. The results of this study are translated into

> **Box 10–1.**
> **NCLEX® RN and PN Domains of Nursing Practice/Client Needs**
>
> Safe and Effective Care Environment
>   Management of Care (RN) or Coordinate Care (PN)
>   Safety and Infection Control
> Health Promotion and Maintenance
> Psychosocial Integrity
> Physiological Integrity
>   Reduction of Risk Potential
>   Pharmacology and Parenterals
>   Basic Care and Comfort
>   Physiological Adaptation

areas of emphasis on the examinations. Each student's examination is computer-adapted to meet the percentages of the current blueprint, and questions are selected based on the student's performance and the indicated level of difficulty. For this section, teaching strategies are recommended for each of the eight major client needs represented on NCLEX®.

Management of Care (RN)/Coordinator of Care (PN)

This section discusses priority setting, delegation, leadership, change, dealing with disasters, organizational issues, and case management. Strategies applicable to this section challenge students to use high-level decision-making skills applicable to nursing practice.

IDEAS

Case Management Case Studies

General Description. Nurses are often called on to anticipate discharge needs, provide discharge education, and establish a plan of care. Although novice nurses are usually not candidates for case management roles, this content area is also part of the NCLEX® Blueprint.

Case Management Case Studies allow students to pinpoint client needs and discuss education, referral, and community resources associated with their care.
Example of the Strategy at Work. I use this in professionalism courses as students anticipate taking the NCLEX® examination. Students work in groups with the following exercises: You are planning the discharge of the following

clients—what is the greatest need in each of these scenarios? If you have more time, students may develop more comprehensive lists of client needs.

Case 1

You are planning the discharge of a 76-year-old woman with osteo-myelitis. The client has type 1 diabetes mellitus. Her hemoglobin A1C is 10.5. She is visually impaired and receives four injections/day.

Case 2

An 83-year-old man has mild dementia, COPD, and a history of smoking 30 pack/years. He is on oxygen continuously and spot-check pulse oximetry. Patient is to receive nebulizer treatments every 4 hours.

Case 3

A 6-month-old child is on an apnea monitor with two near-miss SIDS events. Patient has frequent episodes of apnea and a history of gastroesophageal reflux. Parents need to learn CPR and speak no English. The client is to be discharged on reflux precautions.

Case 4

A 54-year-old woman has chronic pancreatitis and bipolar disorder. Patient has a history of chronic alcoholism. Patient experiences exacerbations with high-fat food or alcohol intake and does not regularly take prescribed medications.

Case 5

Patient is a 38-year-old man with chronic hypertension and substance abuse. Client experiences posttraumatic stress disorder subsequent to war experiences and is periodically homeless. Patient does not have a place to live at this time. This hospitalization is related to facial drooping secondary to a cerebrovascular accident. Patient does not remember when he last took his blood pressure medications prior to admission.

Case 6

Client has delivered a healthy 7-lb 10-oz. baby girl at 39 weeks gestation following a 23-hour labor with pitocin induction. Patient received a fourth-degree episiotomy. During teaching, the mother states she "isn't sure she wants this baby . . ." She is weepy and attempting to breastfeed. She has no visitors postpartum.

Case 7

Client is 14 years old with a diagnosis of depression and is expressing suicidal ideations. The client denies a plan to hurt herself but feels "life is not worth living." This admission was for gastric lavage after the ingestion of 10 valium tablets. The client's mother is a single parent and works two jobs.

Incident Report Exercise

General Description. Completing incident or variance reports is part of nursing practice and is cited as a potential topic being tested on the NCLEX®. Following a discussion of the types of scenarios that might lead to the need for an incident report, the legal precautions related to these documents, and the role of the nurse, students may complete this exercise to be better acquainted with the information included on these reports and the nurse's role in the completion of incident/variance reports.

Example of the Strategy at Work. I use this case study to describe a medication error. After discussion about incident/variance reports, I have groups of students read and appraise the following case. Students are asked to identify the components of the case that should be included in the variance report. Because most reports are online or part of the agency's intranet, the ability to select key information is important for practicing nurses (a similar exercise is described as a medication incident report worksheet).

Incident Report Exercise

You are a new nurse providing care to a client. Your client is ordered to receive D₅/.45 NSS via a peripheral IV at 75 mL/hour. At 0645, a physician prescribes to include 20 mEq of KCl in each 1,000-mL bag of the IV fluids. This order is not transcribed by the night shift nurse. At 1600 in your chart review, you notice the order and realize that the patient has not received the KCl. The physician is called, a serum K level is drawn, and the client's level is 3.0 mEq/dL. The client is ordered a K rider and a new IV solution is hung. Four hours later, the serum K level is 3.9 mEq/dL. The client is asymptomatic and suffered no long-term effects. The family is not notified and the documentation in the medical record is limited to the client's toleration of the K rider and lab results.

Delegation Exercise

General Description. One of the most difficult tasks for new nurses is to delegate tasks to unlicensed assistance personnel, licensed practical nurses, and other registered nurses. Developing a case study that demands that students consider a variety of components, including levels of education, experience, and scope of practice, allows students to practice these skills. *Example of the Strategy at Work.* The complete exercise that I have used for this strategy is found as the **Group Thought** Delegation Case Study. Because that method takes a lot of time in class, it may be used as an **Admit Ticket, Take-Home Quiz**, or **Write to Learn**. The following brief case study may be used instead to reinforce concepts of delegation.

Concepts of Delegation

The charge nurse of a district is establishing the patient assignments for the shift. There are 10 patients in the district. There are two registered nurses (RNs) (one is the charge nurse), one licensed practical nurse (LPN), and one unlicensed assistive personnel (UAP). The charge nurse makes decisions on the following patient variables:

- Three patients are postop: one had an exploratory laparotomy to determine the cause of a bowel obstruction, one had a carotid endarterectomy, and one had an implanted vascular access placed to begin total parenteral nutrition related to Crohn's disease.
- Two patients are admitted for initial chemotherapy protocols.
- One patient was admitted for a fever of unknown origin and had a bone marrow transplant.
- One patient is in the postanesthesia care unit following hip pinning from a fracture.

- Two patients are in isolation for *Clostridium difficile* infections and are on oral vancomycin and metronidazole (IVPB).
- One bed is empty and no admissions are posted.
- All of the personnel are experienced and have worked on the unit for 3 years or more. The UAP is a senior nursing student.

How would you assign the patients to each nurse? What other information would you like to know? Who should receive the first admission?

Nurse Practice Act Write to Learn

General Description. Students often do not know about, nor have they read, the Nurse Practice Act for their state of residence or education. It is important for nursing students to review the act and to understand the role of the nurse as governed by law. The **Write to Learn** strategy is designed to encourage students to reflect on an issue or problem. In this exercise, students consider the act related to components such as the role of the nurse, mandates for delegation, scope of practice, and the role of the act in protecting the public from inappropriate care.

Example of the Strategy at Work. I use this exercise specifically related to delegation. Each state has different language for LPN/LVN and RN roles and delegation. Most laws stipulate that RNs should not delegate their duties in assessment, teaching, and evaluation to someone else. For this assignment, I have students consider these three components as they view the Nursing Practice Act and then reflect on this information in the **Nurse Practice Act Write to Learn.** I also ask students to contemplate their findings and how this knowledge, or lack thereof, may have an impact on their nursing practice.

"Call Bell" Examination Questions

General Description. As we become more sophisticated in testing students to replicate real-life clinical decision making, questions on NCLEX®, standardized testing packages, and our examinations become more valid measures of reasoning and thinking. One important component of this is testing students about how to establish priorities between and among patients. These questions are noted with increasing frequency and offer a challenge to students. I call them "**Call Bell" Examination Questions** because they ask students to imagine that they are standing at the nurses' station and four call bells ring. Based on the information at hand, the students are asked which patient they would attend to first. This resembles the priority setting necessary for nursing practice.

Example of the Strategy at Work. Here's one of the questions I use:

You are standing at the nurses' station and the following four clients' call bells alarm. Which postoperative client would you visit first?

1. A 6-year-old child following an appendectomy
2. **A 6-month-old child who had a cleft palate repair**
3. A 9-year-old child who had a central venous access device inserted in the OR
4. A 16-year-old patient following pinning of a fracture

I think these types of questions are especially important as students near graduation and the NCLEX® examination. These can be used as **Quickie Quizzes**, **In-Class Test Questions**, or **Admit Tickets**.

Other strategies from the book that may be used related to this content:

- **Student Seminars:** A seminar on case management or continuity of care/discharge planning.
- **Setting Priorities Icebreaker:** Use this exercise to open a discussion about decision making related to priorities and how this relates to nursing practice and test taking. Discuss the importance of priority setting for a single patient and among several patients.
- **In-Basket Exercise:** This method allows students to process limited information when all they can work with is what is in their inbox. See the **In-Basket Exercise** for the use of this exercise to set priorities while STUCK on an elevator.
- **What's the Big Deal?:** While lecturing about material, stop and ask, **What's the Big Deal?** Another question might be: "Why is this important?" Students often have difficulty differentiating key information because they lack clinical experience interpreting priorities. This phrase cues students into the importance of information and helps them learn how to identify critical details about content.
- Some of the most difficult questions on NLCEX® relate to priority setting—**In-Class Test Questions** provide the opportunities to practice questions, for example:

A nurse received a report on the assigned patients. Based on the information in each option, which patient should the nurse visit first?

1. A 76-year-old man with DVTs being converted from IV heparin to po warfarin
2. A 45-year-old client with type 1 diabetes mellitus with an FBS of 130 and is hungry

3. **A 60-year-old client who had a tracheostomy placed yesterday and is on a humidivent**

4. A 75-year-old client who had a TURP 2 days ago and has a three-lumen catheter

- **Pass the Problem:** This strategy helps students work together to identify patient outcomes and nursing interventions for each other's assigned clients. This strategy may be adapted for management situations in which students select a conflict, issue, or problem and pass their papers around a small group of classmates. Each student contributes a solution to the issue and passes the paper. After all classmates have completed their additions, one student is provided with several different perspectives on the issue and several options for addressing it.

- **Invented Dialogues:** Students are often perplexed about their personal potential responses to conflicts, issues, or problems in the clinical area. The nurse's potential role of leader or manager demands that professional nurses consider their own communication styles and how to address issues. **Invented Dialogues** provide students with the practice to have "ready answers" to potential statements by others that generate conflict or discussion, or bring forth problems that need to be addressed.

- **Shapes Define Your Personality:** This strategy is effective as an icebreaker and also provides a context within which to build a discussion on team building, personal styles, and the unique talents of individuals. Individuals pick a shape that defines their role as a nurse or their role in this group. These shapes are defined by their strengths and what each set of characteristics contributes to the group or as a team member. Participants then appreciate how each individual brings different qualities and how these various qualities build a team and enhance team productivity and function.

- **Use the Star:** This strategy involves placing a star on important material to assist students to learn priority setting.

Safety and Infection Control

Safety parameters guide all nursing actions and are inherent to clinical practice. The emphasis of NCLEX®, along with accrediting bodies and the QSEN initiative (see later in this chapter) on safety, warrant nursing education strategies that affirm the importance of safety and the basic nature of many safety principles. This section addresses strategies that are valuable for use in teaching infection control, whereas concepts related to safety education will be noted in the section on QSEN.

IDEAS

What Not to Do or Find the Error

General Description. This strategy allows students to evaluate how others carry out procedures to detect breaks in sterile technique, improper procedures, or skills that do not follow concepts of asepsis. Students are asked to watch others practice the skills, view videos, or critique each other for adherence to principles that avoid infection transmission. Instructors may demonstrate skill completion and consciously commit errors, especially in sterile technique, or students may be asked to video each other doing skills incorrectly. Other students may view these and are charged with identifying errors. In **Find the Error,** students need to have a strong knowledge base to be able to complete these tasks. This method should be reserved for more advanced students who have incorporated the skills in their personal repertoire. The risk of doing this strategy with novice students is that they may learn bad habits or the incorrect way to do procedures. Another application of **Find the Error** is to provide a room, picture, or simulated setting/scenario with unsafe practices, errors, and policy infractions. Students are charged with identifying these errors to reinforce safe practices. Examples include a urinary catheter bag on a bed, oxygen tubing wrapped around the neck, siderails down, restraints tied incorrectly, inappropriate techniques, or safety hazards.

Example of the Strategy at Work. I have used this method many times in the clinical area to ensure clinical skill acquisition prior to implementation with a patient. Central line dressing changes, insertion of a nasogastric tube, adherence to isolation precautions, and medication administration and injections are all appropriate skills to carry out. Ask students to identify errors or breaks in sterile technique. This strategy also reinforces the correct order of steps as tested on NCLEX®, foundational elements inherent to all skills, and the importance of checking agency policy prior to completing a procedure. Another example is the use of simulated videos that depict clients with infections and show each healthcare team member's role in infection control. The Centers for Disease Control and Prevention provides a great video showing the transmission of an infection to a vulnerable client and each individual's role in spreading that infection. Here are my instructions for the students.

Go to Healthcare Associated Infections > Partnering to Heal, and see the interactive online simulation at www.hhs.gov/ash/initiatives/hai/training/. Click the Full version. Watch the case introduction. When that is complete, click the picture of Dena, the nurse. Watch through the entire scenario. The quiz during class will relate directly to this exercise. This section takes 50 minutes to complete, so please plan accordingly.

If you go to the website, you will find a great video simulation with several parts showing the nurse, family member, doctor, and infection control practitioner roles in the death of a client as a result of a nosocomial infection. I require students to watch this simulation and focus on the role of the nurse. The students have a **Quiz That Counts** in class and several **Think-Pair-Share** activities to debrief the exercise. The exercise reinforces the role of the nurse in limiting infection transmission and the education of patients, families, and other healthcare professionals.

Other strategies from the book that may be used related to this content:

- **Current Events:** There are always stories in the news about infectious diseases, new cases of antibiotic resistance, epidemics, and immunizations. Use those stories to augment your class content and ground infectious disease issues in reality. Nursing students are often insulated from current events. We have a responsibility to help students stay aware of current issues related to their practice and profession. This may be especially critical with **Current Events** involving infections and infection control.
- **Safety Scavenger Hunt:** Much as with any other hunt, students are asked to find infection hazards or violations.
- **Group Tests: Group Tests** are effective ways to foster test-taking skills and remind students of critical material. Students often forget basic principles of asepsis and isolation precautions. This is a great place to include a review of those precautions needed for individual disease entities, the importance of patient and family education, and the rationale behind such recommendations.
- **In-Class Test Questions:** Students appreciate the opportunity to practice using test questions related to challenging content. Putting test questions on the screen in PowerPoint allows students to select an answer, and educators may use the animation function to add an arrow or other shape to denote the correct answer. This allows for student practice, breaks up lecture content, and

offers the opportunity for instructors to assess the students and their level of knowledge.

- **Self-Learning Modules:** Combining case studies, questions, and psychomotor skills, such as isolation precautions or procedures, may prove a valuable way to reinforce infection control principles.

- **Let's Be Real in Clinical:** This strategy provides a chance for students and educators to explore how concepts learned in class are operationalized in the clinical area. Whether as a preconference or postconference or as a discussion on the unit in a private setting, have students consider the isolation precautions used on the unit. Do not allow the session to turn into a critique of isolation practices on the unit; it should be a constructive appraisal of adherence to isolation dictates. Questions may include the following:
  - How well do the healthcare professionals adhere to the precautions?
  - How well do family and visitors comply?
  - What improvements may be made in carrying out the recommendations?
  - Why are the selected isolation precautions indicated?
  - What impact may the precautions have on the emotional and social aspects of the client and client care?

Health Promotion and Maintenance

Although health promotion and maintenance do not make up a large percentage of NCLEX® content, we often need to emphasize to students the importance of preventive health measures, keeping healthy behaviors and lifestyles, and everyday aspects of attaining and maintaining health across the life span. Students may not find these topics very intriguing to study, and some nursing programs do not focus on wellness and health promotion activities. Teaching strategies that reinforce these principles are critical for personal health, the role of the nurse as teacher, and NCLEX® success.

IDEAS

Basics of Maternity Case Study

General Description. Learning about labor and delivery is often difficult for students. The lack of clinical exposure to a delivery, the unique vocabulary associated with this specialty, and lack of personal interest or experience with this phase of life contribute to the increasing complexity of this content. Providing a **Basics of Maternity Case Study** as a reminder of learned concepts may assist. Such cases may be adapted to meet the objectives of the course and the learning needs of the students.

Example of the Strategy at Work. Here is the case study I wrote for a senior seminar course. The case is found on a single PowerPoint slide, and the questions are on the second slide. I have the students work in groups to answer the questions, and then I show them a third slide with the answers. I follow with a discussion of the vocabulary unique to this and other nursing specialties, the need to remind themselves of such content, and the importance of health promotion in nursing practice.

Basics of Maternity Case Study

A woman enters an ED. She is pregnant but does not know her due date. Her LMP was [adapt this date to be appropriate for your class date]. This is her second pregnancy; she had one therapeutic abortion. Her fundal height is 36 cm. She is found to be Rh-negative, 100% effaced, and 4 cm dilated. The fetus is found to be in an attitude of flexion, longitudinal lie, cephalic presentation, ROA position, and at +2 station.

- Using Nagele's rule, calculate her EDC.
- What is her GTPAL/GP?
- What is the interpretation of her fundal height?
- What are the implications of her Rh-negative status?
- What interpretation can you make of the fetus's location and other assessments?

End-of-Life Case Studies—Documents to Help

General Description. One topic we frequently discuss as part of the students' clinical experiences is the implementation of do not resuscitate orders, end-of-life decision making, and the potential for legal and ethical issues. Using case studies related to the social and emotional components is very common. **End-of-Life Case Studies** provide the forum to address such issues and explore documents that assist us in decision making and supporting clients and families. Because agencies differ in their policies and terminology surrounding resuscitation parameters, it is critical to discuss local practices; nurses need to be aware of agency protocol.

Example of the Strategy at Work. Here are the brief cases that I provide to students. Rather than focusing on solutions, students are asked to consider the procedures; legal tenets; or policies available to support them, clients, and families at this difficult time. Living wills, durable powers of attorney, the Patient Self-Determination Act, agency policies, the state Nurse Practice Act, the nursing Code of Ethics, and other state and federal laws provide dictates for nursing actions. Although only a few pieces of end-of-life care, these cases provide the mechanisms to clarify difficult issues prior to having personal experiences in the clinical arena.

- An 88-year-old woman sustains a head injury after a fall and does not regain consciousness. She is dependent on the ventilator and enteral tube feedings. What documents inform her care?
- A client is end-stage with ALS and asks for the nurse to assist in garnering medications to end his life. What documents inform the nurse's actions?

These may be done as **Email Exercise**, **Think-Pair-Share**, **Group Thought**, or **Write to Learn**.

Other strategies from the book that may be used related to this content:

- **Preclass Case Studies:** These case studies are useful when content exceeds the time available in class to address fundamental knowledge or topics addressed in previous courses or classes. One potential use for **Preclass Case Studies** in health promotion and maintenance is related to developmental differences, expectations, and nursing implications across the life span. Nurses are often called on to provide advice, teaching, and anticipatory guidance about developmental milestones and how health has an impact on development. Teaching young parents about infant care, assisting caregivers in understanding the unique aspects of adolescence, or helping a family deal with an aging grandparent may all be adapted to **Preclass Case Studies.** As indicated in the previous discussion of this strategy, it takes a little work to develop a case and appropriate questions. The beauty of the method is the ability to cover material quickly and then moving on to difficult-to-grasp concepts. Have students read a case study and answer focused questions, and use these as an **Admit Ticket** or other assignment. You may also elect not to grade the assignment but include this information on an examination. These cases may be used again and again.
- **Field Trips:** This strategy may be difficult to implement, but I have used field trips to supplement class material, replace a clinical experience when inclement weather changes our plans, or when I feel that students would benefit from a change of

venue. From a health promotion and maintenance standpoint, **Field Trips** may be conducted in schools, toy stores, child-care centers, primary-care settings, adult day-care settings, or any environment that assists students in meeting course objectives. Students need to have a clear understanding of the potential contribution and objectives of the **Field Trip** (so they don't consider it a day off), establish personal objectives for the experience, and be held accountable for their **Field Trip. Write to Learn** or other assignments may serve to focus the students on set objectives.

- **Imagine:** This method guides students through a story or scenario, allowing students to "live" an experience outside their personal realm. Developing stories from the perspectives of different clients builds empathy and allows students to appreciate challenges confronted by patients, families, and communities. This is important in health promotion and maintenance as nurses work with clients of different ages and circumstances. **Imagine** may detail the experience of hospitalization from the eyes of a child, share the perspectives of a woman in menopause at risk for heart disease, tell the story of a mother who is separated from her child due to illness, the frustrations experienced by a client with Parkinson's disease, or the sorrow felt when an older adult loses a spouse. **Imagine** allows students to step out of their reality and develop an understanding of the experiences felt by our patients. **Short Clips** may be used with this strategy to enhance the personal connection for students. Clips from movies about aging, the birth process, childhood issues, or illness may enhance the emotional connection with material and allow students to develop the empathy so critical to nursing practice.

- **In-Class Test Questions:** Because students often diminish the importance of test questions associated with health and wellness, often considering such issues common sense, it is important to demonstrate in class the potential questions in this arena. Questions related to growth and development, immunizations and health surveillance, health assessment, and nutrition are important to challenge students. Class participants may be encouraged to intervene with the least invasive measure possible, to encourage as much self-care as is feasible, and focus on respect for patients in both the NCLEX® and professional nursing practice. A variation of this strategy is to ask students questions in class. You may choose a student at random; some instructors throw a beach ball into the crowd and seek an answer from the catcher of the ball. Another strategy is to pass out sticky notes and ask the holders of the notes of a certain color to answer an in-class question. You can ask the students to answer a question that is "two seats to the left of the pink sticky note" to keep the students on their toes.

- **Be Prepared:** This strategy encourages students to prepare for classes. In teaching about health promotion, students need to consider developmental characteristics, safety principles, and tasks associated with assorted periods throughout the life span. Providing preclass assignments that demand students prepare and look up age-related facts prepares them for discussion about nursing implications and priorities.

Psychosocial Integrity

Students often find psychosocial nursing intimidating. Some contend that this type of nursing causes us to be introspective about our own thoughts and feelings. Others believe it is feared because of the stigma associated with psychological issues and problems. On the other hand, we all deal and cope with life's challenges, and every patient we connect with may benefit from self-awareness and caring. Because of this, concepts such as therapeutic communication, defense mechanisms, coping, stress, and grief should be addressed at multiple times throughout the educational process. Using strategies throughout the curriculum, in addition to clinical and other experiences, ensures appreciation of the importance of psychosocial concepts in nursing care.

IDEAS

Psychosocial Case Studies

General Description. Case studies, as in other areas, really prove their value in the psychosocial nursing realm. Case studies may humanize a situation, include family and contextual details, note appropriate medications, mention a vocabulary unique to this specialty, and illustrate the role of the nurse. Perhaps most important, they allow students to reflect on their thoughts, emotions, and coping, and on how their feelings have an impact on their interactions with clients.

Example of the Strategy at Work. I used this strategy to elaborate on the issues associated with psychosocial disorders.

Psychosocial Disorders

A 33-year-old woman was diagnosed with schizophrenia at age 22. She takes two medications that decrease her psychotic symptoms, which include hallucinations, paranoia, and delusions. When she stops taking her medications, she does not attend therapy, care for herself, or interact with others. She lives with her parents who are 86 and 87 years old. She enters the partial hospitalization center looking very disheveled and disoriented. She is admitted to an inpatient unit.

1. What are her needs at this time?
2. What needs do you anticipate upon discharge to home?

Students do this exercise as a **Think-Pair-Share** or a **Group Thought** exercise. Another alternative is to ask students to write their own case scenarios, create scripts for a simulation, or create a video. Any strategies that ensure that decision making is rendered safely and sensitively will continue to foster caring nursing practice.

Other strategies from the book that may be used related to this content:

- **Same Information:** This strategy includes the development of two stories or scenarios. One story includes basic details, and the other includes additional information that adds depth and substance to the story. For example, the less comprehensive story may describe a person's erratic behavior, history of substance use, poor hygiene, aggressive ideations, a high blood alcohol content, violent behaviors, and abusive language. The second story may depict the same client but with information about the client's history of schizophrenia, a traumatic childhood, nonadherence to medication, and lack of social or familial support. Armed with these additional details, nurses may better understand the motivations behind a patient's actions and the need to conduct comprehensive histories and assessments in order to make optimal decisions.

- **Continuing or Unfolding Case Studies:** These case studies allow for discourse. After the initial case is presented, more information is added to indicate the effect of interventions and developments in the client's condition. These cases provide a more realistic view of nursing care and clients' outcomes, stimulate critical thinking, and may be expanded for as many iterations as needed to achieve class objectives. I used an unfolding case, which follows.

Unfolding Case

A 14-year-old boy enters the school-based health center asking to meet with someone to discuss "something bothering him." The nurse conducts an intake interview and finds that he is having thoughts of hurting himself, is the subject of ridicule by his classmates, and is questioning his sexual orientation.

1. What is the first priority for this client?
2. What resources are needed immediately?

The nurse asks the student to stay at the wellness center and notifies the office of his need for assistance and to be excused from class. The nurse proceeds to schedule the client to meet with the counselor immediately and completes a medication history for the client. He states that he takes 20 mg/day of fluoxetine and 1 mg of diazepam prn, and he is seeing a psychiatrist weekly. His parents are supportive and he gives permission for the nurse to contact them.

1. What information should the nurse share with the parents?
2. What questions do you have about the client and his medications?
3. What referrals might be made?

- **Why Are You Here?** Some students love psychosocial nursing, anxious to embark on a career in this field. Others proclaim that this is not their favorite area of practice and hope they never have to work in this capacity. What is important to remember is that we all work in psychosocial environments; we work with people and provide care in the context of relationships. Many of our clients, though perhaps seeking care for physical complaints, have significant psychosocial issues. **Why Are You Here?** allows instructors to ask this question and explore students' thoughts about the role of psychosocial content in nursing curricula, the importance of psychosocial concepts in nursing practice, and their personal comfort and skills in providing therapeutic care.
- **When You Think of This, Think of That:** This matching exercise charges students to pair left and right columns of information. For this section, an important set of concepts is the ability to define and recognize common defense mechanisms. Create a PowerPoint slide with the defense mechanisms listed on the left and the definitions on the right. Students can print this as a handout or use arrow

functions to match concepts. Also, **In-Class Applications** may assist in reinforcing principles related to the psychosocial realm.

- **Short Clips:** Several popular movies are valuable in making real the concepts, behaviors, and stress associated with psychosocial illness and mental health issues. As noted previously, film clips are popular with students because they emphasize the reality of symptoms and issues, demonstrate methods of management, and clarify the emotions evoked in "real" client situations. Thinking questions, or objectives, are critical so that students see the learning value of the film clips instead of potentially seeing film clip sessions as time off from learning.
- **Day in the Life of a Patient with . . .** may also assist students to learn empathy, the challenges confronted with mental health issues, and the daily stressors that add to the complexity of psychosocial illness.

Reduction of Risk Potential

Nursing's role in monitoring for and preventing complications is well understood by seasoned nurses but sometimes eludes the novice ones. The active roles of nurses in early detection, education, health promotion, and assessing risk are addressed in this section of NCLEX®. Educational strategies that allow students to relate the cause and effect of interventions to prevention, and assessments to early detection are important to nursing practice.

IDEAS

Perioperative Care Case Study

General Description. Nursing study of the perioperative period provides a great opportunity to explore risk and the role of the nurse. Significant complications are associated with the perioperative period, and nurses, in their assessments and teaching, have a role in monitoring for and preventing such complications. Using a case study allows pairs, trios, or groups to explore the perioperative period, either preparing them for or debriefing their visit to the operating room. A case study promotes discussion about the importance of this type of nursing care. These may be adapted as **Unfolding Cases** or as a **Feedback Lecture**.

Example of the Strategy at Work. Here is the case study I use to drive home the role of the nurse in the Reduction of Risk Potential. Used with **Think-Pair-Share**, **Teaching Trios**, or a **Group Thought** exercise, this strategy was well received by students as they integrated their experiences with clients in the preoperative and postoperative periods on surgical clinical units, in the operating room, and in the postanesthesia care unit.

Perioperative Case Study

You are caring for a 43-year-old client who is having a cholecystectomy. The client's BMI is 31. The client has smoked for 20 pack/years. The client has been vomiting and has had no po intake for 4 days. The client has a history of hypertension, which was treated with atenolol hydrochlorothiazide. In the preop area, the client's BP is 146/96. Other VS include: 120-30-37.8.

1. Discuss the risk factors associated with this surgery.
2. List six topics that would be included in preoperative teaching with this client.
3. Identify 10 things to be checked or confirmed before the patient leaves the preop area and is taken to surgery.
4. Explain the roles of the circulating and scrub nurses.
5. The client is to have an incisional cholecystectomy rather than laparoscopic surgery. What are the implications of this?
6. The client is transferred from the operating room to the postanesthesia care unit. What assessments are key in the immediate postop period?
7. What five complications could you anticipate in the postop period?
8. What discharge instructions would you be sure to emphasize with this client?

Other strategies from the book that may be used related to this content:

- **What's the Big Deal?** Early in their learning, nursing students often memorize laboratory test normal results and note when values are outside the norms. As they progress in their studies, they become more acquainted with the need to focus on critical values. This strategy uses lists of lab values to help familiarize students with normal lab values, abnormal but not critical lab values, and critical values warranting further assessment and intervention.
- **All Things Being Equal:** Students often focus on the norms for lab values and need encouragement to consider critical values for

lab studies. This exercise helps students to make these discrimina-
tions. Students view the three lab values and identify the one that
"worries them the most." This is a critical lab value.
1. Serum pH 7.34
2. Serum K 5.0 mEq/L
3. **Ca 6.5 mg/dL**

- **Write to Learn:** This is a valuable way to have students consider
  all the risks associated with the perioperative period. Combine
  this with an **Unfolding Case Study** and ask students to correlate
  risks and nursing interventions associated with the preoperative,
  perioperative, and postoperative periods.
- **Progressive Quiz:** The sequential nature of the perioperative period makes the **Progressive Quiz** a perfect way to maintain student interest, assess learning, and establish priorities for patients
  during this period.

Pharmacology and Parenterals

This domain of nursing practice probably causes the most angst among
nursing students. The number of medications, the breadth of information
related to medication classes and each medication, dosage calculation,
principles of administration, and nursing implications can be daunting
for novice and seasoned nurses. This strategy emphasizes the imperative
that nurse educators develop creative strategies that enhance learning in
this area.

IDEAS

Pharmacology Field Trip

General Description. As described in the section on **Field Trips**, sending
students to explore the world may add to their learning experiences.
Asking students to investigate their medication cabinet or a pharmacy
adds to their knowledge about medications and their use in today's
healthcare environment.

Example of the Strategy at Work. Below are the descriptions of these
assignments as I used them in a pharmacology course. They can be used
throughout the curriculum if they may meet course objectives. You
may use these as **Admit Tickets**, **Email Exercises**, or **Ah-Ha Journals**.
They may also serve as **Discussion Starters** to generate discourse about
the instructions provided to clients about medications, the keeping of

old medications in a medication cabinet, issues of polypharmacy, the prevalence of antibiotic resistance, and the potential negative effects of inappropriate use of medications.

Pharmacy Field Trip

For this assignment you need to visit any pharmacy. Select an over-the-counter medication. Spend a minute carefully reading the label on the brand-name medication. Find the generic or store-brand medication and read that label carefully.

- Compare and contrast the ingredients, instructions, packaging, and price for both medications.
- What important patient education issues are found on the medication labels concerning the medication? What is the reading level for both sets of instructions?
- Which medication would you purchase? Why?

Medicine Cabinet Assessment

Find a medicine cabinet that has at least four over-the-counter or prescription medications in it. Answer the following concerning those medications:

- List at least four of the medications in the cabinet.
- Are any of these medications in the cabinet expired? What nursing implications are associated with the medication and its expiration?
- Are prescription medications in the originally labeled bottles?
- What specific precautions are noted for any of the medications?
- Imagine that a client was taking all four of these medications. What potential interactions should be part of client instruction?

Pharmacology Critical Thinking Exercises

General Description. As with many areas of nursing practice, eliciting critical thinking in nursing students about pharmacology and medication administration is a valuable element of nursing education. Whether in nursing pharmacology, general specialty classes, or before graduation, **Pharmacology Critical Thinking Exercises** remind students of the thinking involved with medications, their administration, and nursing implications and patient education.

Example of the Strategy at Work. Here are several exercises I use to instill critical thinking and foster decision-making skills. You may develop these "thinking questions" and intersperse them in lectures and other teaching strategies to encourage active involvement with material and encourage students to think carefully about their actions and consequences.

Pharmacology Critical Thinking Exercises

- You are giving a client an injection. You check his name band, and he tells you a different name than is shown on the band. What do you do?
- You are giving an injection to a client. When you insert the needle, it bounces. What do you do?
- You are giving an intravenous medication to a client. Ten minutes after the drug has infused, the client becomes short of breath. What do you do?

Other strategies from the book that may be used related to this content:

- **Unfolding Case Studies:** These cases may be developed to include care of a client receiving a blood transfusion, care of the client on total parenteral nutrition, titration of a medication, or any course of medication therapy that has extensive nursing care. The unfolding nature of these cases allows students to see the effects of nursing interventions and evaluate next steps in care.
- **Quizzes That Count/Quickie Quiz:** Ongoing quizzes on medication administration, calculations, drug classes, and specific medications allow students to practice skills with less stress than an examination. Some agencies require students to pass medication quizzes before employment or clinical experiences. Frequent quizzes will reassure students of their skills.
- **Legal Cheat Sheet/Worksheet:** Have students make their own or complete faculty-generated worksheets to reinforce principles of pharmacology. Much like drug cards and others tools, these worksheets encourage **Active Reading** and **Write to Learn** about medications.

Basic Care and Comfort

Sometimes students are surprised by the importance of the fundamentals of basic nursing practice. Seasoned nurses appreciate that it is often the most basic of nursing interventions and principles that make the most difference in patients' lives and their ability to heal. Concepts such as pain, comfort, skin integrity, hygiene, nutrition, hydration, positioning, basic care, fundamental skills, assistive devices, and other measures should be presented within the context of important nursing care.

IDEAS

Pain Continuing Case Study

General Description. Students benefit from seeing the effect of basic nursing measures. Framing a real-life client situation within a case study about pain reinforces the role of the nurse in pain assessment and management. *Example of the Strategy at Work.* This case study allows students to progress with a patient throughout a portion of the pain experience. By following the nursing process, students can see pain as a key factor in nursing practice and identify nursing's critical role in pain management. I use this case study as part of a discussion on the importance of the basics in nursing practice and the emphasis on basic care and comfort on NCLEX®.

Other strategies from the book that may be used related to this content:

- **Imagine:** Visualizing the client is especially valuable when positioning clients; using assistive devices, including crutches, walkers, and wheelchairs; assessing client comfort; and assessing a client's basic need.
- **Group Test:** Because students are often surprised by content related to basic skills and principles on NCLEX®, providing a **Group Test** is a way for students to practice with potential test items, to remind them of basic principles, and to start group discussion of ideas and experiences.
- **Think-Pair-Share/Equipment Conference:** Students may want to review psychomotor skills and procedures (insertion of a nasogastric tube, injections, tracheostomy care/suctioning, use of equipment, and others). For students who have established a baseline level of skills, working together in pairs to reinforce best practices and proper procedures may be an important means to ensure a high level of care. **Active Reading Conference** may also support agency adherence and best practices. **Ah-Ha Journal** and **Let's Discuss** may further promote learning of the principles behind psychomotor skills.

Physiological Integrity

The final major domain of nursing practice represented by items on NCLEX® is the physiological status of patients, pathophysiology, and the effect of nursing measures on the human body. These questions may relate to acute and chronic conditions, the signs and symptoms associated with pathophysiological changes, and lab and other studies that are manifested by changes in body functioning.

IDEAS

Two Truths and a Lie

General Description. A common parlor game is providing three facts to students and having them identify two statements that are true or correct and one that is incorrect or false. This type of game allows students to fine-tune their skills. The three facts may be placed on papers around the room, and students or groups of students may be given stickers to indicate true or false statements. Another way to use this strategy is by making a PowerPoint slide and using animated arrows to indicate the true and false statements. This is a great strategy to use with a large group and asking students to **Think-Pair-Share** each set of statements.

Example of the Strategy at Work. I use this strategy as a way to reinforce data, lab values, assessment criteria, signs/symptoms, or any other information that needs to be memorized. It is also very effective when addressing epidemiology and population-related data.

What's the Big Deal and How Is It Treated?

General Description. This strategy builds on a previous teaching tool (**What's the Big Deal?**). This strategy asks students to identify the significance of the physiological changes leading to signs or symptoms and goes the next step by challenging students to delineate the appropriate treatment for the conditions or illnesses.

Example of the Strategy at Work. This strategy works well with diabetes and its management.

What's the Big Deal? How Is It Treated? A Client With . . .

- A blood sugar of 75 mg/dL
- A blood sugar of 440 mg/dL, positive ketones, a pH of 7.3, and lethargic
- Vomiting and diarrhea for 2 days, no oral intake, and questioning his need for insulin
- A blood sugar of 70 mg/dL complaining of a headache and tremors
- Kussmaul respirations, ketotic breath, and is unconscious
- A blood sugar at 0700 of 340 mg/dL and given a.m. insulin. Then a blood sugar at 1000 of 50 mg/dL

- A client with diabetes needing surgery, NPO for 8 hours, and pending insulin dosing
- A patient with a blood sugar of 38 mg/dL
- A pregnant woman whose blood sugar is above 300 mg/dL throughout her pregnancy
- A client with an Hgb A1C of 9%
- A man with a blood sugar of 450 mg/dL with positive ketones in his urine, demonstrating signs of abdominal pain and dehydration
- A patient whose blood sugar is 200 mg/dL at 0900 and 40 mg/dL at 1000, and is demonstrating lethargy and sweating

Other strategies from the book that may be used related to this content:

- **Write to Learn:** Have students do a **Write to Learn** about physiological concepts. One example I use is: *You are caring for a client having major abdominal surgery. Name three postop complications of the procedure for which nurses provide preoperative teaching and postop monitoring.* This exercise asks students not only to identify the complications but also to consider the role of prevention through teaching.
- **In-Basket Exercise:** Using the previously discussed exercise, the students are asked to adapt their nursing care and anticipate the needs of a client with diabetes as follows:
- You are stuck on an elevator with a 16-year-old young woman with type 1 diabetes. You will be stuck on the elevator for 24 hours. Write down 20 items you need to assist to keep this young woman safe and normoglycemic for that time period. The security guard will contact you in 5 minutes.
- You can then have the students further refine their priority-setting skills by ask them to narrow their list to three to five items.

NCLEX® Integrated Processes

Teaching and Learning
- **Teaching Trios:** Teaching trios provide an opportunity for one group member to teach another group member while a third student observes teaching style, barriers and facilitators for understanding, and potential issues as they arise in teaching.
- **Teaching Tools:** This strategy provides students with knowledge about teaching patients and a way to enhance learning in patient education.

- **Invented Dialogues:** This strategy offers students the opportunity to practice teaching skills by having the clients pose a question or statement and the students form a response or invent a dialogue. These statements then become part of their repertoire and are available when needed to confront teaching challenges as they arise. These may be reinforced using **Let's Discuss**.
- **Self-Learning Mini-Modules:** Patient characteristics related to education may be presented in a case study and questions asked about ways to teach clients and plan teaching methods.

Communication and Documentation

- **Documentation Case Study:** This strategy offers students experiences in using a flow sheet or electronic record to document information presented in a case study. Students troubleshoot how to write a note, where to document, the components of the flow sheet, and the nuances of documentation. This may also be a great opportunity to attend to the agency-related policies and customs related to documentation.
- **Speak Up:** This strategy reinforces assertiveness as a patient advocate and reinforces the need for appropriate handoff. This exercise uses status, background, assessment, and recommendation (SBAR) to design a handoff report and serves as a way to ensure that information is communicated appropriately. **Write to Learn** activities may also be used to simulate an SBAR exercise.
- **Mock Trials:** Allowing students to demonstrate and defend communication styles, statements, and components of documentation may assist students in differentiating between positive and negative elements of therapeutic communication. Similarly, **Invented Dialogues** allow students to practice responses to selected statements or questions and encourage students to have "ready answers" when confronting difficult situations.

Nursing Process

- **One-Minute Care Plan:** This brief care plan format allows students to plan their care for a client. It may be expanded to a **One-Minute Class** as students share their plan of care and evaluation of interventions with fellow students, a clinical group, or an orientation class.
- **Pass the Problem:** This strategy allows students to contribute to each other's work by passing a paper around a group. The paper starts with one student's summary of a patient's status, nursing diagnosis or problem list, and background information. It then

fosters teamwork when it is passed around to fellow classmates, who give ideas for client outcomes, strategies, and evaluation criteria.

- **Nuts and Bolts:** This strategy is a short, quick way to reinforce the components of the nursing process and enables students to learn about nursing interventions and the difference a nurse can make in the life of a patient.
- **Put It All Together:** This strategy has students collate data and **Put It All Together** by using the nursing process to develop a comprehensive view of the patient and the plan of care. **Jigsaw** and **Clinical Puzzle** offer similar opportunities to reinforce the steps of the nursing process.
- **Grand Rounds:** This strategy may be used to gain a clearer understanding of patient care and nursing intervention.

Caring

- **Imagine, Remember When,** and **Past Experiences with . . .:** These strategies challenge students to remember, reflect upon, and learn from past or imagined experiences wherein caring was exemplified and then use these memories or thoughts to inform future caring behaviors.
- **Ah-Ha Journals:** Ask students to reflect on experiences in these journals and focus on the concept of caring. Students may comment on caring episodes they have witnessed, the emotions these behaviors evoked, and general reflections for future experience.
- **The Six Hats:** This strategy asks students to take different perspectives, including the logical, optimistic, emotional, pessimistic, creative, and values-based views of a situation. The sharing of points of view and stepping outside usual response patterns may foster caring behaviors. Students may then use **Let's Discuss** to reflect on this experience.

IDEAS TO REINFORCE QSEN PRINCIPLES

QSEN principles reflect an ongoing focus on safety and represent best practices in nursing to maximize patient safety outcomes. The QSEN website (www.qsen.org) provides myriad resources highlighting the history and progress of QSEN, potential teaching methods, learning modules, and means to evaluate safety education in nursing education. Selected strategies from this text that may also assist nursing instructors to include QSEN in their teaching repertoire are presented.

Patient- and Family-Centered Care

- **Imagine, Remember When,** and **Past Experiences with . . .:** These encourage students to see a situation or experience from the past or the patient's or family's point of view.
- **Same Information:** This strategy may encourage students to delve for more information and better understand situations when they don't have all or the same information.
- **Grand Rounds/Bedside Report: Grand Rounds** is a popular clinical education strategy wherein students present their patients to each other. A spin on this is to involve the patient and family in the rounds to ensure a focus on patient priorities, get their input, and allow for assessment of the client at the bedside. A newer twist on this has been adopted by clinical agencies where the shift-to-shift report happens at the bedside and fosters communication and family- and patient-centered care. Incorporate the **Clinical Quick Write** strategy to ensure reflection about the activity.
- **One-Minute Care Plan:** In this exercise, students may be encouraged to add the family concerns and patient priorities into the plan of care.
- **The Right Thing to Do:** In this strategy, students are asked to analyze a situation and develop a list of the correct or appropriate actions. Soliciting students' responses about the **Right Thing to Do** related to patient- and family-centered care grounds nursing care in this foundation of practice. An **Ah-Ha Journal** provides the forum to record the responses and reflections.

Teamwork and Collaboration

- **Titanic 2.0:** This is a team-building strategy in which students are provided six to 10 pictures of people who the class participants may identify as famous or well known. Students or groups of students are asked to build a team so that five of the individuals can be "on the island" or survive the sinking of **Titanic 2.0**. Students build a team based on individual and group characteristics with an eye on survival, skills, and needs. Students then present the rationales for their choices and explore characteristics of effective teams based on the traits of individual team members.
- **Group Thought/Group Work in Clinical/Group Concept Mapping/Think-Pair-Share/Teaching Trios/Group Tests/ Six Hats/Cooperative Strategies:** These strategies provide a

self-explanatory introduction to teamwork. Although nurses often prefer individual work, I would encourage you to foster team skills in nursing students to prepare them for a team-oriented and collaborative workforce.

- **Student Seminars:** Have the students conduct seminars on teamwork, the transdisciplinary team, the team members, and/or the healthcare team.
- **The Six Hats:** As noted previously, this strategy enables students to discuss a situation as a team and take different perspectives based on their "hat." Allowing students to take a variety of perspectives, which may be different from their customary vantage point, enables individuals to empathize, fostering collaboration and teamwork.
- **Debate:** Asking students to take stands on issues may foster cooperation skills and emphasize that cooperation does not always imply agreement or consensus. The realities of the working world and the need for leadership may be reinforced by this exercise.
- **Icebreakers: Icebreakers** are important methods to set the tone for an experience and establish a community of learning based on cooperation and teamwork. **Shapes Define Your Personality** exemplifies a great icebreaker to foster team-building skills.
- **Learn from Each Other/Team Leading Experience:** Leadership, delegation, and supervisory skills are associated with this exercise. Both **Clinical Puzzle** and **Jigsaw** may also augment these strategies as students are required to anticipate the holistic needs of the patient.

Safety

- **Field Trips:** Students are asked to find homes in their community or clinical experiences and assess for safety issues. Criteria to be assessed include the walkways and stairways, floors and rugs, furniture, bathroom, kitchen, refrigeration, bedrooms, electrical system, fire protection (smoke alarms, sprinklers, fire escapes, exits, extinguishers, heating sources), toxic substances/potential for ingestion, communication devices, pets/animals, medications, and age-related hazards. These may be combined with a **Write to Learn**, **Ah-Ha Journal**, or **Critical Thinking Exercise**.
- **Find the Error:** Creating a room or scenario depicting safety hazards is a useful teaching tool. **Active Reading Conferences, Equipment Review Conferences, Games,** and **Creative Lab Skills** provide additional strategies to reinforce safety principles.

- **What's the Big Deal?:** Safety should always be paramount for patients. Asking **What's the Big Deal?** while addressing specific patient conditions, ages, or situations may highlight key components of safe nursing care.
- **Current Events:** The news is replete with examples of medication errors, practice infractions, operative events, and poor patient outcomes related to safety issues. Use these news stories to drive home points about the importance of safe nursing care.
- **Case Study:** Case studies are great ways to drive home the point of safety. An example is provided in the next case.

Safety Case Study

You are a home care nurse. Your client is a 12-year-old male who was discharged yesterday from the hospital with a diagnosis of Lyme's disease. You are visiting him in 1 hour. The client has a peripherally inserted (PICC) IV, and you are administering antibiotics every day. The client's family is close-knit, the father works at a nearby factory, and the mother is the primary caregiver. The family has four other children ages 10, 8, 6, and 3.

- What roles would the nurse assume in providing care to this client?
- What would be your priorities for this client and family?
- What issues should the nurse consider related to the ages of the client's siblings?

Quality Improvement (QI)

- **Debate:** Having students compare, contrast, and debate selected agency practices may highlight potential improvements in practice. This may be used as an **Admit Ticket**.
- **Nurse Interviews:** These interviews assist students to explore agency practices and professional nurses' thoughts on quality and quality improvement, and to determine agency priorities and investment in such practices.
- **The Right Thing to Do:** This strategy asks students to identify recommended nursing actions based on evidence and quality improvement initiatives.
- **Write to Learn:** During clinical rotations, have students research an agency quality improvement initiative. Students may also do an **Ah-Ha Journal** or **V-8 Conference** as they build their skills in

identifying potential issues and knowledge about quality improvement (QI) projects.

- **In the Know:** This strategy asks students to assemble the data or evidence associated with specific nursing practices. As nurses become more accomplished at quality and evidence-based practices, these exercises may highlight areas that need review and ways to streamline or inform nursing practice.

- **Guided Discussion Groups:** These discussion forums may provide a great means to explore quality improvement initiatives or to develop potential projects.

Evidence-Based Practices

- **Campus/Agency Research, Mock Studies, Faculty Sharing, Group Research Critique, Poster Sessions, Research Concept Maps, Applications of Findings, Research Moments,** and **Bring on the Evidence:** This book is filled with strategies to reinforce evidence-based practice, nursing research, and practical application to nursing practice. These exercises may be adapted to illustrate levels of evidence and ways of knowing, and to compare and contrast evidence-based practices from research.

- **Clinical Area Questioning:** The questions an instructor poses to students often assess their critical thinking, application of classroom information to the clinical setting, and preparation for the clinical area. Students may also be questioned about their knowledge of evidence-based practices, where to find such information, and the importance of evidence-based practices in today's healthcare environment.

- **What's the Point:** Students often need to explore the ability to apply research findings in the clinical area. Learning the agency processes to analyze evidence, research policies, and revise nursing practices helps teach students about **What's the Point?** of nursing and other research. Connecting students with agency policies or evidence-based practice committees fosters ongoing exploration of best practices.

- **Let's Be Real:** Similar to the previous strategy, students discuss the realistic applications of research studies in nursing practice. More focused on the information than on process, nursing students or novice nurses in groups discuss and hypothesize how collected research sources may be used to inform nursing practices.

Informatics

- **e-Journaling:** By using **Ah-Ha Journal** formats, blogs, or other journal methods, students' awareness of electronic communications is increased.

- **e-Portfolios:** Use the **Condensed Portfolio** to create a format for an electronic platform for students' or new professionals' portfolios related to schoolwork, professional experiences, or creative work in nursing.

- **Computer Scavenger Hunt:** Just like the **Scavenger Hunt** strategy, this allows students to explore the electronic health record. Instructors should ensure that students either do not have entry access or use a training simulation "hospital" to ensure that there are no inappropriate entries. Students may search for lab results, information from past hospitalizations, operative reports, and other information to facilitate future chart searches.

- **Email Assignments:** These and **Web Assignments** encourage students to use electronic platforms, the assignment function of electronic classroom management systems, or other routes to connect with instructors or answer class-related questions.

- **In-Class Test Questions:** In addition to using PowerPoint slides to display questions for the class, **Text Polling** and **Clicker** methods are now available to allow for classroom assessment and technology-based questions in the classroom. Students use their personal cell phone to text a specific number with varying number messages to indicate answers to questions. The website creates a graph of responses and reveals class aggregate answers. Instructors should note that fees and minute usage of personal phone plans must be considered.

- **Documentation Case Study:** This approach may provide a means to teach students about the electronic health record.

- **Scavenger Hunt:** This strategy may be adapted to allow students to search through the electronic health record for specific information.

- **Online Discussion Groups:** As noted in the **Guided Discussion** strategy, this evolving method of teaching is highly popular in online teaching. As part of class requirements, students respond to discussion questions, contemplate fellow students' responses, work to provide unique responses to discussion strings, reflect on the impact of discussion questions to nursing practice, and use critical thinking skills to reason through professional issues. Web-based classroom management systems enable educators to create a system for students to complete assignments at convenient times and locations and, many say, provide superior opportunities to engage students because of convenience and assurance that every student or participant is active rather than passive in the process, as in traditional classrooms.

CONCLUSION: A CHARGE TO NURSE EDUCATORS

This chapter provided additional ideas to enhance nursing education. Using lecture and traditional teaching methods provides a sound foundation that is both cost- and learning-effective. The incorporation of creative teaching strategies into these traditional methods in any setting, including small groups, large groups, discussion groups, orientation groups, units, or clinical experiences, may enhance enjoyment of learning, reinforce priority concepts such as safety and patient outcomes, and create a love of learning that will last a lifetime. Integration of these methods into newer models such as the NCLEX® Blueprint, NCLEX® Integrated Processes, QSEN, and Next Generation NCLEX® enhances nursing education and reinforces safe and professional nursing practice.

References
1. Dickison P, Luo X, Kim D, et al. Assessing higher order cognitive constructs by using an information-processing framework. Journal of Applied Testing Technology, 17(1): 1–19, 2016.
2. Sutherland K, Schwartz J, and Dickison P. Best practices for writing test items. Journal of Nursing Regulation 3(2): 35–39, 2012.
3. National Council of State Boards of Nursing. Next Generation NCLEX® Project. https://www.ncsbn.org/next-generation-nclex.htm, 2019.
4. Peck SD, Werner J, and Raleigh DM. Improved class preparation and learning through immediate feedback in group testing for undergraduate nursing students. Nursing Education Perspectives 34(6): 400–404, 2013.

Chapter 11

Creative Evaluation Strategies

> *"Everything that can be counted does not necessarily count; and everything that counts cannot necessarily be counted."*
>
> —Albert Einstein

Challenges

- Just like teaching styles, the way we evaluate students is often the same as the way we were evaluated. As students have changed and we have progressed in our teaching careers, so should our evaluation methods.

- Evaluation can often be laborious, especially with large classes and classes with a high credit load, or when workload requires that you teach several courses.

- Sometimes it is difficult to know when to teach and when to evaluate—at what point are students still learning and require nurturing and when can they be held accountable for independent functioning? This is especially difficult in the clinical area.

- Evaluation strategies are often needed to determine if students prepared for class or clinical.

- Evaluation may be class-, course-, curriculum-, or program-specific and measure student learning and achievement, professionalism, clinical decision making and performance, and values.

- As we evaluate students and staff members, they also evaluate us, and others evaluate our ability to evaluate our students and staff members. Evaluation and assessment are critical for nursing education and practice.

Not only are creative teaching strategies critical in our teaching methods, but we also need to infuse our evaluation of students with creative innovations. Lecture is a tried-and-true teaching method that may benefit from creative strategies, and our means of evaluation are often sound but may benefit from new and innovative evaluation tools. Classroom assessments, clinical evaluation, end-of-program assessments, and student self-appraisals are critical elements of the evaluation process. The concepts of formative and summative evaluation provide the foundation for sound student appraisals. These assessments are paramount as we prepare students for graduation, the NCLEX® examination, and professional nursing practice. This chapter discusses principles and strategies to foster test-taking skills, with the goal of NCLEX® success. In this chapter, other evaluation methods are addressed as we consider the breadth of nursing, as both an art and a science, and the scope of nursing practice.

BASICS OF EVALUATION

FORMATIVE EVALUATION

Teaching and evaluation are held in balance in classroom, clinical, and other settings as students are assessed in formative evaluation. Using a variety of media, formative evaluation is:

- Learner-centered
- Ungraded
- Focused on nurturing and achievement of outcomes
- Known for providing ongoing feedback to learners
- A measurement method to assess progress toward outcomes

SUMMATIVE EVALUATION

Launching students into their next steps mandates that instructors evaluate achievement of course objectives. Each course may also be formative as students strive toward the summative completion of their program or course of study. Summative evaluation:

- Is achievement oriented
- Is focused on abilities, accomplishment, competencies, and outcomes
- May occur at the end of a course or the end of a program
- Is usually graded.

ASSESSING OUR STUDENTS

Assessment is the collection of data about the learner over a period of time. Good assessment includes multiple measures as we measure achievement of outcomes and nursing competency. Keep an eye on your student learning objectives as you build evaluation measures.

CLASSROOM ASSESSMENT

Instructors often know when students reach the **Muddiest Parts** in their classroom lecture and other teaching methods. Questioning looks, murmurs among students, a flurry of questions, or students craning their necks to view other students' notes often let educators know that they need to pause, conduct a classroom assessment, and explain a concept or set of concepts again. The following methods of classroom assessment may prove valuable for determining when additional explanations are needed and when other creative teaching strategies are warranted to clarify or reinforce concepts. Creative strategies also provide the mechanism to evaluate students in multiple learning styles, fostering a more comprehensive picture of the students' abilities than relying on a single method.

IDEAS

It Starts With the Syllabus

General Description. Your syllabus is your contract with students about the expectations of the class. In the syllabus, students learn about the course requirements, logistics, and the grading scale. Other components should include policies related to classroom behavior, plagiarism, and lateness. Also included are school-related policies and available academic services. Students should be referred to the syllabus often, and they need to see the syllabus as a tool rather than asking you or other students to answer their questions.

Example of the Strategy at Work. As a faculty member, it is very discouraging to have multiple students ask questions about topics that are addressed in the syllabus or when students recount, 6 weeks into a class, that they still have not read the syllabus. A great way to reinforce this concept and make sure that students use the syllabus is to provide a quiz about the syllabus during the first day of class. Students need to be warned about this in advance. The quiz may be "open book" (using the syllabus) or closed. I have found the open-book method is a great way to allow students the opportunity to look up material and locate important facts for future reference because it is not necessary for them to memorize information. Questions about due dates, required books and readings, and other facts make this quiz a valuable way to see the syllabus as a vital resource for class success.

Other strategies from the book that may be used related to this content:

- **In-Class Test Questions, Clickers, Text Polling**
- **Write to Learn**
- **Admit Tickets/Exit Tickets**
- **FYI—Classroom Questioning**
- **Group Tests**
- **Quickie Quizzes**
- **Unfolding Cases**

A Word About Examinations

Although an in-depth discussion of writing and creating multiple-choice examinations, the gold standard for preparing students for the NCLEX® examination, is beyond the scope of this text, several hints I have found helpful to ensure reliable and valid tests follow:

- Make sure that test questions are at the applying, analyzing, or synthesizing level. Critical thinking is not measured with remembering or comprehending questions, and these higher-level questions are represented on NCLEX®.
- Make sure tests evenly represent your class discussions or course objectives. Even distribution of test items to represent class sessions or topics ensures that tests have content validity. Provide students with examination breakdowns a few classes before the examination.
- NCLEX® policies dictate that each question stands alone (no case scenarios or linked questions), no proper names are used, no multiple-multiples are included, and questions cannot be in the "all of the following except" format. These may change with the Next Generation NCLEX®.
- Tests need to be proofread carefully and be presented in an easy-to-read format. Questions should not span two pages, include typographical errors, or be difficult to read.
- Make sure 25% of your questions (excluding alternative items) represent each response (for example, for A, B, C, and D, all are

represented as answer choices). Students quickly learn that educators may gravitate to the same answer choice.

- Ensure content validity of your exam by blueprinting the exam. Items may be blueprinted based on topic, course objective, question type, cognitive level and other parameters such as QSEN competencies, NCLEX® client needs, or program framework.
- Use caution when using test banks. Such questions are often not at the application level and above, and may not represent content as discussed in your class or the text. If questions from test banks are used, make sure that you review each question carefully and revise as needed to match class content and the areas you emphasize in your teaching.
- Limit the ability of students to ask questions during the examination. Not only does it enable students to get an unfair advantage and additional information, but it is also distracting to other students.
- These is some evidence that all objective items should end with a question mark (not sentence completion) to avoid potential misunderstanding or bias.
- You may want to refer to the National Council of State Boards of Nursing (NCSBN) website for terminology guidelines. Terms such as *healthcare provider, unlicensed assistive personnel, prescriptions* (not *orders*), *presents with* (rather than *complains of*), and generic names of medications only are used on the NCLEX® exam.
- Use exam and item analysis and other statistical measures to ensure a valid and reliable examination. Remember, you are a critical piece of this analysis. If statistics indicate a poorly performing item, analyze the data carefully to determine if the item or grading needs to be changed.
- See the NCSBN website for the alternative items and try to incorporate those in your exams.
- Newer trends in collaborative testing may assist in building student skills. Students take the test individually and these individual tests are submitted. Students then get into assigned groups. These groups are given one test form, and students retake the test as a group. You can decide how to score this strategy. One formula is that the group grades dictate points be added to individual scores. If the group gets an A, each individual gets 3 points added to her or his test. A B receives 2 points, and a C gets 1 point. Research indicates a high level of student satisfaction and retention with better test scores and outcomes as a result of collaborative testing.[1]

- Research continues to build the nursing and non-nursing literature related to effective testing practices. Several quality journal articles may further assist with item writing and test administration.[2–6]

CLINICAL ASSESSMENT

Clinical instructors are often puzzled about how to assess student preparation before a clinical day and whether students have the level of knowledge and skills to care for clients safely in the clinical area. Challenges include: getting a comprehensive review of all students when groups number seven to 10 students, using preceptor and other nurse feedback, using pass-fail versus graded clinical, and alleviating the stress associated with clinical for both students and instructors. These strategies may help in both formative and summative evaluation of students in the clinical arena. Some schools assign clients to students the day or so before clinical, especially in earlier courses. Others provide general recommendations for clinical preparation or may use these strategies to ensure preparation and to evaluate the quality of this preparation.

IDEAS

Preclinical Case Studies

General Description. Similar to the strategy discussed previously concerning **Preclass Case Studies**, one way to ensure that students are prepared for clinical or that nurse orientees are ready to practice is to have them complete case studies on clients that are typical of the unit or agency. Case studies frame a scenario that the students may encounter and include data and questions for students and orientees to consider prior to caring for clients. Questions may include: What additional data do you need? What precautions are indicated? What interventions do you anticipate? What complications and issues do you anticipate?

Example of the Strategy at Work. Our unit cared for children across the pediatric spectrum who were newly diagnosed with type 1 diabetes. I developed a case study discussing the management, teaching aspects, nursing implications, and developmental aspects. This case study allowed students to be prepared for this diagnosis and in tune with the developmental aspects of the care of all pediatric clients. I have also had students complete the case in pairs, with each pair receiving a different diagnosis, and share with classmates during a preconference or postconference.

Type 1 Diabetes Case Study

You are caring for a 3-year-old client who was admitted from the ED with a blood sugar of 475 mg/dL. He came to the ED with his mom who reported that he was wetting his pants, drinking lots of fluids, eating a lot, and sleeping more than usual. She stated that he vomited three times on the morning of admission and that his breath smelled "funny." He is diagnosed with type 1 diabetes. You are the nurse caring for this client. Answer the following questions:

1. What are the key physiological needs at this time?
2. What lab studies and other data do you need to provide holistic patient care?
3. How will these physical symptoms be treated?
4. What aspects of the care of a child with type 1 diabetes should the nurse anticipate?
5. List five aspects of teaching that need to be covered with the client's mom. Describe how those may best be taught.
6. What developmental aspects should be considered with this 3-year-old client? What would be different if the client were 1 year old? 5 years old? 10 years old? 15 years old?
7. What equipment will be needed for the client to manage his illness at home?
8. What responses would you anticipate from the client's mother and other family members?
9. What aspects of safety do you believe are a priority with this client?
10. How would this client look if his blood sugar were low? What would you do? How would he look if it were high? What would you do?

Other strategies from the book that may be used related to this content:

- **Clinical Questioning**
- **Pass the Problem**
- **Clinical Quick Write**
- **Clinical Puzzle**
- **V-8 Conferences**
- **One-Minute Care Plan/One-Minute Class**
- **Group Concept Maps**

Other ways to assess clinical behaviors include written work; staff and preceptor feedback; skills checklists; and the use of simulations, standardized patients, and skills labs to provide a summative view of clinical performance. Written papers, such as care plans and patient profiles, ensure research and thinking about client care and indicate depth of understanding. Postconferences, presentations, and student self-assessments may also be used to assess performance.

A Word About Assigning and Grading Written Work

In both the classroom and the clinical area, papers, research assignments, and concept maps are often assigned to assess student knowledge and application of critical thinking. Here are some hints to make the use of these approaches easier on educators, to make assignments evaluated more fairly, and to facilitate student success:

- Try using rubrics. These grading scales assign points based on paper sections or expectations and provide guidelines for both instructors and students. Sections of the paper should clearly delineate the expected components, and these sections should clarify the level of research, the length, and thesis of the paper. Assigning number of points to each section and a certain amount to formatting, spelling, and grammar clarifies grading methods and expectations.
- Consider the amount of feedback that you can give each student. Make sure you are consistent in giving both positive and negative feedback. Use the rubric to highlight standard errors and issues.
- Consider peer critiquing of student works, especially those with low point values in the class grades.
- You may want to try group written assignments. Not only does this reduce the number of final papers to be graded, but it also enhances group work, collaboration, and teamwork.
- More and more programs are using concept maps to assess thinking and decision making. Students may use computer software to design concept maps. Several resources are available to assist with evaluating these to ensure that educators assess causal relationships, making connections, and critical thinking rather than grading artistic talent.

A Word About Clinical Evaluation Tools

Clinical evaluation tools (CETs) have been around for a long time. Although they remain the primary means to evaluate students in the clinical area, they may be enhanced to ensure effective use in nursing education. These tools provide objective assessments of clinical abilities and professionalism, and they are usually formative and summative. They should be developed specific to your program outcomes, focus on competencies and behaviors, and include the opportunity for faculty *and* student evaluation. Many forms include the ability to rate behaviors as satisfactory, unsatisfactory, and no opportunity. CET templates are available on the internet, but make sure that they include course- and program-specific objectives referring to:

- Safety
- Concepts and knowledge for practice
- Evidence-based practice
- Nursing process
- Psychomotor skills
- Communication and teaching
- Ethically and culturally competent care
- Leadership
- Self-awareness and personal responsibility for learning
- Other parameters depending on your program's objectives

Students and instructors should use CETs almost daily to assess performance and to determine learning needs and experiences for the clinical day, and tools should reflect increasingly complex care and greater levels of independence throughout the course or program. Most nursing programs have automated or computerized CETs to foster communication and develop an electronic record of student performance.

To ensure that CETs evaluate student performance in a valid manner, instructors should use and collect appropriate data about a student. Some basic principles apply:

- When observing students, make sure you note patterns rather than isolated experiences. Everyone may be a little awkward or less efficient when starting out. It is just as important to "catch students doing something right" as "catching students doing something wrong."
- Put aside any biases when evaluating students in clinical. Many of us have had students who are strong in test taking or paperwork yet need extra assistance in the clinical area, and vice versa.
- Be systematic. View all students for the same time and doing equally challenging tasks. Sometimes we tend to spend more time with the weaker students (because patient safety is our priority), but we also need to make sure we see all students meeting objectives. Some students are extra skilled at "flying under the radar." Make sure you use **Clinical Questioning** and other methods to assess student knowledge and preparation.
- Keep detailed anecdotal notes on each student. These may be done on clinical worksheets, on the CETs, electronically via

smartphones or other devices, or as needed to meet the needs of the individual instructor. I found that anecdotal notes needed to be written during or immediately after the clinical experience to ensure comprehensiveness, and I frequently referred to the CET to ensure that my observations were based on expected behaviors. Sometimes we say things in our anecdotal notes like "good job" or "good day." Instead we need clear and concise statements based on the CET to ensure objective evaluation criteria.

- Experts recommend that CETs be reviewed annually to ensure that the meaning of each competency is agreed upon by all instructors, means to assess behaviors are understood, pass-fail performance behaviors are clearly delineated, and some methods exist to support interrater reliability of the CET. Oermann et al. suggested that simulations of student behaviors be conducted with instructors rating their performance.[7] Ongoing debriefing may assess for reliability. Other issues with CETs to be addressed by educators include limited opportunity for students to demonstrate performance, rater drift, tools not relevant for clinical practice, and CETs that are too long to be practical for student rotations.

END-OF-PROGRAM ASSESSMENT

Student assessment at the end of a program may be very difficult as many different pieces of evaluation come together to ensure that students meet program outcomes. Several methods are used to evaluate students' abilities to assess priorities, individuals' rationales for nursing actions, capacity to respond to changes in patient status, and clinical reasoning skills. Current concerns about the clinical judgment skills and safety of patient care by novice practitioners reinforces our need to engage in rigorous evaluation methods. Using both formative and summative evaluations is common as students prepare to complete the program.

IDEAS

Clinical Preceptorships or Clinical Capstones

General Description. Many programs include a preceptorship program during which nursing students are paired with a staff nurse and provide highly independent levels of care. School policies and board of nursing mandates may define the parameters of this experience as students are able to bridge nursing school experiences with real-world practice.

Example of the Strategy at Work. Our nursing program provides an 84-hour clinical practicum in cooperation with area nurses and agencies. Students rank this experience as one of the greatest components of our curriculum as they transition to professional practice. Schools are also starting to use a final simulation experience that tests patient care, prioritizing, delegating, judgment, and psychomotor skills to assess end-of-program attainment of outcomes.[8]

Other strategies from the book that may be used related to this content:

- **Portfolios and e-Portfolios**
- **Final Simulation Experience/Out of the Hat**
- **Poster Sessions**

STUDENT SELF-ASSESSMENT

An important part of learning in nursing education is reflection on lessons learned and considering what could be done differently. Students often need to be encouraged to think of these elements. They need to be provided the opportunity to consider their personal performance and compare it to the competencies expected of nursing practice.

IDEAS

Reflective Journaling

General Description. Journaling provides students with the forum for assessing their own performance and developing insights into their strengths and weaknesses. Students may reflect upon the following:

- What do I do very well?
- What do I do well and could do better?
- In what areas do I need the most improvement?
- What other experiences do I need?

Example of the Strategy at Work. This journaling accompanies student appraisal of their CET. Although some students are more detailed in their journaling and in their appreciation of the qualitative and quantitative natures of evaluation than others, this self-reflection ensures that students see their personal role in their own learning and prepares them for the workforce in which personal appraisal is a critical component of the annual evaluation. Students are sometimes reluctant to identify areas for improvement, believing they will provide "ammunition" to instructors. Nursing instructors would do well to reward students who self-assess accurately and assist students to identify means to identify strategies for growth.

We developed a unique strategy to ensure that students self-evaluated their completion of program outcomes and readiness for NCLEX®. We had the students do a study plan assessing their personal study habits; areas needing concerted study efforts; and plan for study, including a calendar. They compared their own study needs with the NCLEX® blueprint to develop their personal areas of concern. This assignment provided important preparation for students.[9] We also asked the students, in some administrations of this assignment, to explore their achievement of the program outcomes.

Other strategies from the book that may be used related to this content:

- **Assessing Learning Style**
- **Ah-Ha Journals**
- **Self-Assessment Write to Learn**

CONCLUSION: NEWER TRENDS IN STUDENT ASSESSMENT

Evaluation as a field continues to grow with new and different ideas. Current trends focus on self-evaluation as a critical piece of student-led and student-centered evaluation. Learner-centered strategies include reflective commentaries on practice, learning logs, program-to-workplace projects and papers, and the use of simulation and debriefing experiences to assess skills and critical thinking. Student projects designed to meet both the needs of their education and of the clinical agency are common in community and clinical settings when related to quality assurance and improvement activities. Additional school-to-work activities may add to the value of the student in the clinical arena and build key workplace skills. The sharing of school evaluations with employers may provide an ability to show experience for a new job. Newer models call for the increasing emphasis of nursing education to evaluate for elements of social justice, ethical principles, cultural competence, and the role of primary healthcare.

Some ideas about new trends in evaluation:

- **Viva/Think Aloud Evaluation/Oral Exams:** With rubrics to assess decision making, reflection, integration of knowledge, and innovative action, oral examinations are being used to assess student accomplishments.[10]

- **Objective Structured Clinical Experiences (OSCE):** Although not a new concept, OSCE is now being used to assess skills in distance education using objective scoring and rubrics.[11]
- **Nursing Competency Scale (NCS):** The NCS assesses the helping role, therapeutic interventions, work role, diagnostic functions, teaching/coaching, assurance of quality, and the management of selected situations.[12] This scale has been used to evaluate students in academic and practice settings and is gaining traction as a way to evaluate nursing performance holistically.
- An increased focus on mentoring and preceptor evaluation may accompany changes in clinical education models. Nurses in these roles need education on how to evaluate and the expectations of the experience. The preceptor and educator, in consultation with each other, need to focus on context-required competencies and means to foster student growth.

As nursing, nursing education, practice training, and other elements evolve, so too will the means available to assess students and practicing nurses. Because our ultimate goals are safe patient care, professionalism, and the health of society, our tools to evaluate will reinforce these elements and increase our ability to assess growth and achievement accurately.

References

1. Green R, Worthey T, and Kerven J. Collaborative testing: An effective invitational strategy for high stakes testing in nursing. Journal of Nursing Education 57(5): 291–295, 2018.
2. Dickison P, Luo X, Kim D, et al. Assessing higher order cognitive constructs by using an information-processing framework. Journal of Applied Testing Technology 17(1): 1–19, 2016.
3. Sutherland K, Schwartz J, and Dickison P. Best practices for writing test items. Journal of Nursing Regulation 3(2): 35–39, 2012.
4. Kantar LD. Assessment and instruction to promote higher order thinking in nursing students. Nurse Education Today 34: 789–794, 2013.
5. Coughlin PA and Featherstone CR. How to write a high-quality multiple-choice questions: A guide for clinicians. European Journal of Vascular Surgery 54: 654–658, 2017.
6. Bristol T and Brett A. Test item writing: 3 Cs for successful tests. Teaching and Learning in Nursing 10: 100–103, 2015.
7. Oermann MH, Yarbrough SS, Ard N, et al. Clinical evaluation and grading practices in schools of nursing: Findings of the Evaluation of Learning Advisory Council Survey. Nursing Education Perspectives 30: 352–357, 2009.
8. Sideras S, McKenzie G, Noone J, et al. Making simulation come alive: Standardized patients in undergraduate education. Nursing Education Perspectives 24: 421–424, 2013.

9. Herrman JW and Johnson A. From beta-blockers to boot camp: A nursing course approach to NCLEX® success. Nursing Education Perspectives 30(6): 384–388, 2009.

10. Roberts D. The clinical viva: An assessment of clinical thinking. Nurse Education Today 33: 402–406, 2013.

11. Oranye NO, Ahmad C, Ahmad N, et al. Assessing nursing clinical skills competence through objective structured clinical examination for open distance learning students in Open University Malaysia. Contemporary Nurse 41(2): 233–241, 2012.

12. Kajander-Unkuri S, Meretoja R, Katajisto J, et al. Self-assessed level of competence of graduating nursing students and factors related to it. Nurse Education Today 34: 795–801, 2014.

Chapter 12

Creative Strategies for Concept-Based Curricula

> "Concept-based teaching [demonstrates] the difference between memorizing facts related to the American Revolution and developing and sharing ideas related to the concepts of freedom and independence as a result of studying the Revolution."
>
> —H. L Erikson

Challenges

- Students may find concept-based learning very different from what they expected in nursing school. They probably anticipated hearing about medical diagnoses and working in environments similar to those depicted on television hospital shows, and they may be impatient with learning concepts rather than about cutting-edge diseases. Students may be reassured with the following phrase: "When you hear hoofbeats, think horses, not zebras." In this sense, we need to focus on common concepts and their nursing care rather than on the unusual, yet perhaps intriguing, presentations of human health and illness.

- Instructors may struggle with the transition to a concept-based curriculum. We tend to teach the way we were taught—many of us remember long lectures with or without PowerPoint support. Change may be hard. Authors discuss instructors' reluctance to give up traditional specialities, and personal identification with a specialty, to the more general approach to concepts.[1]

- Faculty development, which involves investments of time, money, and effort, is critical to ensuring smooth transition to this new curricular model. Searching the literature, networking with other schools, and seeking consultation may assist in curricular revision or enhancement.[2]

- Clinical agencies may find concepts rhetorical and not applicable to client care. When agencies are acquainted with the deep learning and applicability of concepts, they may be more receptive to this new curricular change.

- Creative strategies cannot be created quickly or implemented without deliberate selection, design, and planning. Strategies must be objective-driven, connected with evaluation measures (including examination questions), and perceived as valuable to student understanding.

- Instructors need to have a thorough understanding of concepts and exemplars as a foundation for implementing creative teaching methods. These active strategies generate conversation, thought, and student questions. Students will often ask really complex questions as a result of this active engagement and thinking. Instructors should anticipate such questions and foster this spirit of inquiry in their classroom.

- Evaluation of concept-based curricula may be slightly different and may require a variety of methods to assess program and student-learning outcomes. Several studies discuss the nuances of evaluating a concept-based curriculum.[3–6] Again, seeking expertise both within and outside the program is warranted.

Nursing schools have always grappled with curriculum development. Some curricula are based on the NCLEX® blueprint, the Quality Safety Education for Nurses (QSEN) competencies, nursing theories, or other frameworks. A revolutionary model of curricula was needed to deal with content saturation in nursing education. As is sometimes said, "We keep adding information to nursing education, and we don't take anything out. We just talk faster." Concept-based curricula have become highly prominent across the country and represent a student-centered approach to learning. Some states have adopted curricula for all their programs. Concept-based curricula provide instruction based on a list of concepts adopted by the individual program or from selected models in the literature. The emphasis is on concepts and learning rather than on continuing to add endless content. These concepts may be related to health and wellness, healthcare provision, professionalism, population health, collaboration, nursing roles, and other categories. The major premise behind these concepts articulates that nurses provide care based on common presentations or concepts that inform specific nursing assessments and interventions. Instruction is driven by major nursing issues and client needs rather than long lists of facts or lectures that reinforce memorization, regurgitation, and forgetting. Nursing instructors discriminate among what students "need to know," what is "nice to know," and what is "nuts to know."

For example, a client enters the emergency department presenting with severe pain in the right ankle and reports an injury while participating in a sports event. Even though the medical treatment is focused on diagnosing and managing the potential fracture, nursing emphasizes comfort, pain, perfusion, and inflammation (these are concepts). Nursing care includes pain management, ice and elevation of the effected limb, assessing perfusion, and assessing responses to treatment. We may also extend our care to safety and injury prevention, emotional responses, and teaching. Should we encounter another client with an injury, we can use our knowledge of concepts to determine our care. How does the new client compare and contrast with a previous client? How will this inform our nursing practice?

Concept-based curricula have been linked with positive student outcomes, including higher-order thinking and deeper understanding of nursing practice, with some studies indicating higher NCLEX-RN® success rates and graduation rates, higher critical thinking skills, and higher program satisfaction.[3–5] As noted in Chapter 3, deep learning is needed to ensure retrieval for later practice, passing the licensure exam, and dealing with the challenges of nursing care. Deep learning is characterized by personal intrinsic motivation, engagement in learning, and a zest for learning that results in thorough understanding of information.[7] This is in contrast to superficial learning, which is best described as the "learn it, spit it, forget it" phenomenon.

Qualitative and quantitative studies, although limited by small sample sizes and descriptive methods, demonstrate promising results, especially when concept-based curricula are combined with engaging teaching methods.[3–5] In fact, creative teaching and active learning strategies go hand-in-hand with concept-based learning. Concept-based curricula built on conceptual learning is defined as a process in which students develop high-level skills and the ability to apply knowledge within and between concepts.[7] Concepts are presented in class, illustrated with exemplars, and operationalized in clinical settings. As instructors present concepts, with associated and deliberately selected exemplars, active teaching strategies are woven in to provide emphasis, reinforcement, and active engagement opportunities.

Active learning strategies may be used to supplement lecture material, provide valuable experiences in the flipped classroom (see Chapter 13), or add to other teaching methods to enhance deep learning. These strategies also allow students to practice problem solving and clinical judgment, which are critical to successful nursing practice. Instructors are charged with being thoroughly familiar with concepts, leveling the concepts across the curriculum, in-depth discussion of concepts, ensuring the building of concepts in depth, ensuring breadth and complexity across the courses, and establishing common definitions of attributes and characteristics.

This book is not meant to be a manual for revising a concept-based curriculum. Works by Giddens;[7] Giddens, Caputi, and Rodgers;[8] and other sources in the literature may provide guidance to this major curricular change. Instead, this chapter is designed to build on concept-based learning and combine them with some new strategies and others already discussed in this book to demonstrate the clear linkage between creative strategies and concept-based instruction.

Building Blocks of Concept-Based Teaching

Concepts
Exemplars
Compare and contrast
Reflection
Clinical application

IDEAS

Here I present strategies that I have implemented, with a brief description of how each may work for you. See the index to find the original description of each strategy that appears in bold and, as always, mold the strategies to your personal teaching preferences and needs.

Concepts

Definition. Concepts are elements of care that are described by attributes. They are used to organize or frame information, skills, knowledge, and facts as they may be applied to situations and assorted contexts.[7] As we teach about concepts, we relate them to clinical practice, providing a reality-based model for students to find relationships. For example, if a nurse is providing care to a client with immunosuppression secondary to steroid use, the student will be able to identify characteristics and nursing care associated with protection from infection and transfer application of this knowledge to care of the client experiencing neutropenia secondary to chemotherapy.

Strategies

- **Getting Carded:** Bristol[9] discusses the importance of memory tools and brain organizers in learning nursing information, including concepts. He suggests that students write important information, like concepts and attributes, on index cards. These cards are punched with a single hole and are linked with a metal ring. Students add to these cards during class, lab, and clinical, and they can carry these cards with them to provide a study resource. In clinical, students may refer to concept cards during client care to ensure comprehensive assessments and reinforcement of learned information.

- **When You Think of This, Think of That:** This matching exercise is effective in the initial stages of presenting a concept. Concepts in the left column are matched with attributes in the right column. Some attributes are noted as applicable to more than one concept.

- **Pass the Problem:** Students write a concept at the top of a piece of paper and a brief description of a clinical or case study client. Each student can explore the same or different concepts. Then the paper is passed around the group and fellow students provide their input about relevant attributes, assessments, and interventions. Each student in the group makes a contribution to other students' papers. Once the paper has made the rounds of the room, students have a document that provides a guide for client care. This can be done in a preconference to plan care, in postconference to reflect on care, or in a didactic class to explore exemplars.

- **Short Clips:** Use brief film clips to exemplify larger concepts or highlight attributes. Remember the value of thinking questions when implementing **Short Clips**. Provide the questions before the clip to ensure that students are focused on the objectives of the exercise. Then review the questions following the clip. Questions may refer to the concept and prompt students to watch for specific information about the discussion of the concept and attributes.

- **Admit Ticket/Exit Ticket:** Students are required to complete a brief exercise or assignment in order to enter or exit class. There are logistical issues associated with this strategy that were addressed earlier with the description of this method. It is helpful with concept-based learning to reinforce concepts or to ensure completion of preparatory assignments. Students can write a test question, indicate a **Muddiest Part or Point**, complete a **Nuts and Bolts,** do a **Write to Learn** or **Clinical Quick Write,** or answer questions about a case study.

- **All Things Being Equal:** This strategy includes writing selected assessment findings, laboratory results, or other manifestations on a PowerPoint slide. Students are asked to identify those that are most "worrisome," thereby learning to set priorities. These slides may also be made with attributes of concepts, and then students are asked to prioritize them and indicate appropriate nursing interventions.
- **Nuts and Bolts:** This strategy, as discussed previously, has students fill in the blanks of a premade case study with components of the nursing process. Such cases may be adapted to provide further description of a concept. For example, the following **Nuts and Bolts** was used during discussion of respiration/oxygenation.

Nuts and Bolts

A 14-year-old client has cystic fibrosis and is congested with increased work of breathing; pulse ox = 85%. The nurse assesses the patient and determines he has increased mucus buildup and decreased oxygenation. The nurse provides chest PT, administers a mucolytic, and encourages coughing. As a result of the actions, the patient is breathing easier, and pulse ox = 92%.

Exemplars

Definition. Exemplars are cases and stories that allow for application of concepts, in turn allowing students to make cognitive connections between concepts, attributes, and clinical pictures or presentations.[7] Exemplars are developed about health-related situations experienced by clients or gleaned from nursing practice. The most representative exemplars are developed and distributed throughout the curriculum. They are selected because they represent essential content and may be health-related situations experienced by clients, or they may be part of nursing practice. The most representative information should be chosen to represent exemplars. These may be repeated as the breadth, depth, and complexity of the exemplars increase. Exemplars should be deliberately selected and spread throughout the curriculum. Instructors need to emphasize the representative nature of exemplars. Students need to appreciate the broad scope of the human experience and that exemplars provide a common understanding of that experience, not an exhaustive representation or the finite rules concerning the concept or exemplar.

You probably noted when reading other chapters in this book how many strategies are based on stories. Nursing students find that these cases and war stories provide mechanisms to connect with information; put information on a human plane; and help them to relate to information, learn, and apply concepts later.

Strategies

- **Short Clips:** Use popular film clips to demonstrate or augment an exemplar discussed in class. In the concept of Adaptation, a clip from a popular movie or a YouTube video may demonstrate domestic violence. Students may independently complete an exercise or be guided through exploration of the concept, attributes, and exemplar as demonstrated in the video. Remember the value of thinking questions prior to and after the clip to ensure active thinking and engagement in the **Short Clip.**

- **Continuing Case Studies:** While presenting an exemplar, present a piece of the case study or exemplar. Then provide discussion with increased detail about the case intermittently throughout the class. **Continuing Case Studies** provide the opportunity to revisit material throughout the class and presentation of the exemplar, reinforcing key information and ensuring that students understand the importance of this key information.

- **Clinical Didactic Connect:** One of the greatest assets of the concept-based curriculum is the ability to present concepts and exemplars in a didactic class and then see clients, real or simulated in the lab or clinical area, that exemplify learned material. Instructors across the educational experience need to be aware of concepts being addressed in the classroom and clients being encountered in clinical. Instructors need to communicate often, perhaps developing formal communication mechanisms, so that students can benefit from the ability to learn across the curriculum. Bringing clinical to the classroom and ensuring that clinical sites reinforce classroom material are critical to deep learning of concepts and exemplars. Guide students to correlate theory with practice, but also hold students accountable for applying concepts across settings and engaging in comprehensive preparation for both classroom and clinical experiences.

- **Unfolding Case Studies:** As previously discussed, case studies that replicate reality, slowly unfold, provide additional information, continue to develop over time, and demonstrate the unpredictability of client responses are valuable for student learning. A case is presented, and students analyze key data and selected interventions. The client response is discussed, along with other new information, and further assessments and interventions are planned. Students may be asked to consider other variables affecting care (culture, family, age, previous health history, or lifestyle) and the case study continues to unfold. Complex cases may be developed so that correct and incorrect interpretations or interventions may lead to different outcomes, much like a simulation activity. The dynamic nature of exemplars and deviation from the perfect prototype are important so that students learn about the variability of individual care and client outcomes.

- **Pause for Priority Setting/What's the Big Deal/What Would You Do?:** These are more approaches than strategies. While presenting an exemplar, pause and ask a question. Ask students to consider or discuss selected attributes of the concept or other information that delineates the exemplar as a priority or identifies key information as critical to client care.

  Questions may include the following: What is the big deal? Why is this so important? What is the first nursing priority? What do you need to assess first? How would a nurse respond to this client statement? What laboratory studies would validate your conclusions? The next feature is an example of this strategy as I have used it with the concept of perfusion and in the context of discussing an exemplar of postpartum care and the potential for postpartum hemorrhage.

What's the big deal? What do you need to assess? What do you do?

- A woman who is one day postpartum and has soaked through a peri-pad in 3 hours.
- A client who is 2 hours postdelivery. During fundal massage, the client passes an egg-sized clot.
- During vital signs assessment, the nurse notes that there are bloody stains on the top sheet of a client who is 6 hours post–vaginal delivery.
- The unlicensed assistive personnel (UAP) reports that a postpartum client is difficult to arouse and that her blood pressure is 86/52 and heart rate is 124 beats per minute.

In this next example, several concepts and examples are provided. Students are asked to consider and establish priorities of each situation, and then distinguish between them. This is similar to the decision making needed to care for multiple clients:

What's the big deal? What do you need to assess? What do you do?

- A 10-year-old with decreased <u>oxygenation</u> as a result of acute asthma.
- A 65-year-old with decreased coronary <u>perfusion</u> secondary to an acute myocardial infarction.
- A 24-year-old woman in preterm labor at 30 weeks' gestation and experiencing <u>stress</u> with decreased coping.
- A 46-year-old who has experienced a significant loss and is <u>grieving</u>, and has mood changes related to depression.

- **Reverse Case Studies:** This strategy can be very valuable in clinical and the classroom. As published by Beyer,[10] students are given a list of the home medications and a short synopsis of the client situation or exemplar. Students are then charged with fleshing out the rest of the case study and providing details to meet the needs of the class topic. In this case, students can use introductory information to meet the attributes of the concept and the details of the exemplar. This exercise may be both creative or more prescribed, as needs dictate.

Compare and Contrast

Definition. A key element of concept-based teaching is the reinforcement of comparing and contrasting new clients and events with previously learned content and experiences. Students are introduced with the acts of comparing and contrasting as exemplars are introduced. Students can compare and contrast exemplars while considering how other concepts are also related and involved in client care. Allowing students to consider how an infection looks the same or different in two clients, how two children of different ages react to a therapeutic procedure, and how an adult or an older adult's reaction to a medication is similar or different, or having them compare the assessment of respiratory distress and cyanosis in clients with a variety of skin colors may all exemplify comparing and contrasting.

Strategies

- **Worksheets:** One creative worksheet I came across is called the Daily Compare and Contrast Sheet. The sheet includes a grid that delineates the concept or exemplar being discussed. Students are asked to discuss the risk factors, assessments, and interventions indicated for different populations or ages. For example, perfusion may be assessed for a woman experiencing postpartum hemorrhage, a child in septic shock subsequent to meningitis, and an elder adult client in cardiogenic shock following an exacerbation of heart failure. Students are asked to compare and contrast these states and come to conclusions about similarities and differences, which provides a great forum for learning and application of conceptual information. Another example of **Worksheets** is to Compare and Contrast Patients with an Infection.[8] Patients with infections are compared on criteria such as type of infection, age-related consider-ations, preexisting conditions, prescribed medications, attributes of the concept of infection, and related concepts. Students are then asked to review the concepts of care coordination, patient education, developmental level, healthcare environment, health promotion, and ethics as they may relate to this infection. Shaffer et al[11] describe the use of a **Worksheet** to guide a clinical reasoning exercise related to emerging technologies in the healthcare environ-ment. The structure of this exercise allows students to engage in meaningful examination of technology in healthcare.
- **Pharmacology Compare and Contrast:** Bristol[9] designed this worksheet, which is much like medication sheets used traditionally by students to prepare for medication administration, to include the following: the classification of medications, specific examples of the medication class, the relationship to the concept, specific nursing concerns, lifespan considerations, and common nursing concerns.
- **Debate:** As discussed, students present different perspectives of a viewpoint and how this may affect nursing care. Within a concept-based curriculum, students present each concept as it relates to an exemplar or case study patient. Students debate to compare and contrast how the concept relates with other con-cepts in a single client or how the client is the same or different from other clients. Students may also debate priorities, methods of care, healthcare practices, evidence basis for nursing actions, and current versus past practices in providing nursing care.
- **Compare and Contrast Write to Learn:** Giddens, Caputi, and Rodgers.[8] developed a medication administration written exercise that focuses on the healthcare organization. Two students shadow

the medication nurses or several nurses as they pass medications. Students then compare and contrast different nurses' techniques or different patient experiences, create concept maps or written organizers of the medication administration process, reflect on the potential for errors from individual and organizational perspectives, share experiences in postconferences, and consider medication administration systems of other agencies and how organizations work to ensure safe practices.

- **Interspersed Case Studies:** As you present an exemplar representing a concept, additional case studies or manifestations are added to the presentation. Each is compared and contrasted with those previously presented. In this method, students gain an understanding of the breadth of scope of each concept and the individual differences that may exist. Cases are revisited or new cases are developed as exemplars increase in breadth, depth, and/ or complexity.

- **Clinical Judgment Exercise:** Another exercise designed by Giddens, Caputi, and Rodgers[8] uses the compare-and-contrast theme to provide students with exposure to conducting assessments or procedures with clients, such as taking vital signs, and then comparing and contrasting findings, illness states, concepts, and individual client variables. Students may discuss the need for larger blood pressure cuffs, gaining cooperation of a client, how preexisting and current conditions affect vital signs, and other client data. Students conference about each client's set of vital signs to determine their comparison with norms, the impact of each client's condition on findings, and nursing implications. Students then compare vital signs between clients to learn about norms and variations. This exercise may be expanded to other assessments and circumstances.

Reflection

Definition. Reflective practice and reflection as a teaching strategy are gaining momentum as we appreciate how people learn and how to reinforce learning for later retrieval. Reviewing experiences, considering additional information needed, addressing additional potential actions that may affect the situation, and anticipating how new knowledge may inform future practice are all components of reflection.

Strategies
- **Ah-Ha Journals:** These journals, as previously described, inherently provide for reflection. The new twist for concept-based curricula is to add the focus on concepts. Students identify

the critical concepts associated with the experience, client, or assignment; compare and contrast with classroom and previous connections; and then reflect using the journal format. This includes describing the events, persons, and issues; describing the individual's reactions, feelings, and any contributing factors; and then generalizing about lessons learned from the experience and how these lessons may prove useful in future practice. Authors reinforce the value of journaling and debriefing as a means of reflecting on practice and decision making.[13]

- **V-8 Conference:** In this clinical strategy, students share their **Ah-Ha Journals** and reflections related to concepts and clinical experiences. Students do most of the talking and share information, with less input from instructors. Students reflect on each other's insights while building connections with previous experiences.

- **One Minute Class:** Within the classroom, students share clinical **Ah-Ha Journals** as they connect with classroom exemplars and clinical experiences. These are limited to one minute and require students to prioritize information to be shared. This is a great lesson in concise reporting and expressing needs, skills that will prove useful in handoff and end-of-shift reports. You may assign these in advance or, if you have students in both class and clinical, you can identify clinical events that may be presented in the classroom.

- **Community-Based Concepts/Teaching About Poverty:** Decker et al.[12] describe implementation of a concept-based unit on social determinants and poverty as part of a community nursing course. Students are shown videos depicting poverty and social disadvantage, engage in debriefing discussions, participate in a poverty simulation, and measure attitudes toward poverty using a reliable evaluation tool. In addition, other concepts are interwoven to address community and family violence, community health, vulnerable populations, and the role of the nurse. Reflective journals demonstrate increases in understanding of the role of social determinants in health and the value of the concept framework to transfer knowledge to nursing practice.[12]

- **Clinical Quick Write/Write to Learn:** These exercises provide spontaneous and planned reinforcement of current material. During class or in clinical, ask students to reflect on current topics or experiences, as in the following examples. How would it feel to be a client going through what the client you are caring for is going through? A nurse comes upon a client with these symptoms [list symptoms here]; what would the nurse do first? A client states that he or she is leaving the hospital; how would you respond based on what you know about the client? The client you are assigned to care for experiences a rapid change in status; how would you respond? The number of questions is limited only by your experience and imagination. Choose critical concepts or information and have students spend just a minute reflecting on the material to reinforce engagement and learning. Have students write a narrative format, bulleted comments, or identify and write down a few words to engage in thinking about the exercise. These brief notes may jog the memory later. Students can also be asked to integrate current concepts with previous experiences in a **Write to Learn,** comparing previous characteristics with current discussions and reflecting on the meaning of these differences.

- **Think-Pair-Share:** As discussed, this strategy can be used frequently to ensure that more students have a voice in class. Discuss important concepts in pairs. This is especially effective for larger classes where students may be reluctant to participate, but it can also be used in small groups like clinical groups. Have students reflect on material and share with each other or with the larger group. Students can consider issues related to cultural sensitivity, clinical reasoning, and care coordination. For example, following a discussing on nursing care of the client with burns, ask students to consider the issues of pain, infection, fluid resuscitation/homeostasis, body image, and regulation/nutrition/elimination. Have students reflect on potential problems in each area and correlating nursing interventions.

- **Day in the Life of a Client With . . .:** Students are asked to consider how a condition or illness may affect selected issues in a client's life. Students conjecture how a client's day progresses, aspects of the client's daily routine, how the client may interact or rely on family members and the social environment, and how the illness or condition may affect functioning. They are encouraged to contemplate the challenges the client may confront and nursing implications. Students reflect on the major concepts relevant to the client, how nurses may assist to make the client's days easier, what community resources may be involved, and what gaps may exist that may lead to future problems or complications.

Clinical Application

Definition. Clinical experiences in a concept-based curriculum have similarities and differences compared to traditional clinicals. Students in hospital, home, and community settings learn total patient care, the means to manage priorities within a client assignment (whether with one or more clients), and how to provide care within the healthcare setting. In addition, concept-based curricula provide the impetus to attend to concepts that transcend the health and wellness continuum. These may deal with the concepts associated with healthcare delivery, the role of the nurse, and professionalism. Assign two or three students to other projects related to the healthcare system, workplace environment, healthcare organization, or other concepts. Students may compare and contrast experiences between clients, and demonstrate team leading and delegation in exercises. These experiences are rotated among the students throughout the clinical session and shared in postconference to reinforce group learning. In concept-based curricula, postconferences are essential to provide the opportunity to allow students to compare and contrast experiences and learn vicariously from each other. Nuances related to the care of clients in the home and community may also be addressed. Clinical experiences are designed to exemplify and make "real" the concepts discussed in didactic class.

Strategies

- **Clinical Huddle:** An instructor once told me about this clinical strategy to address concepts in the clinical area. Early in the clinical shift, the instructor would "huddle" with each student to discuss the top concepts with their patient or patients and the assessments and interventions associated with these concepts. Later in the clinical shift, the instructor again "huddled" with the students to determine if the interventions were implemented and to evaluate their effectiveness. By keeping the focus on these concepts, the students can then be challenged to compare and contrast and to engage in reflection.
- **Reverse Case Studies:** This strategy can be very valuable in clinical and the classroom (see the discussion about Beyer's work[10] earlier in this chapter). Using these in preconference and postconference to reinforce concepts can be very effective. One instructor told me how they provided students with client information in postconference. The instructor gave each student a list of medications that the client was on and a list of the diagnostic tests with their findings. The students needed to determine the medical

diagnosis and the associated critical concepts involved in each client's plans of care. This provided a unique way to then compare and contrast each student's clients and reinforce students' knowledge of pathologies. Subsequent discussion may then ensue about nursing priorities and nursing care.

- **Group Concept Mapping:** In this strategy, the clinical group is divided into smaller groups, and each group creates a concept map for common problems, nursing diagnoses, or medical diagnoses on the unit or at the agency. This strategy may be tailored to a concept-focused experience by creating the map on certain attributes of a selected concept. Shaffer and colleagues[11] describe an adaptation of this as "Ask Why? Three to Five Times." Their concept map identifies the concept and the exemplar, client history, client assessments, interventions, and evaluation. Students "Ask Why?" about several components of each map in order to develop a deeper understanding of the concept. This strategy may be used in the classroom or clinical area to encourage thorough understanding of concepts. Bristol[9] calls a similar exercise Critical Thinking Maps. The top three assessments, risk factors, pathophysiological changes, laboratory and diagnostic tests and findings, interventions, potential and actual complications, medications, and elements of client or discharge teaching are linked with concepts and exemplars as a way to clarify and broaden the understanding of the concept.

- **Clinical Questioning:** Consider again what questions you ask to ensure that students are knowledgeable, are prepared, meet objectives, and are safe. To foster conceptual learning, the instructor may ask students about applicable concepts and the priorities for the day, and use other strategies (compare and contrast or reflection) to further investigate student awareness. Focusing on higher-level questions (for example, What could be done differently? What complications may be anticipated? What if the intervention doesn't work? What else do you need to know?) ensures deeper thinking.

- **Patient Safety Goals Clinical Assignment:** Giddens and colleagues designed an assignment for students in the clinical area. They use the patient safety goals to assess the environment and three clients. Students assess clients' priority safety needs, the precautions indicated, how these are implemented for this client, aspects that need to be communicated to the next shift, and any gaps in care that may be remediated.[8]

- **Clinical Puzzle:** A puzzle with eight to 10 pieces is used. Each puzzle piece has a concept written on it, and one puzzle piece is given to each student. Throughout the clinical day, students review the electronic health record or chart of the client and collect data relative to that concept. One student conducts a thorough assessment of the client. In postconference, students convene to share information and place their piece on the table. As the puzzle nears completion, students see the critical nature of concepts in providing holistic client care.

- **Preclinical/Preclass Case Studies:** In preparation for class or clinical, have students complete a designed exercise. Students analyze critical concepts for the clinical agency or those covered as exemplars in class. You can use any format for the output, either a care plan, concept map, or question and answer. Independently or in pairs, students explore the care of a client, and their determinations are reviewed in class or clinical. Asking higher-order questions of the data (for example, What additional data do you need? What precautions are indicated? What interventions do you anticipate?) ensures higher-order thinking in these assignments.

- **Grand Concept Rounds:** Employing **Grand Rounds** is a common strategy to allow students to present their clients to their group. The presentation may include the client and family members as indicated. For **Grand Concept Rounds,** students are asked to focus on variables of selected concepts, which may be the focus for the day or the semester, or topics that are currently being addressed in the didactic class. They then compare and contrast with didactic class exemplars, develop insights on the priorities of care, and reflect on the experience. Neilsen[13] described having students informally visiting each other's clients as part of a clinical rotation and observing asepsis precautions, privacy, and personal issues. This allowed students to compare and contrast client assessments and responses to treatment, noting individual differences in how a concept manifests itself in a variety of clients.

- **One-Minute Care Plan:** Students identify major concepts of concern for clients and plan care accordingly. Client assessments, planned interventions, and evaluation of effectiveness of strategies are part of this written or electronic document, with emphasis on addressing identified concepts (see the previous discussion in this chapter for formats and suggestions).

CONCLUSION

Remember, it is up to you to change any of the strategies in this text for your personal use in a concept-based curriculum. Refer to previous chapters and use the strategies to reinforce key concepts, attributes, and exemplars or to allow students the opportunity to compare and contrast, explore, and reflect on nursing care.

References

1. Erikson HL. Concept-based curriculum and instruction: Teaching beyond the facts. Sage, 2002

2. Hendricks S and Wangerin V. Concept-based curriculum: Changing attitudes and overcoming barriers. Nurse Educator 42(3): 136–142, 2017.

3. Duncan K and Schulz PS. Impact of change to a concept-based baccalaureate nursing curriculum on student and program outcomes. Journal of Nursing Education 54(3): S16–S19, 2015.

4. Getha-Eby TJ, Beery T, O'Brien B, et al. Student learning outcomes in response to concept-based teaching. Journal of Nursing Education 54(4): 193–199, 2015.

5. Harrison CV. Predicting success for associate degree nursing students in a concept-based curriculum. Teaching and Learning in Nursing 13: 135–140, 2018.

6. Murray S, Laurent K, and Gontarz J. Evaluation of a concept-based curriculum. Teaching and Learning in Nursing 10: 169–175, 2015.

7. Giddens JF. Concepts for nursing practice. Elsevier, 2017.

8. Giddens JF, Caputi L, and Rodgers B. Mastering concept-based teaching. Elsevier, 2015.

9. Bristol T. Conceptual learning for all: Begin today. Presentation, 2016.

10. Beyer DA. Reverse case study: To think like a nurse. Journal of Nursing Education 50(1): 48–50, 2011.

11. Shaffer K, Swan A, and Bouchard M. Designing a new model for clinical education: An innovative approach. Nurse Educator 43(3): 145–148, 2018.

12. Decker KA, Hensel D, Kuhn TM, and Priest C. Innovative implementation of social determinants of health in a new concept-based curriculum. Nurse Educator 42(3): 115–116, 2017.

13. Neilsen A. Concept-based learning activities using the clinical judgment model as a foundation for clinical learning. Journal of Nursing Education 48(6): 350–354, 2009.

Creative Strategies for the Flipped Classroom

"Every one of us is both a student and a teacher."

—S. Johnson and C. Johnson

Challenges

- Students often do not embrace flipped classrooms at first. Students prefer passive learning to the work involved in flipped methods. Instructors need to reinforce the perseverance involved in true, deep learning and the value of effort, repetition, retrieval practice, and spacing in learning and retaining information for use later in nursing practice. From another perspective, the skills learned in this student-centered method foster self-accountability and professionalism. Students may also see the repetition of content as redundant rather than as reinforcing the application of knowledge. Instructors can emphasize the value of this repetition in the learning process. They also need to be ready for this resistance, and armed with information, because students may encourage them to return to the traditional lecture format. Learning, studying, and nursing education are *hard*. My personal belief is that we need to reinforce the difficulty of nursing school, uphold the high standards of the nursing profession, and hold students accountable for lessons learned prior to their participation in our courses. Again, communication and sound rationales for the increased levels of work and the need for teaching method transition are critical.
- Instructors may find the change to the flipped classroom quite distressing. The perceived increase in faculty preparation time, class time, and time with students may be an obstacle. On

the other hand, once a flipped classroom has been developed, resources may be reused and the preparation time may be less.

- It may be especially difficult if you are the only instructor within your organization to lead a flipped classroom. The method is more readily embraced if it is implemented throughout a program. Students begin to see it as the status quo, and instructors can support each other throughout the transition.

- Flipped methods often require a knowledge of technology and their implementation in both the preparatory materials and the didactic/working classes. This may be a challenge for students and instructors. Resources emphasize that flipped classrooms work with both low- and high-technology methods, allowing instructors to "grow into" their facilitation of the flipped classroom.[5]

Implementation of the Flipped Classroom

- As noted above, the transition to this method may be distressing. Resources suggest that instructors should make this transition slowly, perhaps with part of a course at first or one course at a time, allowing time for the positive outcomes to become apparent.[5]

- There is the potential for multiple assignments in this method, producing lots of moving parts that instructors need to grade. In your planning the flipped classroom, consider your own time when deciding how many assignments, quizzes, and exercises require grading. Instructors should also consider student workload when designing assignments.

- In addition, instructors must ensure that the transition is smooth and that communication is transparent for team players, especially students. Students may not embrace this change and the perception of increased workload. Communicating both the assets of this format and the potential outcomes, along with all logistical details, increases the chance of successful implementation. Reinforcing that the flipped classroom is a shared responsibility, making instructors and students jointly accountable for learning, may allay some resistance.

- Make sure your content, methods, and evaluation components all mesh with the student learning objectives. Ensuring alignment of all these pieces enhances the positive outcomes of the flipped classroom. These must also be clearly communicated to students via the syllabus, learning management system, and other class policies.

- Barbour cautions that instructors who embrace the flipped classroom must be ready for and able to tolerate "controlled chaos."[5] As will be noted in Chapter 15, creative classrooms are not quiet, often breeding discourse, debate, and difficult questions. Instructors who are content experts and are enthusiastic for new ways of teaching may be the best candidates to implement the flipped classroom.

Current innovations in nursing education, such as the flipped classroom, provide powerful mechanisms to reach students. First implemented in a 2007 chemistry classroom by Bermann and Sams,[1] the flipped classroom is a student-centered, active learning, and technology-supported teaching strategy. The developers described flipped classroom methods wherein "that which is traditionally done in class is now done at home, that which is traditionally done as homework is now completed in class."[1] Knowledge is obtained outside the classroom and applied in real-life situations in the classroom, thereby enhancing critical thinking and clinical judgement. Also called flipping, inverted, or blended classrooms, flipped classrooms are thought to bridge the education-practice gap in nursing by fostering decision-making, problem-solving, and reasoning skills. The flipped classroom method encourages individual engagement while also reinforcing teamwork and collaboration.

Flipped classrooms create partnerships between students and instructors, cultivating professionalism and accountability in the learning process.[4] Instead of instructor-centered, instructor-led lecture and learning experiences, the content is provided to students prior to class, and formal class time is used to reinforce, repeat, and reiterate content and to assess learning. The instructor moves from being the "sage on the stage" to the "guide on the side." Authors herald the flipped classroom because it embraces heutagogical learning, wherein learners and learners' needs drive the learning.[2,3]

This class format requires knowledge and skill on the part of instructors to ensure effective implementation. Barbour differentiated the time periods of the flipped classroom as the (1) Preclass, (2) In Class, and (3) After Class phases.[5] Creative teaching strategies ensure that class preparation is beneficial and engaging; classroom time is valuable and reinforces content; and after-class time offers the opportunity for reflection, retention, and retrieval. Instructors design the learning experience by carefully crafting each phase of the process. Preclass exercises are designed to provide self-directed learning through instructor-developed didactic content. Such content ensures that students are prepared for class, enhances learner engagement, and promotes learner accountability in accessing information. These exercises may or may not be graded, and students can pace their learning by pausing videos and planning their completion of preparatory tasks. The flexibility while learning is a benefit. The In Class phase continues to engage the learner in high-level thinking, critical thinking, problem solving, and review of content while providing the mechanism for immediate assessment and feedback. This segment allows for application, analysis, and synthesis of the content presented prior to class. The After Class component allows for scaffolding of the learning experience, providing opportunities for reinforcement and reflection about content learned. It also reveals areas of confusion and provides a way to continue the learning process and address critical gaps in learning. The very deliberate learning process capitalizes on what we know about learning, harkening back to *Making Nursing Stick,* through spaced retrieval, calibration, interleaving, elaboration, reinforcement, and effortful practice. Boxes 13–1, 13–2, and 13–3 note common Preclass, In Class, and After Class activities, respectively.

OUTCOMES

The flipped classroom appears to enhance the quality of education; however, the empirical research validating this premise is somewhat limited. Several studies, integrative reviews, and systematic reviews indicate that the research findings are mixed. More extensive research is found in non-nursing use of the flipped classroom, demonstrating positive

Box 13–1.
Preclass Phase

- Taped or voice-over PowerPoint lectures
- Podcasts/Wiki's/web-based assignments
- Screen capture software recordings
- Interactive online modules
- Quizzes embedded in videos/before-class quizzes
- Incomplete worksheets
- Study guides
- Modules in standardized learning and testing packages
- Film clips or videos on YouTube
- Directed readings
- YouTube patient case studies and debriefing
- Team quizzes at achieved mastery levels
- Mini-lectures
- Learning management system assignments
- Practice of psychomotor skills
- Concept maps/learning mapping
- Graded **Admit Ticket** worksheets
- **Pause and Do** (time-stamped questions)

outcomes in the learning environments for pharmacy, medicine, audiology, and public health education.[6–9]

In nursing education, there appears to be some positive outcomes, that is, higher scores on tests and other performance measures.[2,10–12] Several studies noted that the flipped classroom demonstrated similar outcomes to traditional methods of teaching (lecture, discussion).[5-6,9–10] Others reported higher levels of student satisfaction with the flipped classroom, although this was often tempered by the quality of the preparatory videos, the length of the videos, and the amount of preparation time.[5,7,9–12] Several studies revealed that the flipped classroom method yielded higher scores in critical thinking measures[11–13] and higher levels of student engagement and attentiveness in class.[5,10,11] Other studies noted improved instructor–student interaction.[8,10]

Perhaps the greatest dissatisfaction with flipped classrooms is the perceptions of the increased workload associated with the method. It was found that instructors perceived the flipped classroom increased their workload by increasing preparation time; time in class; and time in addressing student concerns, questions, and problems.[11,12] Students

Box 13–2.
In Class Phase

- Discussion of preparatory work
- In-class, in-lab, videotaped, or podcast simulation
- Reinforcement of psychomotor skills
- Group exercises
- Group and individual presentations
- Case studies
- Test questions and review
- Quizzes/group testing/team quizzing/quiz discussion
- Using mobile devices for polling, searches, and quizzes
- Role play
- Debates
- Infographics
- Mind mapping/whiteboard debriefing
- Crossword puzzles
- Mini-lectures
- Assessment of content requiring clarification
- Peer education opportunities
- Movie clip analysis
- Calling on students/question-and-answer session
- Activity stations or **Activity Carousel**

Box 13–3.
After Class Phase

- Tip folder in learning management system
- Online fast facts (click to reveal)
- Crossword puzzles to reinforce content
- Virtual communities
- Reinforcement of difficult content
- Readings
- Test questions as practice for exam
- Self-developed videos
- Journals
- Organization of class notes (personal or group exercise)
- Social media test questions (writing and/or answering)

were similarly disgruntled by the work associated with the flipped class-room, expressing frustration over the need to teach themselves or teach their peers rather than being taught by an instructor.[12] Others expressed dissatisfaction with the stress associated with the workload.[10–12] Even when students performed better on learning measures with the flipped classroom method, they continued to express concern and were resistant to these effort-filled methods.[12]

Because flipped classrooms are implemented differently in each setting and because studies measuring their effectiveness use very different methods in assessing outcomes, more research is needed to determine the value of the flipped classroom in nursing education.[5,9,11,12] Nonetheless, researchers indicate that active learning strategies, which are the inherent foundation of the flipped classroom, support the vast diversity of learning styles and substantiate the value of the flipped classroom method.[6,12]

IDEAS

In the flipped classroom environment, students watch taped or streaming classes at home, attend classes for application exercises, and complete after-class exercises. There is a natural connection between the flipped classroom and active learning strategies. Many of the strategies in this text can be used at each of these three phases to ensure enhancement of the educational experience. In this chapter, I present strategies that I have implemented at these different phases, and I include a brief description of how each strategy may work for you. See the index to find the original description of each strategy that is bolded and, as always, you can mold the strategies to your personal teaching preferences and needs.

Preclass Strategies

- **Worksheets:** Worksheets provide guidance for students as they complete readings and view recorded lectures or mini-lectures. Providing case studies, narratives with blanks to be filled in, blanks next to vital sign and lab data findings, and questions allows students to begin to apply lecture content. These may be graded, be used as a **Quickie Quiz,** or serve as an **Admit Ticket.** **Worksheets** should be provided with blanks and incomplete information to allow students to actively engage in the material. You can post the answers to these in the learning management system or provide and discuss answers in class as a way to encourage students to attend class. Search the internet for interesting and appealing graphics that can be scanned or imbedded into worksheets. These graphics can include decision trees, plans of care, illustrated study guides, and other valuable tools.

- **Preclass Case Studies:** Preclass case studies offer students a guided walk through lecture content by applying content to case studies in preparation for class. Preclass case studies may be used for the most common issues, problems, or diagnoses, or they may serve as the discussion of a typical client for less complex cases. See the previous discussion of Preclass case studies for more details. These may be graded or not.

- **Preparation:** As discussed in Chapter 4, it is essential that you guide students through preparation for the class content by providing clear guidelines and instructions, ensuring that readings are pared down to the most critical content (rather than simply assigning entire chapters), listing specific exercises, clarifying expectations, making the most of video times, and ensuring that preparation is directly applicable to class content. Well-designed Preclass work helps students to see the value of preparation. Remembering to follow through your focus on objectives and ensuring that exercises and exam questions synchronize with these objectives provides important messages to students about critical material.

- **Critical Thinking Exercises/Clinical Decision-Making Exercises: Critical Thinking Exercises** and **Clinical Decision-Making Exercises** allow students to focus their study efforts and appreciate critical aspects of class content. These exercises are developed by instructors and may be used for **Quickie Quizzes** or with other strategies to prime learners. These exercises may be answered informally, written and collected as an assignment, or submitted via the learning management system. Remember that these exercises should reflect class objectives and that students should be tested on them to ensure their learning of key information.

- **Setting the Stage:** This strategy sets the tone for the content to be presented through the flipped classroom experience. The exercises you develop for the preparatory time set up an atmosphere of excitement and spirit of inquiry. Using interesting case studies, videos, stories, and other information assists in creating this interest prior to class so that students are excited to come to class and to apply content to real-world situations.

- **Discussion Starters:** Discussion starters may be used for the video lectures and mini-lectures and for in-class time. Using a phrase that signals class is about to begin provides an introduction to the students and indicates that it is time to focus. You can develop your own statement that triggers learning. Students learn that when they hear those **Discussion Starters**, it is time to start class and engage their brain!

- **Getting Carded:** This strategy, designed by Bristol,[4] helps students learn crucial facts and develop a personal learning resource. Students are coached to write these facts and information on cards and connect them with a metal ring. Students carry the deck of cards from class to clinical to lab, providing a mechanism for study and easy reference. Part of class preparation may be to have students make these cards, answer questions that can serve as cards, or check these cards to complete other exercises. Card content may include lab norms, vital sign values, decision trees or algorithms, terminology, mnemonics, assessment criteria, mini concept maps, and other useful information.

- **When You Think of This, Think of That:** Preparatory work provides the foundation for class work. This matching exercise assists students in learning terminology and basic facts so that they then can apply this information in class.

- **All Things Being Equal:** This strategy provides several signs and/or symptoms, laboratory values, or other data and students are asked to select the one they are the most "concerned" about. This exercise can assist students to prioritize information both within an assessment for a single patient or for many patients. This can reinforce information prior to and after class applications.

Class Strategies

- **Use the Book:** Students benefit from seeing that instructors **Use the Book** in the classroom. It is believed that students see higher value in the readings, and perhaps complete them more, when the class preparation lecture and the active learning in the class are based on information in their text. Using pictures, charts, and test questions from the book in the preparatory lecture, while also using questions as **In Class Test Questions** during discussion, may prove valuable. Textbooks may have exercises, case studies, and quizzes that can be used during class to further reinforce information.

- **Keep 'Em Awake Quizzes, Quickie Quizzes, Quizzes That Count: Keep 'Em Awake Quizzes** are questions asked during class to increase attentiveness and reinforce material. These questions usually don't count toward a grade. **Quickie Quizzes** are done at the beginning of class and do not count. They are simply designed to open up the class and prime the students for learning. **Quizzes That Count** may be done in the learning management system prior to class, with paper and pencil in class, or after class as an **Email Exercise** or entered in the learning management system. They may also serve as **Admit Tickets** or **Exit Tickets**. Another quiz mechanism is the **Progressive Quiz**. While they are in class, students are asked a question at intervals throughout and then submit their answers at the end of class. These quizzes ensure attendance throughout class while increasing attentiveness. **In Class Test Questions** may also be entered into a PowerPoint to reinforce content and test-taking strategies. Students may **Write Their Own Test Questions**, and selected questions may be used in class as examples.

- **Case Studies (Interspersed, Intro, Quickie, Continuing):** I encourage you to return to Chapter 5 to see all the ways case studies can be used in the classroom. Creating case studies to open up class, provide transitions between exercises, reinforce lecture and preparatory content, or merge several topics may prove useful here. Often we discuss diagnoses and issues as if they occur in isolation. Case studies that discuss a client with chronic obstructive pulmonary disease, glaucoma, heart failure, type 2 diabetes, and cellulitis of the right big toe assist students to establish priorities between problems in a single client, learn the interrelationships between diagnoses, and develop nursing interventions with the knowledge that complexities in this client's condition have significant physiological and psycho-emotional impacts.

- **Group Concept Mapping:** Concept mapping organizes information to allow better understanding of material. Completing this strategy in groups can encourage peer teaching, informed discussion, and practicing concepts in class while students are supervised and guided by the instructor. Mapping may be done on paper, on a tablet or computer, or on large or small dry-erase whiteboards. The whiteboards allow for trial-and-error concept mapping, discussion and revision, and group debriefing of concept maps.

- **Guided Discussion Groups: Guided Discussion Groups** provide specific guidelines to allow students to reinforce and use content learned during lectures and preparatory work. **Guided Discussion Groups** are structured to allow students to self-assess or assess others, analyze data, engage in group discussion, and develop a plan of care or a list of potential solutions. Chapter 8 provides guidelines for class participants' self-assessment of stress and resilience, interpretation of the stress resistance measurement, peer discussion, and developing a **One-Minute Care Plan** with their peers to assist in dealing with stress. You may also use **Think-Pair-Share** to reinforce the care plan, and other strategies can guide each class discussion time. Although these discussions may take some time to prepare, they may be adapted for other classes and used several times in one semester. They may also be used semester after semester with minor tweaks to ensure currency. **FYI: Classroom Questioning** can be used to assess learning and to provide the spaced retrieval so important for learning and retention.

- **Student-Led Seminars:** Many flipped classroom models include an individual or group presentation component. In **Student-Led Seminars**, students are assigned to explore the care of a client with a problem, issue, disorder, or diagnosis. Students are graded, in part, on the creative nature of the presentation. Developing a skit, creating a newspaper or newsletter to elaborate on the care of a client, interviewing someone in front of the class with the disorder, collecting the health history of a client through the use of an actor or standardized patient, developing an exercise to allow students to meet class objectives, making a YouTube video, or cooking food that highlights aspects of care all augment other presentation components.

- **One-Minute Class:** Class presentations may be limited to (around) one minute to ensure that students include only critical components. These may reflect an ah-ha idea about the care of a client and may also be operationalized via the **Ah-Ha Journal**.

- **Short Clips:** Providing short clips of videos or videos from **YouTube** in class provides appealing ways to demonstrate signs and symptoms, show psychomotor skills in action, attend to the affective realm of nursing care, and entice learners to consider the human aspects of nursing practice. Remember the value of thinking questions wherein you ask students objective-driven questions prior to watching the clip to give students an idea of what to watch for in the clip. Then discuss those questions after the clip to reinforce class objectives.

- **Current Events:** Consider current issues in the news, on social media, or in healthcare research that align with class objectives. Briefly summarizing these at the beginning of class or when relevant to class content can reinforce key concepts. Providing **Research Moments** may assist students to see the importance of evidence-based practices and its relevance to clinical issues.

- **In-Class Applications: In-Class Applications** apply concepts as they were learned in preparatory work. Exercises designed to expand on learned concepts and then to be applied immediately to a real-world exercise may be used to reinforce key concepts and focus study efforts. Exercises such as **Pause for Priority Setting/What's the Big Deal/What Would You Do?, Imagine/ Remember When, Same Information, Invented Dialogs,** and **Admit/Exit Ticket** may be used to provide diversity in your teaching methods and offer fun and effective ways to reinforce preparatory work. Invented dialogs may provide a more acceptable way to manage a role-play exercise. Consider this strategy when using with safety-oriented communication strategies identified by the Agency for Healthcare Research and Quality, including SBAR, CUS, and Check Back.[14] Have these **Invented Dialogs** simulate the clinical environment and address the clinical conditions or concepts addressed in the preparatory work and In Class topics. See Table 13–1 for definitions of these concepts.

Table 13–1. **SBAR, CUS, and Check Back**

SBAR	Used to develop and refine handoff or interprofessional communication	Situation: A statement of what is happening right now that needs attention. Background: Puts the situation into context, clarifies the circumstances that have led to this situation. Assessment: Conveys thoughts about the situation. Recommendation: Explains what should be done, indicating when and by whom.
CUS	Used to raise safety concerns; each statement indicates a higher level of concern	C: I am concerned. U: I am uncomfortable. S: I think this is a safety issue (if no action, move up chain of command for help).
Check back	Used to clarify communication	Repeat a healthcare provider's prescription, request, or other clinical information to be sure message was received as intended.

Source: Adapted from Agency for Healthcare Research and Quality (AHRQ), https://www.ahrq.gov/ 2018.

- **Group Thought Exercises:** Group exercises are pillars of the flipped classroom. Consider group exercises to vary the methods in class, and use the principles discussed in this book for selecting and managing groups. Group discussion of case studies and completion of **Worksheets** or other exercises allow for discourse and learning the perspectives of others. **Group Tests** provide mechanisms for students to reach consensus on the correct answer, discover why the incorrect answers are wrong, and share thought processes among group members. Other interactive methods in class, like **Think-Pair-Share** and **Teaching Trios**, can offer additional changes in class configuration. Group exercises like the **Six Hats Exercise, In-Basket Exercise, In Class Debate, Gaming,** and **Jigsaw** are optimal to implement in the flipped classroom. Review these methods as presented in this text for further details and then mold them to make them work in your classroom.
- **Creative Lab Skills:** Simulations both in the lab and in the classroom are also critical elements of class activities. Integration of clinical simulations into didactic content ensures contextual learning and repetition of content from a variety of modalities. These simulations may be followed with **Group Thought Exercises** like briefings, huddles, and debriefings as identified by the Agency for Healthcare Research and Quality to ensure safe communication and group learning.[14] Table 13–2 defines these concepts, which may be adapted for didactic content, specific simulations, and class topics or focus areas.

Table 13–2.   Briefings, Huddles, and Debriefing

Briefings	To plan care	What is the most important thing this patient needs? What are the safety issues? What are the benchmarks and/or evidence for the care interventions?
Huddles	Problem-solve or clarify strategy; get everyone on the same page	What is the priority? What else could it be? What was done well? What could be done differently?
Debriefing	Review and feedback	What was done well? What did not go well? What could be done differently?

Source: Adapted from Agency for Healthcare Research and Quality (AHRQ), https://www.ahrq.gov/ 2018.

After Class Strategies

- **Ah-Ha Journals:** As discussed previously, these scripted journals give students the opportunity to consider ah-ha events and describe them. They then debrief in the journal about the contributing factors, emotions, and contextual factors related to the event, and then they come to some conclusions about this event and how lessons learned may affect future nursing practice. **Ah-Ha Journals** may explore what it is like to live a **Day in the Life of the Patient With. . . .** In this exercise, students examine how a day is spent with alterations in concepts or illnesses. For example, a journal may be submitted discussing living with type 1 diabetes. How the client spends the day, including meeting her or his personal and professional needs while checking blood sugar levels; planning diet; exercising; administering insulin; and dealing with daily stressors, illness, and care, would be a great learning experience. Students may also engage in **Reflective Journaling,** where they reflect and debrief on content presented in class. Perhaps they compare and contrast clients from the classroom discussion as they relate to clients encountered in clinical. Debriefing after simulations can then be compared to classroom case studies and submitted in the After Class period as a **Reflective Journal**. Another journal may include **Imagine When** or **Remember When** exercises. Either the students can imagine what it would be like to deal with a diagnosis, condition, or threat to a concept, or they can contemplate a time when they dealt with stressors similar to those discussed in class. Providing opportunities to explore client issues may foster empathy and caring in personal nursing practice.
- **Muddiest Part** or **Muddiest Point:** These exercises are key to identifying students' misconceptions and areas of confusion. With this information, you can design further learning experiences to assist students. These experiences may include directed readings, videos, exercises, and test questions to allow students to revisit and reinforce information.
- **Email Exercises:** Following your class, whether via email or as an assignment in your learning management system, have students consider questions posed in class or posted in the class web platform. Students may also write test items, as in **Write Your Own Test Questions**, because I believe that writing test questions is actually a great study strategy. These exercises can sometimes be graded and count as a quiz grade. At other times,

they may serve to simply reinforce material without an accompanying grade. These may be done individually, in pairs, or in groups and may assist in focusing study efforts. Make sure these assignments focus on study objectives and future evaluation via testing.

- **Case Studies (Unfolding, Reverse, Case Management):**
  Consider the value of After Class activities, such as case studies, to reinforce learned concepts. Use these case studies to reinforce client concepts and conditions, or merge them to add contextual factors affecting clinical judgment. For instance, have the case study include discussed topics and add other factors, such as environmental, social, or individual traits, that may offer a new twist to problem solving.

- **Writing exercises** may offer chances to continue learning and appeal to kinesthetic learners. Have students develop a **Legal Cheat Sheet** based on preparatory work and class reinforcements. These sheets serve as study guides and assist students in establishing learning priorities while exploring class content on a different plane. As discussed in Chapter 12, the **Clinical Quick Write** may appear in many versions and allows students to describe clinical experiences and reflect on how those experiences may be viewed when placed in the class context. These may be one-word or one-sentence descriptions of the clinical comparison experience or a letter written to a real or fictional client, or they may focus on what differences were detected when applying classroom learning to the clinical picture. **Write to Learn** exercises may be sent via email to students, may be assignments in the learning management system, or may be assigned in class as **Admit Tickets** and due the subsequent class meeting. Students may be asked to assess the **Muddiest Part**, build on classroom case studies with additional twists and turns in care as assigned by instructors, or answer higher-level questions related to case studies. See Box 13–4 for examples of higher-level questions.

Answers to these questions may be submitted as **Admit Tickets** or as **Email Exercises**, or they may be used as **Discussion Starters** for subsequent classes and or to provide segue between previous and subsequent classes. Have students do a written SBAR (see Table 13–1) and submit it as a writing assignment. Bristol[4] suggests that the first SBAR could be "SBAR Your Car." The students use the SBAR framework to discuss an issue with their car as the initial introduction to the SBAR format, its components, and the critical nature of this information. Then they can

> Box 13–4.
> ## Higher-Level Questions
>
> - What complications do you anticipate?
> - What additional data do you need to care for this client?
> - What equipment do you need to provide care for this client?
> - What isolation precautions are warranted?
> - What needs do you foresee for this client at discharge?
> - What issues could be addressed by a case manager in coordinating this client's care?
> - What other healthcare professionals will be integral in coordinating this client's care?
> - What challenges might this client encounter in the future?

move on to more complex, clinical written SBAR assignments once they master the format. Finally, a **One-Minute Care Plan** may be written and submitted about the contents of previous classes, thus allowing students to gather or organize nursing assessments, analyze data from classes, establish client outcomes, develop nursing interventions, and anticipate evaluation criteria. This **One-Minute Care Plan** may also be taken to clinical or the simulation lab should the opportunity be available for direct application of content.

CONCLUSION

Flipped classrooms increase the workload for students and educators as they design and complete exercises and learning strategies discussed in this chapter. Evidence is favorable, however, about the value of the flipped classroom and the assets of this method in educating clinical professions for problem solving, clinical judgment, and real-world application of knowledge. Use the strategies in this chapter to develop this rich learning environment and continue to explore others throughout the text.

References
1. Bergmann J and Sams A: Flip your classroom: Reach every student in every class every day. International Society for Technology in Education, 2012.
2. Green R and Schlairet MC: Moving toward heutagogical learning: Illuminating undergraduate nursing students' experiences in a flipped classroom. Nurse Education Today, 49: 122–128, 2017.
3. Schlairet M, Green RD, Benton M: The flipped classroom: Strategies for an undergraduate nursing course. Nurse Educator, 39(6): 321–325, 2014.
4. Bristol T: Flipping the classroom. Teaching and Learning in Nursing, 9: 43–46, 2014.
5. Barbour C and Schuessler JB: A preliminary framework to guide implementation of the flipped classroom method in nursing education. Nursing Education in Practice, 34: 36–42, 2019.
6. Harrington SA, Bosch MV, Schoofs N, et al. Quantitative outcomes for nursing students in the flipped classroom. Nursing Education Perspectives, 36(3): 179–181, 2015.
7. Telford M and Senior E: Healthcare students' experiences when integrating e-learning and flipped classroom instructional approaches. British Journal of Nursing, 26(11): 617–622, 2017.
8. Berg A, Ibrahim H, Magaster S, et al. Flipping over the flipped classroom. Contemporary Issues in Communication Science and Disorders, 42: 16–25, 2015.
9. Chen F, Lui A, and Martinelli SM: A systematic review of the effectiveness of flipped classrooms in medical education. Medical Education in Review, 51: 585–597, 2017.

10. El-Banna MM, Whitlow M, and McNelis AM: Flipping the classroom: Accelerated Bachelor of Science in Nursing students' satisfaction and achievement. Nursing Education Today, 56: 41–46, 2017.

11. Njie-Carr V, Ludeman E, Lee MC, et al. An integrative review of flipped classroom teaching models in nursing education. Journal of Professional Nursing, 33(2): 133–144, 2016.

12. Betihavas V, Bridgman H, Kornhaber R, et al. The evidence for "flipping out": A systematic review of the flipped classroom in nursing education. Nursing Education Today, 38: 15–21, 2016.

13. Dehghanzadeh S and Jafaraghaee F: Comparing the effects of traditional lecture and flipped classroom on nursing students' critical thinking disposition: A quasi-experimental study. Nurse Education Today, 71: 151–156, 2018.

14. Agency for Healthcare Research and Quality. Pocket Guide for TeamSTEPPS. Accessed from https://www.ahrq.gov/teamstepps/index.html, 2018.

Chapter 14

Creative Strategies for Technology and Online and Distance Education

"Teaching Digital Natives proposes that educators focus on verbs (essential skills) and nouns (tools to learn skills). Teachers own the verbs; students own the nouns."—Marc Prensky[1]

Challenges

- Instructors have inherent talents, biases, and desires to use technology in their teaching. Depending on the teaching assignment and learning objectives, the most integral tool in teaching is the teachers themselves. Technology allows us to reach more students, personalize the teaching environment, organize the teaching experience, and integrate new methods. With support, teachers can grow and learn how to use these methods to enhance their personal style and impact.[2,6,11,14]

- Our students also have varied experiences with technology. Some are those digital natives who have always lived in a socially connected world. Others are digital immigrants and find themselves learning both the process and content of what we teach.[1–2,7] As with varied learning styles, teachers must design experiences that meet all of these needs. This is a real challenge!

- The capacities and "cooperation" of the technology differ on campuses, in regions, and even in classrooms and other settings. Many of us have taught a class when the computer doesn't "cooperate," the internet doesn't work, or that great video doesn't play. As with all teaching, the key is to have an alternate plan and be flexible about meeting needs in other ways while focusing on student outcomes.

- Technology is ever-evolving. This in an area where we as educators should continue to grow and capitalize on our resources—those in information technology, computer manufacturers, and our peers—to be the best teachers we can be.
- Individuals across the technology-skills continuum may find websites, information, and "facts" in print on the internet all considered "truth." As educators, we need to teach critical consumer skills; the need for valid, evidence-based science; and the plethora of false or less-then-accurate information available to us through the internet on seemingly credible websites and on social media. Like research consumerism, internet usage for professional purposes must be deliberate and questioning. Here is where creative teaching strategies may prove useful.

As in most aspects of our lives, technology is having an impact on teaching and learning and is changing our methods, capacities, and daily operations. Technology is no longer an elective component of the teaching environment; it is an integral component to ensure that our students learn clinical judgment and critical thinking for a technology-based world. Skiba, in 2018, conducted a survey of students that revealed that they *want* instructors to use more technology in the classroom.[2] In contrast, faculty members' self-efficacy and confidence, along with the supports needed, are less known.[3] Not only is technology an effective way to integrate and convey information, it is also an imperative as nursing students launch into an information-rich, technology-based healthcare world. Myriad studies reflect the successes and challenges associated with e-learning, online teaching, and the use of technology.[4–16]

For our purposes, we will address digital teaching and learning from four perspectives: engaging students in e-learning to prepare for class, using technology and e-learning in the traditional classroom, using technology in online and distance education, and interfacing with technology and informatics in the clinical arena. We also polled educators about their use of creative strategies in the classroom and in clinical and online education; these will be noted throughout this chapter. These technologies may also be used in laboratory settings, although I will not discuss the high-fidelity mannequins or digital technology available to support labs and simulation. Nonetheless, many of the strategies discussed thus far have practical applications in the lab setting.

There are certainly generational aspects to the use of technology. We know that many of our instructors and some of our learners are digital immigrants for whom technology was introduced after learning foundations had been established; for them, using technology adds some burden because they have to both learn the process of using technology and attend to the content to be learned. A digital immigrant often learns from written text, whether from books, writing themselves, or other print media (remember the blackboard?). Learning was focused on single, goal-directed tasks in which there was a finite, but adequate, set of resources to be consulted and synthesized (perhaps you remember the household encyclopedia). Learning was sequential, organized, and based on a tangible and embraceable array of information.

In contrast, some of our learners, if not most, and many educators are digital natives. Digital natives learn through multimedia resources and are able to multi-task during the learning experience. Although much literature has been devoted to the assets and challenges of multi-tasking and the propensity for multi-tasking to yield mediocre results in all areas upon which an individual focuses their attention, we do believe that digital natives are better able than ever to focus and attend to multiple sets of stimuli. In addition, digital natives have had the internet at their fingertips for most of their learning years. The Web provides an almost limitless source of information that allows for parallel thinking; attending to several tasks at once; seeking information from multiple resources; using simultaneous sources of media concurrently; and mining information to extract priorities, current truths, and validity.[1]

Within this limitless world, nursing instructors can and should function with and use technology. Our learners have vast capacities for learning and growing. Our responsibility is to teach the art and science of nursing within this technology-based world of information. We should teach students to be critical consumers; focus on the outcomes of safety and patient-focused care; maintain caring in an era of technological advances; and use technology as a tool to better care, not distract from that care. Here, technology, or e-learning, intersects with creative teaching strategies. This chapter retrieves strategies from throughout the book, provides some new ones, and puts them in the context of e-learning or technology preparing for and in the traditional classroom, in online and distance education, and in the clinical arena. As with other chapters, this one begins with some of the challenges posed by technology and e-learning and then focuses on the strategies discussed throughout the book and how to mold or implement them in these environments.

IDEAS

Engaging Students in e-Learning to Prepare for Class

Student preparation for class is a much discussed and agonized-over issue in nursing education. Providing meaningful and useful assignments for students to ensure that they are prepared to attend to and comprehend class material is just part of the issue. Educators are cautioned that the grading of these types of assignments, especially if designed for every class meeting, may be labor- and time-intensive. Instructors must judiciously create these assignments to ensure that they do not exceed their personal grading burden. Experienced educators have suggested strategies such as random checking of assignment completion, having students peer-grade their assignments, or making assignments pass-fail based simply on assignment completion. Herrman and Waterhouse discussed the assets of an undergraduate teaching assistant program to provide for grading of these more simplistic assignments through the use of well-designed rubrics.[17] Again, educators need to ensure that they are making good use of their time. Nonetheless, preparation prior to class increases learning through spaced retrieval, repetition, and active engagement. Here are some strategies to foster effective preparation skills, provide valuable incentives to students, and stimulate preclass curiosity to see the foundation for subsequent learning experiences.

- **Electronic Admit Ticket:** Students submit the response to a faculty-driven query via email, via text, or in the learning management system (LMS). Students must do this assignment prior to class as a way to prepare for class. As discussed previously, the responses may be in the form of answers to questions, answers to items about case studies, a **Worksheet,** the writing of a test question, or exploration of a previous class's **Muddiest Part.** Educators may post a test question and ask students to create the right answer and three distractors as part of the **Electronic Admit Ticket.** Instructors review these prior to class and generate class discussion based on these preparatory assignments.
- **Electronic Quizzing:** Frequent quizzing is an important component of learning and retrieval practice. Many LMSs and software packages provide mechanisms to conduct preclass

quizzing of students. Also commonly used to ensure preparation for simulations and lab exercises, **Electronic Quizzing** ensures that students meet a certain level of mastery prior to receiving credit for assignment completion. Educators may also make up their own quizzes to be administered via the LMS prior to class.

- **Student Puzzle Creation:** Several websites provide the means for students to develop crossword and other puzzles about class content. One I have used is www.puzzle-maker.com/CW/. Building on this, students may also develop quizzes and surveys with or without software. Students may use tools such as Survey Monkey to assist with writing and disseminating surveys. These puzzles, quizzes, and surveys may be exchanged among students for completion prior to class. Students are accountable for both the creation of and the completion of a puzzle, quiz, or survey prior to class.

- **Preclass/Preclinical Case Studies:** These assignments are discussed more completely in previous chapters of this book. They may be adapted through the use of technology to be submitted electronically to the LMS for tracking and grading. Completion of these case studies prior to class or clinical ensures that students have a strong foundation in class to build on basic concepts, explore nursing care, and understand real-life circumstances, such as comorbidities, social determinants, or condition deterioration or exacerbations. Ensure that high-level questions, such as those listed below, are included in these case studies:
  - **What additional data do you need?**
  - **What precautions are indicated?**
  - **What interventions do you anticipate?**
  - **What complications and issues do you anticipate?**
  - **What teaching issues do you anticipate?**
  - **What web-based resources might be helpful in the care of this client?**

- **Email/Learning Management System (LMS) Assignments:** As noted previously, email and LMS assignments charge students with answering questions prior to discussing the material in class. These questions may be somewhat brief and may pertain to a specific component in class that is more complex or may have proved to be a **Muddiest Part** in the past. Again, grading may be simplified by making these assignments pass-fail. It is important to discuss these aspects in class and ensure that critical components are in line with class objectives and appear on tests or evaluations, thus helping students understand priorities of care.

Technology and e-Learning in the Classroom

You, as an educator, need to assess your classroom when using technology and e-learning in this environment. Does every student have a device in class? Is it the same device? Instruction methods may need to be adapted because some students use their smartphones, while others use tablets or laptops. It is important to consider that technology use in the classroom is more than just using PowerPoint. It is using social media, the internet, simulation, videos, smartphones, and other devices to introduce and access information while assisting students to learn, analyze, synthesize, and prioritize information. As noted by Benner and colleagues, we need to "step out from behind the screen full of slides and engage students in clinic-like learning experiences" (p. 14).[18] Here are some strategies to assist you:

- **Apps in the Classroom:** Many students are aware of the capacities of their smartphones and use them to aid in learning. Others may benefit from instruction. Apps to record class, develop quizzes based on learning needs, search information, and provide circumscribed information (about drugs, lab studies, or diagnostics) may be useful. Bristol[19] explored the use of apps in clinical nursing education, including using them for audio recording teaching sessions, access to e-books, feedback and grading, clinical reference tools, communication tools, and prevention services. Apps may also be used in providing client care and education; tracking health practices such as exercise, nutrition, and education; raising awareness about diseases and conditions; and even in reminding clients and healthcare professionals when to use the restroom (RunPee)!

- **In-Class Test Questions:** Using PowerPoint to present test questions in class allows students to test their own knowledge and offers the opportunity for instructors to assess the students' level of knowledge. It also provides students with valuable information about your test items. Using application and analysis level questions in class ensures that students understand the need to use higher-order thinking as they are studying. Providing examples of your style of questions in class prepares them for the level and type of questions on the exam. Using the animation function in PowerPoint with arrows and exclamation points provides a little reward for students getting the right answer and helps you assess the percentage of students that may need more information or tools for learning. Phone polling websites or clickers may also be used to pose questions to the class and assess the group's level of understanding. Try www.Polleverywhere.com, www.Socrative .com, or https://create.kahoot.it/for some ideas. (*Note:* Minutes, charges, or data usage may apply.)

- **Short Clips:** We previously discussed the value of showing clips from popular movies, commercials, or YouTube as a means to cultivate thought and engage learners. These may be referenced in the LMS and used as part of the class discussion in online learning experiences, or they may be using during live class along with other reflection exercises (**Quick Write, Think-Pair-Share, Imagine/Remember When,** and **Common and Different**) to reinforce connections to class objectives. The true value of **Short Clips** is the use of thinking questions to focus students on critical information.

- **YouTube Projects:** These assignments, implemented in a pharma-cology class, used YouTube videos as part of a group assignment.[20] Students were split into groups and assigned a class of medica-tions. Students developed videos to advertise or provide patient teaching appropriate to these medications. Students used sock puppets, animations, flip-book drawings, infomercials, music video, and television spoofs to relay information to their class-mates about this class of drugs. The finished products were shown in the class, and videos were graded on validity, creativity, and meeting assignment objectives.

- **Quick Write via Tablet/Device:** As you provide content, wheth-er during a lecture, mini-lecture, or class discussion, engage the learners by asking them to answer a question, identify a **Muddiest Part,** write a test question, or solve a problem using their phone or device. Tablets and handheld portable devices offer convenience, accessibility of apps, greater size of workspace than a phone, and portability for classroom and clinical environments.[21] Students may be charged with offering their own perspective, thoughts, or alternatives via this route. These can be shared via text, email, or the LMS. Students can share their **Quick Write** with a colleague to compare their thoughts. They also may be loaded to a cloud-based system for instructors to monitor an ongoing discussion. The **Quick Write** exercises attend to multiple senses and modes of learning, and implement the principles of repetition and reflection in learning.

- **Think-Pair-Share via a Tablet/Device:** This provides the means for students to think on their own and then pair with another stu-dent in the classroom to compare and contrast their thoughts and perspectives with each other. Writing or texting it into a phone or device may increase personal engagement in the exercise and ensure that all students really think about the subject of the exercise. This approach may also be more acceptable to some students than the traditional way of writing down answers and thoughts on paper.

- **Classroom Simulations: Classroom Simulations** are gaining popularity as instructors haul mannequin, supplies, and equipment into class. Walters and colleagues noted that students' knowledge levels and perceptions of satisfaction with the learning experience were increased following **Classroom Simulations.**[22] These are generally considered low-fidelity simulations, based on the classroom environment, but with experience they may become more reality based. Tables are transformed to stretchers or beds, PowerPoint presentations become the electronic health record, and students are guided to engage in the simulation in a variety of ways. Sources indicate that voice-over PowerPoint may provide the client's history and use several voices to depict the client, nurse, and family member in obtaining a health history or course of events. When this client backstory ends, patient care begins. Then, you can show the slides with the medication administration record, the vital signs, results of diagnostic tests, healthcare provider prescriptions, and other relevant information. Some instructors implement classroom simulations by having one group of students in the front of the room engaging in the simulation while others watch. Others conduct several simulations around the room or rotate students through a simulation as different events occur. Students may engage in creative strategies during the simulation to maintain attentiveness, including developing a situation, background, assessment, recommendation (SBAR) or handoff report of the events in the simulation; completing a provided **Worksheet;** writing a narrative note about the simulation; completing drug calculations; interpreting cardiac rhythm strips; establishing priorities; or engaging in **Think-Pair-Share** with colleagues. Proponents of **Classroom Simulations** contend that this method replaces most lecture, instead providing active learning in real-time with mini-lectures or building on students' completion of preparatory work prior to class. Continued research about the use of virtual reality simulation, virtual reality software, the use of avatars in the classroom, and other technologies continues to emerge.[23,24]
- **Electronic In-Basket Exercise:** As discussed, this exercise challenges students to solve a problem with only the information provided in the introduction to the exercise. Although discussed previously, let me share with you an exercise I presented in class:

You are part of a group of four nursing students on your way up in the elevator to your clinical experience. On the elevator with you is a woman who appears to be pregnant. The woman appears to be uncomfortable. Suddenly, the elevator stops. The voice of the security guard announces to you that you will be stuck on the elevator for 24 hours. In the next instant, the woman gasps and it seems that her water has broken. She doubles over and begins to yell and moan loudly. She holds her abdomen, looks at you in fear, and says "I think I am in labor." The security guard announces that they will be able to lower plastic grocery bags full of supplies down to you: One for the four students and one for the woman. In three minutes, the security guard will call you back for your list. You have enough oxygen, heat, light, and space to be comfortable.

Students work together to make up this list. You can add to the challenge by saying that, instead of as many items that will fit in the bag, you are now only allowed three items for the young woman and three items for your peers. This exercise is great at establishing priorities and may be adapted for any client situation. It may be adapted to incorporate technology by using tablets to record items, posting lists to the LMS for comparison, and using search engines to determine best practices and needed supplies. A recording of the woman's voice and her story may be taped and played for students to supplement the exercise. In this case, the gestation of the pregnancy, the potential for a multiple birth, whether the mother is a primipara or multipara, whether the woman received prenatal care, and pertinent facts of her health history may be valuable in assisting with the outcome of the exercise.

- **Same Information: Same Information** provides two different sets of information or two different perspectives to separate groups of students. Students must analyze the data they are given and determine a course of action. When students reconvene, they discover that the two groups received different amounts of information. This strategy is made even more valuable with the use of tablets or laptops. Students receiving different levels of information develop their plan of care and then switch with other students. Students compare and contrast their course of action, at some point realizing that the students had different information. The true value of this exercise is the realization of the power of comprehensive information and the need to always ask "Why?" when attempting to trudge through difficult situations. This strategy is most effective when implemented the first time and loses its element of surprise if used again.

- **Case Studies With Technology:** I encourage you to peruse previous discussions of case studies in this book. Consider for yourself: "How can I incorporate technology into this assignment?" "How does electronic assignment completion ease my grading burden, cut down on paper waste, and meet the digital natives' learning styles?" **Quick Writes, Think-Pair-Share, e-Journaling,** and other assignments can be adapted for use with technology and thus create e-learning adaptations of traditional assignments and teaching approaches.

Technology and e-Learning in Online and Distance Education

Online education and distance modes have become quite prevalent in nursing education, especially at the graduate level and for baccalaureate programs for current registered nurses. Schools, programs, and individuals implement these learning experiences in numerous and highly effective ways. Our survey respondents discussed several tools that assisted with organizing and implementing online education. See Table 14–1 for ideas.

One major difference between online and traditional learning is whether classes, lectures, group work, or experiences are synchronous or asynchronous. In the asynchronous mode, these experiences are prepared and delivered for use at the students' discretion. This provides flexibility for both the students and instructors, and the learning experiences are enriched by multiple exercises designed to broaden the learning environment. In the synchronous environment, all the students sign on for the learning experience at the same time and meet as a large community. This allows for "in-time" questions and answers but reduces the convenience and flexibility for learners. Discussion sessions, along with lectures, mini-lectures, and students' presentations, may occur in the synchronous or asynchronous modes. Courses may also be totally online or a hybrid of several learning platforms and modalities.

Online courses may breed feelings of isolation among the students and perhaps the instructors. This is where creative strategies may be most needed for instructors and students to build a sense of community, engage in interactions, and respect the needs and priorities of all involved in the online experience.[14,25]

- **Guided Discussion Groups:** The reader is encouraged to review this strategy earlier in this book. This mechanism is perhaps most common among distance educators and generally reflects a very deliberate and designed learning experience for students. Readings and internet searches provide a foundation for mini-lectures, videos, and presentations. Scripted exercises that are carefully

Table 14–1.　Online Teaching Resources

Name	Purpose	URL
Live Binder	To organize materials and portfolios	www.livebinders.com
Moovly	To create videos	www.moovly.com/
Nearpod	To engage technology in the classroom and among devices	https://nearpod.com/
Shadowhealth	To provide web-based, digital clinical experiences	https://shadowhealth.com/
Goose Chase	To create scavenger hunts	www.goosechase.com/
iHuman	To provide virtual simulations for medical education	www.i-human.com/
Smartphone polling sites	To provide classroom polling	https://create.kahoot.it/ www.Polleverywhere.com www.Socrative.com
WebQuests	To provide tools to create and implement WebQuests	http://zunal.com/ www.kn.pacbell.com/wired/fil/ http://questgarden.com
Puzzle Maker	To create puzzles and crossword puzzles	www.puzzle-maker.com/CW/
vSim	To provide virtual simulations and scenarios	http://nursingeducation.lww.com/our-solutions/clinical-simulation/vsim-for-nursing.html
Journey Cloud	To provide access to cloud-based journaling	https://journey.cloud
Bubbl	To provide concept and mind map development	www.bubbl.us

constructed from class objectives work together to further ensure that students meet those objectives. Evaluative mechanisms assess learning. Online teaching provides the forum for discussion groups, postings, chats, and peer- and/or instructor-reviewed discussion. Students are evaluated on a minimum number of posts that are rich, meaningful, and reflect knowledge and thought. Students interact with one another and develop a sense of community through these online forums. Following the principles of **Guided Discussion Groups** ensures adhering to the rules of netiquette, individual learning and growth, and group collaboration in this media-based community. Social media and other internet-based resources may further expand the capacities of these strategies.

- **Evidence-Based Practice Searches/The Great Confession:** This exercise, adapted from Bristol and Zerwekh,[26] has the students email or write a letter to a client's daughter or son. The students may be assigned a client with a specific condition, alteration in a concept, or issue. In this letter, the student explains why they have not accessed evidenced-based information in the last 30 days, the possible impact of this decision, and what they will do to remedy this situation. Students are challenged to consider the value of evidence-based practice from the client perspective while also investigating potentially valuable websites for the client's needs. This may also be implemented in the clinical area where students write this letter about a client for whom they provided care.

- **Imagine/Remember When:** In this exercise, students are charged to **Imagine** a situation from the client's perspective. They use mental imagery to consider what it would be like to be going through what a client is experiencing. With **Remember When,** students are asked to remember a time during which they were confronted with a difficult, painful, or stressful experience. These exercises are adapted to technology by having students text or email reflections or enter them into the LMS. Here is a fun **Imagine** exercise I have instructors do during conferences. Instructors **Imagine** what is going on in the student's head and then text or email their responses to me (if you have students text to you, make sure you have enough data).

You are a nursing student on your first day of clinical. You have never worked in a hospital before and have been to visit someone in a hospital only twice in your life. You'd rather be at the nurse's station looking at the computer chart than go in and greet your patient. And what's wrong with that? You need to get information for your paper. Why is it so important to go meet your patient?

In class, we then discuss how we as nursing instructors could address this situation and how to best meet the needs of the student while ensuring safe and diligent patient care. In the distance environment, students post their perceptions to the group discussion board and comment on each other's responses, potentially incorporating best practices and evidence from the literature.

- **Telehealth SBAR:** In this strategy, students are introduced to the concept of SBAR while playing the role of a telehealth nurse. Students are given a client situation that meets the class objectives. Then students develop an SBAR to hand off information to another healthcare professional while in the role of the telehealth nurse. Video technology may replicate telehealth capacities and students must deliver a succinct and relevant handoff while ensuring that information is individualized for the current client.

- **Eight Slides in Eight Minutes:** One conference participant told me about this creative method. Students are charged with a topic and to develop an eight-slide presentation that takes eight minutes to present. Students prepare the voice-over PowerPoint or use another recording mechanism and upload to the common class site for the rest of the class to use. Exam questions may be taken directly from these presentations. The eight-minute limit ensures that presentations include only priority information and attend to the anticipated attention spans of our learners. Presentations are graded on the ability to delineate priority information and on the quality of the presentation.

- **Google Docs Unfolding Cases:** The **Unfolding Cases** (and other case studies noted in this book) provide a great mechanism for exploring the nursing process, complex client situations, and the relationship of circumstances and context in interpreting client issues. The ability to use **Google Docs** or another common workspace platform allows students to collaborate on a case study from any location. I have used this strategy to provide group learning for students who may never actually meet in person. You load the case study into the platform and direct students to work on this one document to build on the case study. As an educator, you need to establish ground rules, such as:
  - Always save when you exit the platform (if this is not automatic)
  - Never erase someone else's post but build on it
  - If a student feels someone has gone down a "slippery path" with his or her suggested course of action, other students can suggest other assessments, diagnostics, or interventions.

- Ensure that netiquette is adhered to by all members of the group
- Clarify grading—is it on the final product in the form of a group grade or is each group member assigned an individual grade?
- Ensure that there is a reflection component to the project so that students are able to select other courses of action, discuss the group process, and reflect on the exercise.

- **Short Clips:** We previously discussed the value of showing clips from popular movies, commercials, and YouTube as a means of cultivating thought and engaging learners. These may be referenced in the LMS and used as part of the class discussion in online learning experiences along with other reflection exercises (**Quick Write, Think-Pair-Share, Imagine/Remember When,** or **Common and Different**) to reinforce connections to class objectives.

- **Think-Pair-Share:** This may be done with distance classes. Students are provided an assignment to consider and then email each other to discuss the answers. Instructors are carbon-copied on these emails but do not interact or reply. The students think about the issue independently, pair up, and share with each other. Instructors can peruse these emails and comment on them on the common class discussion board or during class sessions, whether synchronous or asynchronous. This exercise may prove valuable as instructors assess class learning, explore the **Muddiest Parts,** or determine the "pulse" of the class. Students may also use **Common and Different** in this strategy to address class discussion topics.

Technology and e-Learning in the Clinical Area

Technology is part of the healthcare arena, and our teaching is augmented by our ability to use the technology in those agencies and by using e-learning exercises to assist learning. Perhaps one of the greatest tools is the electronic health record (EHR), which provides a learning platform for nursing care, knowledge about documentation, and integration of informatics into our teaching. Educators discuss how they incorporate the EHR in their students' clinical education[27] and the use of mobile technology in clinical teaching.[28] In addition, the incorporation of artificial intelligence, large amounts of data, and advances in healthcare make this even more of a complex a world for students and novice and experienced nurses to function professionally, critically, and with full awareness.[29] Instructors are cautioned to ensure that students remember principles of confidentiality, privacy, and respect and the need to adhere to principles of HIPAA and agency policy while learning in the clinical arena.

- **Pass the Problem via Tablets:** In this strategy, students input the basic history of their client, in two or three sentences, and the concept, client need, nursing diagnosis, medical diagnosis, or challenge they are addressing. Students then pass each of their tablets around the table to their fellow clinical group members. Each member is asked to add to the plan of care; address the challenge; or provide information, questions, assessments, or other data related to the concept or need. The tablets are passed to the entire group, and each passing requires that the information is saved. By the time **Pass the Problem** has been completed, students have suggestions for care or further topics to research from many perspectives and are able to launch into care of their client. This may also provide a springboard for their working on their care plans or their **Electronic One-Minute Care Plan** (which follows).

- **Electronic One-Minute Care Plan:** This strategy, using tablets or laptop computers, has students develop brief and focused plans of care to guide clinical experiences. Readers are welcome to see previous references to this strategy and adapt it to an electronic format. The document can be created as a form with type-in screens that students complete on their devices. This may be a working document that is carried throughout clinical and added to during and after care. The **Electronic One-Minute Care Plan** is then submitted as a written assignment via the LMS, or it may be downloaded and printed to be handed in as a hard copy. Key to this strategy is the ongoing nature of the document that evolves as client care and condition change and interventions are implemented and evaluated. These can also be discussed in preconference and postconference and can provide the context for **Clinical Ah-Ha's, One Minute Classes,** and rich discussion about clients and care.

- **Online or e-Group Concept Mapping:** Concept mapping exercises are replete in the literature and are noted throughout this text. This strategy is easily adapted to electronic means and may be shared among several users via a website; LMS; or a social media, class-specific site. There are many software packages (some are free and others must be purchased) that allow students to develop concept maps and focus on the components of the concept map rather than the artwork (try www.bubbl.us). They focus their efforts on the components and the relationships of these components by plugging them into software packages that build the concept map.

- **Homeward Bound SBAR:** This creative strategy has students develop an SBAR (see previous references in this book) for a client who is about to be discharged. Students may provide an electronic handoff to home care nurses and/or others in the interprofessional team using the SBAR format. It may also be used to provide transfer information to an accepting facility. The SBAR or other handoff format may be augmented to provide a comprehensive transfer summary to another agency. For example, an electronic report may be provided for a postoperative client following a hip replacement who is being transferred to a rehabilitation facility. Students may anticipate postoperative needs, including positioning, toileting, transferring, pain management, patient preferences, facts about the patient's history and hospital course, and incorporation and adaptation of activities of daily living. This is a great exercise in building skills in discharge planning and case management.

- **Ah-Ha Journals/e- or Cloud-Journaling/Social Media Posting:** Journals are valuable learning resources and are discussed frequently throughout this book. They promote reflection and deep thinking. One instructor responding to our survey discussed the use of journals for students to reflect on lessons and responses after listening to a TED Talk. These journals may be emailed, uploaded to the LMS, or posted to a class-specific social media site. There are also cloud-based journaling sites that I have used (you may want to review https://journey.cloud/). Some have the capacity to review these as a third party and evaluate the journals after students text their journals to the free cloud-based site. Instructors can provide feedback via the LMS and assess students' abilities to self-evaluate in this student-friendly journaling method.

- **Computer Scavenger Hunts:** Some clinical agencies have developed training hospitals that mirror the agency EHRs. Educators may develop a scavenger hunt with items for students to search for in this training platform. For example, students may seek, find, and review laboratory data, videos of surgical procedures or wound care, selected aspects of the client history, and other data. This exercise is quite valuable, as are all **Scavenger Hunts,** to alleviate some of the mystery of documentation and finding components of the EHR. If this mechanism is not available, you may also seek out commercially prepared documentation/health record products to help alleviate some student angst about documentation and agency-specific nuances about charting. In addition, the website Goose Chase (www.goosechase.com/) was cited by one of our survey respondents as a nimble resource in creating scavenger hunts of all kinds.

- **Create a Client in the EHR:** With the training platform noted above or the commercial products available, students may benefit from developing a client within the EHR. Much like the **Reverse Case Study** discussed previously, students are given limited information and then develop a client within the training or commercial record. Instructors may stipulate which details are to be developed, including past medical history; allergies; social, family, environmental, and developmental details; assessments; medications; laboratory studies and diagnostics; collaborative interventions; potential and actual complications; teaching needs; nursing implications; and other components. Student assignments are evaluated on alignment of EHR components, soundness of information, breadth and evidence of research into client details, evidence of clinical judgment, and creativity. A reverse of this procedure could be implemented in the **EHR Case Study.** Instructors develop the case study, and students search a simulated patient's record for information. Then students operationalize critical thinking and priority-setting skills as they complete case study exercises.

- **Evidence-Based Practice Search/Smartphones in Clinical:** Much controversy exists related to smartphones in the clinical area. Some clinical agencies have strict policies about the personal use of smartphones by staff members and students in the clinical area. Others allow them with restrictions on the use of some sites or social media sites. Some agencies limit smartphone use to facility-owned smartphones with controlled accessibility to apps and the internet. Many nursing professional groups established social media policies, and schools of nursing have responded in kind to the potential for smartphone misuse by students and personnel. Clinical instructors are encouraged to instruct students on the proper use of smartphones, if they are allowed, in the clinical arena and provide guidance about how they may be used to search for answers to clinical questions, research evidence-based practices, and seek resources to teach clients since tablets and mobile phones may prove valuable patient education resources.[28,30] Also, students may be able to search instructional websites, access e-textbooks, watch instructional videos, and then sign on to the LMS to enhance their ability to provide client care.

- Instructors answering our survey discussed the use of **WebQuests,** wherein students search the internet for information and answers to questions (see www.webquest.org). **WebQuests** are web-based tasks using instructor-made web pages where students search the internet for answers and evidence-based practices, and learn to discriminate valid information within the realm of knowledge of nursing and other sciences. These exercises are thought to stimulation higher-order thinking and problem solving, encourage interactive engagement, and build communication and patient interaction skills.[31]

CONCLUSION

We have discussed several strategies to augment e-learning and technology in the nursing classroom, online and in distance education, and in the clinical arena. To reiterate previous discussions of student assessment, I want to close with a reminder that many of the strategies in this text may be adapted for electronic use and may augment your ability to evaluate student learning in the classroom, clinical, and e-learning experiences. Some suggestions include:

- **Pause for Priority Setting/Prioritization Power**
- **In-Class Test Questions/Polling/Clickers**
- **Electronic Exit Ticket**
- **Progressive Quiz**
- **Group Testing**

You can review these in previous chapters of this book.

I wish you well in your incorporation of technology into your teaching repertoire!

References
1. Prensky M. Digital natives, digital immigrants. On the Horizon 9(5): 1–6, 2001.
2. Skiba D. Student and faculty views of technology and academic success. Nursing Education Perspectives 39(2): 126–127, 2018.
3. Roney L, Westrick SJ, Acri MC, et al. Technology use and technological self-efficacy among undergraduate nursing faculty. Nursing Education Perspectives 38(3): 113–118, 2017.

4. Breytenbach C, Ham-Baloyi W, and Jordan PJ. An integrative literature review of evidence-based teaching strategies for nurse educators. Nursing Education Perspective 38(4): 193–197, 2017.

5. Lahti M, Kontio R, Pitkanen A, et al. Knowledge transfer from an e-learning course to clinical practice. Nurse Education Today 34: 842–847, 2014.

6. Koch LF. The nursing educator's role in e-learning: A literature review. Nurse Education Today 34: 1382–1387, 2014.

7. Lahti M, Hatonen H, and Valimaki M. Impact of e-learning on nurses' and student nurses' knowledge, skills, and satisfaction: A systematic review and meta-analysis. International Journal of Nursing Studies 51: 136–149, 2014.

8. Abdelaziz M, Samel SS, Karem O, et al. Evaluation of e-learning program versus traditional lecture instruction for undergraduate nursing students in a faculty of nursing. Teaching and Learning in Nursing 6: 50–58, 2011.

9. Sung YH, Kwon IG, and Ryu E. Blended learning on medication administration for new nurses: Integration of e-learning and face-to-face instruction in the classroom. Nurse Education Today 28: 943–952, 2008.

10. Voutilainen A, Saaranen T, and Surmunen M. Conventional vs. e-learning in nursing education: A systematic review and meta-analysis. Nurse Education Today 50: 97–103, 2017.

11. Fiedler R, Giddens J, and North S. Faculty experience of a technological innovation in nursing education. Nursing Education Perspectives 35(6): 387–391, 2014.

12. Wolf A and Peyre SE. Student satisfaction with blackboard-style videos. Nursing Education Perspectives 39(4): 244–246, 2018.

13. Blum CA. Does Podcast use enhance critical thinking in nursing education? Nursing Education Perspectives 39(2): 91–93, 2018.

14. Broussard L and Wilson K. Nursing faculty attitudes and practices related to online teaching. Nursing Education Perspectives 39(1): 40–42, 2018.

15. Hara CYN, Aredes NDA, Fonseca LMM, et al. Clinical case in digital technology for nursing students' learning: An integrative review. Nurse Education Today 38: 119–125, 2016.

16. Perfetto L. Preparing the nurse of the future: Emergent themes in online RN-BSN education. Nursing Education Perspectives 40(1): 18–24, 2019.

17. Herrman JW and Waterhouse J. Benefits of using undergraduate teaching assistants throughout a baccalaureate nursing curriculum. Journal of Nursing Education 49(2): 72–77, 2010.

18. Benner P, Sutphen M, Leonard V, et al. Educating nurses: A call for radical transformation. Jossey-Bass, 2010.

19. Bristol T. Nursing school? There's an app for that! Teaching and Learning in Nursing 9: 203–206, 2014.

20. Zamora Z, Sarpy N, and Kittipha P. Using YouTube in teaching pharmacology to nursing students. Nursing Education Perspectives 38(4): 218–219, 2017.

21. Bristol T. Tablets in nursing education. Teaching and Learning in Nursing 8: 164–167, 2013.

22. Walters B, Potetz J, and Fedesco H. Simulations in the classroom: An innovative active learning experience. Clinical Simulation in Nursing 13: 609–615, 2017.
23. Farra SL, Smith SJ, and Ulrich DL. The student experience with varying immersion levels of virtual reality simulation. Nursing Education Perspectives 39(2): 99–101, 2018.
24. Miller M and Jensen R: Avatars in nursing: An integrative review. Nurse Educator 39(1): 38–41, 2014.
25. Bristol T. Building community in the online course. Teaching and Learning in Nursing 14: 72–74, 2019.
26. Bristol TJ and Zerwekh J. Essentials of e-Learning for nurse educators. Davis, 2011.
27. Baxter PM and Andrew LA Successful integration of an academic electronic health record into the curriculum of an Associate Degree nursing program, Nursing Education Perspectives 39(4): 250–251, 2018.
28. Mackay BJ, Anderson J, and Harding T. Mobile technology in clinical teaching. Nurse Education in Practice 22: 1–6, 2017.
29. Skiba DJ. The invisible health care professional: Exploring the intersection of data, devices, and artificial intelligence. Nursing Education Perspectives 39(4): 264–265, 2018.
30. Day-Black C. Minorities in nursing education: Using smartphones. The ABNF Journal 26(4): 85–89, 2015.
31. Leibold N and Schwarz LM. WebQuests in family nursing education: The learner's perspective. International Journal of Nursing 1(1): 39–47, 2014.

Chapter 15
Conclusion

GENERAL HINTS FOR USING CREATIVE STRATEGIES

Start Slowly

This book is full of ideas that you can add to your personal teaching style and the content of your class. Always use creative strategies in moderation. The class that's barraged with too many strategies and innovative methods will experience "creativity fatigue." One to three strategies per class or session is probably enough to introduce the concept of collaborative learning.

Small doses of creative strategy will also keep you from forcing uncomfortable learning styles on your students. This caution is especially important for students accustomed to passive learning styles and noninteractive teaching. Your students may need time to get comfortable with their own involvement and their need to participate actively in the teaching-learning process. If students are reluctant to transform their own learning practices, you can choose some of the more personal and less collaborative teaching strategies, such as those that involve personal introspection and writing. By beginning with less threatening strategies, you may eventually progress to more active ones. Remember to use any kind of strategy sparingly to keep methods innovative and fun.

Active learning methods can be difficult to introduce into a nursing curriculum. Students used to academic settings may prefer a passive, spoon-feeding approach to learning. "Just tell

"Teaching was the hardest work I have ever done, and it remains the hardest work I have done to date."—Ann Richards

"My joy in learning is partly that it enables me to teach."—Seneca

me what's on the test" is the motto for some of these students. Professional nursing groups may be fatigued and regard class time as a reprieve from the demands of client care. They may prefer listening to participating in a creative strategy. Again, choose your strategies judiciously and add them sparingly.

More Ideas for Groups

Nurse learners may or may not be responsive to working in groups. One of the biggest hurdles in such work is to assign the groups initially. If your class time is limited, you may choose to establish the groups in advance. This approach gives you a chance to split up cliques and ensure the same skill and experience level in each group. Also, students who don't know each other are spared the embarrassment of grouping themselves. You can often facilitate small-group work simply by using seat placement in the room. See **Group Thought** for more hints on group work.

Set the Rules

Not only do creative teaching strategies stimulate learning, they also engender activity, excitement, and discussion. At the outset, you need to establish ground rules that specify how to carry out each strategy, the time frame for each activity, and your expectations for student participation and behavior. You'll need signals to initiate creative strategies and to indicate a return to more traditional methods, which call for quiet listening. Some instructors use a whistle or some other sound to signal transitions. You must also allow time for transitions between strategies. Some spontaneous conversation and activity during the transitions is to be expected.

Not all strategies will be well received or embraced by every student. Learning style, generation, cultural norms, and personality traits all influence a student's response to teaching strategies. Encourage total participation, but respect your students by trying to make your teaching comfortable for all of them.

Develop Your Style

Make sure you are knowledgeable and well versed in the content before you integrate creative teaching strategies. The first time you present a topic may not be the time to implement elaborate strategies. Creative teaching strategies often stimulate deep thinking and inquiring minds. Students immersed in innovative and engaging strategies may think of really difficult questions. Instructors need to be well informed on the topic and also willing to admit that they don't know something. Allow time to search for answers and for class deliberation; this approach recognizes the breadth of knowledge related to nursing and healthcare and the need to know how to find answers. It may also provide a good opportunity for assessing the quality of internet resources and the need to be a discriminating consumer.

Until you feel really comfortable, engage students by using one or two simple collaborative strategies. Focus on delivering organized content that your students can understand. Subsequent teaching will provide more opportunities to use creative methods.

Most important, as you add strategies to your teaching portfolio, you'll develop a teaching style unique to your personality. You must be comfortable with your methods to convey an active learning message to the class. Use the strategies in this book as a springboard to creating new and different teaching methods. Students should have fun with creative strategies, and you should, too. If teaching becomes laborious, it's time to reenergize yourself by assessing your methods and possibly revising your strategies.

MAKE LEARNING FUN

Humor needs to be funny—obviously. As a teacher, you carry the burden of making sure that everybody can laugh at your humor. It must be politically correct, without offensive words or connotations, culturally appropriate, and generally understandable to the class. If you aren't sure whether something is offensive, don't use it. Chances are that you'll offend someone if you do.

Humor changes the pace in a teaching session, reinforces ideas, promotes retention, and puts content on a human plane. When class content is fun to learn and to teach, your students get the idea that you like to teach and are excited to be doing so.

ADVANTAGES AND DISADVANTAGES OF CREATIVE STRATEGIES

The major advantage of creative teaching strategies is the ability to reel in the students and get them to enjoy learning. An instructor can best reach a student by combining creativity, teaching skills, and knowledge of the content. Creative strategies facilitate transitions from one topic to another and appeal to diverse learning styles. They help students connect their knowledge with their experience, encourage lasting retention of material, and stimulate discussion and reflection. But keep your mind on the class objectives. Never let humor derail you from your purpose: great teaching and sharing knowledge to elevate nursing practice!

Creative strategies have their disadvantages. You take a risk with each method: it may work well or it may "crash and burn." Planning and preparation time may be significant. Also, creative strategies can drain the class time needed to cover content.

Some students may prefer more passive learning methods. Others may not connect the purpose of the exercise with the class content. They may misconstrue information, not appreciate its significance, or neglect to apply lessons from the exercise to their theoretical knowledge base and nursing practice. Some students may regard creative strategies as unprofessional or childish, unrelated to the knowledge they need to function as professional nurses.

Your greatest challenge may be the time and effort required to change your teaching habits and launch your students outside their comfort zone. You as the instructor have the choice of using as many creative strategies as you feel comfortable with. You're not trying to overhaul your entire way of teaching, just to spice it up a little. That's the beauty of this book. It's up to you whether to employ one or 100 strategies in your years as a teacher.

FINDING THE "TEACHING FUEL"

You will be able to find teaching fuel (motivation) in some of the most unexpected places. Quotations and stories may come from social media, the internet, magazines, books, calendars, email, quotation anthologies, or colleagues. Ideas will come to you in the shower, at a stoplight, while you are perusing one of your news sites, when you are binge-watching your favorite show, or when you're falling asleep at night. Anything thought-provoking, funny, or relevant, or any **Ah-Ha Journal** is potential class material.

When looking for teaching fuel, keep your professionalism in mind. Remember the key rules of borrowing from others: adhere to fair use laws and cite known sources to give credit where it's due. Seek strategies in unlikely places and share them with others.

GUIDELINES FOR POWERPOINT

PowerPoint has changed the way we teach, especially in the lecture format. It lets teachers connect with the internet during a lecture, linking to websites, YouTube and other online resources. We all know a picture is worth a thousand words. Scanning in photographs, drawings, charts, and other graphics from articles or textbooks helps us appeal to the visual learner. We can also incorporate movie clips, YouTube videos, clip art, and animation. Downloading songs and subject-specific sounds, such as heart and breath sounds, provides a valuable experience for the whole class and especially for auditory learners.

Using PowerPoint, we can download handouts from a remote source or through web-based educational platforms. Handout formats vary (one, two, three, four, six, or nine slides per page), so you can choose the ones you prefer. Blank formats save printer ink and download time. Many campuses are "green," as our many of today's learners, and all handouts are accessed electronically, sent via email, or posted on learning management systems (LMSs). The use of computer and LCD technology provides audiovisual materials that many students can access simultaneously. This method, which is usually reliable, frees students from the burden of taking copious notes. Slide-based notes appeal especially to auditory learners, who can focus on listening rather than writing furiously and perhaps not taking in the material.

A PowerPoint presentation helps you steer the course of your class, keep the lecture on track, and maintain the pace. It can guide both you and your students by highlighting key areas within the class content. In contrast, PowerPoint must be used judiciously and with some caution. The class or lecture is only as good as the instructor. No amount of fancy graphics will compensate for a teacher who doesn't know the subject well. PowerPoint is an instructional tool, not a crutch to get teachers through unfamiliar material. Here are some hints to make PowerPoint an even more effective tool in your teaching portfolio:

- Make sure you use at least a 24-point font on your slides.
- Use a single font throughout a presentation. For emphasis, use upper- and lowercase letters, bold type, underlining, shading, and italics.
- Use the custom animation function to focus on key words. Animation can be used at the beginning or end of a presentation or to emphasize a word at any point. You can change settings to vary any available effects, including animation and the prompt to start it. Be careful not to overuse this function.
- Slide transition animation, used when you advance to the next slide, offers interesting formats. Use the random transition setting for a different type of transition with each slide.
- Use dark backgrounds with light lettering for larger classes. Experiment with different slide designs and color schemes to find what works best with specific class content.

- Don't use too many slides. As a general rule, you should lecture at least 1 to 2 minutes for every slide. For complex or technical topics, one slide every 4 to 5 minutes may be the guideline to use in your lecture.
- When writing a class lecture, use caution if you're making the slides concurrently. The temptation is to write all the lecture content on the slide. Instead, use the Note Page function for your lecture; the actual slides include only integral information.
- Slides should include prompts and bullet lists of ideas, not every fact discussed in class. The general rule is to limit a slide to six bullet points, with no more than six words per bullet. Include graphics and animation to increase interest (discussed above). Keep students actively engaged by leaving blanks in the slides for them to fill in during the presentation.
- For some students, PowerPoint handouts have replaced in-class note taking. Encourage your students to take notes related to class discussions, their questions, or interesting points used to augment the slides. For students who have trouble knowing what to write, suggest that they take class notes in their usual way. Then have them incorporate the PowerPoint notes into their written notes after class. This revisiting of material is especially helpful for visual and kinesthetic learners. Make sure you leave blanks, have questions without answers, provide comments outside the outline format, or include only some of the information on your slides. Although it is not always popular with students, they need to actively engage by attending class, listening attentively, and taking notes on information. If we give students all of the information, some students will choose to study only the slides, may not attend class, or may be passive in class. Make deliberate decisions about your slides while preparing your classes to enhance active learning.
- Control the pace of your class. Allow for questions and pauses by not using automatic timing for slide transitions.
- Don't forget that a well-informed, experienced, and engaging teacher is worth far more than an elaborate slide presentation. The value of teacher-student interchange, class discussion, and class attendance cannot be overemphasized.

EVALUATE YOUR STRATEGIES

We need a research foundation to support evidence-based nursing education. In the early years of nursing research, interest focused on how nurses learned and how to enhance learning. As research priorities became more focused on the client outcomes, funding for and emphasis on nursing education research diminished. Now the earlier interest has been renewed. The emphasis is on developing a better understanding of what works in nursing education and on carrying evidence-based nursing focus from the practice setting into the nursing educational arena.

Readers are charged with conducting evaluative research as they use the creative strategies found in this book. Much of the evidence so far is anecdotal, based on instructor and student satisfaction with a teaching method. The strategies in this book have all succeeded and appear intuitively to have a positive impact on learning. Some have been studied, but only a few have undergone rigorous research to determine their true value.

Most educational research includes small studies of students' responses to classroom innovations, pre- and post-intervention knowledge assessments, and retrospective measures associated with nursing program completion and NCLEX® success. To validate the infusion of new strategies into traditional methods, we need designs that go beyond personal satisfaction or individual perceptions of learning. Solid research designs, including quasi-experimental studies with equivalent control and treatment groups, may best determine the effectiveness of creative teaching methods.

SOME WORDS ABOUT MOTIVATION

An appropriate way to close this book is with a common saying and a not-so-common addition to that phrase. In this book, I've tried to capture the art of innovative teaching. All of these creative strategies are intended to motivate learners and learning.

The old adage contends that "You can lead a horse to water, but you can't make it drink." This phrase has been expanded: "but you can feed it salty oats to make it thirsty" (Figure 15–1).

I hope the creative teaching strategies in this book will stimulate your students' thirst for knowledge and skills. I wish you well as you continue to teach and to enhance learning in today's and tomorrow's nursing professionals.

Fig. 15–1. You can lead a horse to water, but you can't make it drink.

Strategy Locator

Strategy	Chapter
Active Reading Conference	7
Admit Ticket	8
Ah-Ha Journal	7
All Things Being Equal	5
Apps in the Classroom	14
Assess Your Own Learning Style	10
Assessing the Learner	10
Author Guidelines	9
Basics of Maternity Case Study	10
Be Prepared	4
Bring in the Reinforcements [and] In-class Applications	5
Bring on the Evidence	9
A Brush With Fame	4
"Call Bell" Examination Questions	10
Campus or Unit Research and Nurse Interviews	9
Case Management Case Studies	10
Case Studies:	5
Quickie	
Preclass/Preclinical	
Interspersed	
Continuing	
Unfolding	
Reverse	
Case Studies With Technology	14
Classroom Simulations	14
Clinical Application of Findings to Case Studies	9
Clinical Area Questioning—Research at Work	9
Clinical Decision-Making Exercises	6
Clinical Didactic Connect	12
Clinical Huddle	12
Clinical Judgement Exercise	12
Clinical Preceptorships or Clinical Capstones	11
Clinical Puzzle	12
Clinical Questioning	7
Clinical Quick Write	7

Strategy	Chapter
Common and Different	4
Community-Based Concepts/Teaching About Poverty	12
Compare and Contrast Write to Learn	12
Computer Scavenger Hunt	14
Condensed Portfolios	6
Cooperative Strategies	7
Create a Client in the EHR	14
Creative Lab Skills	7
Critical Thinking Exercises (CTEs)	4
Current Events	5
Day in the Life of a Client With	8
Debate	10
Delegation Exercise	10
Developmental Jeopardy	6
Discussion Starters	4
Documentation Case Study	7
Dress-up or Skits	4
Eight Slides in Eight Minutes	14
Electronic Admit Ticket	14
Electronic In-Basket Exercise	14
Electronic One-Minute Care Plan	14
Electronic Quizzing	14
Email Exercises	6
End-of-Life Case Studies	10
Engaging Students in e-Learning to Prepare for Class	14
e-Journaling	10
e-Portfolios	10
Equipment Conference	7
Evidence-Based Practices	10
Evidence-Based Practice Searches	14
Faculty Research Sharing	9
Feedback Lecture	5
Field Trips	7
Film Clips in Clinical	7
Film Clips in Nursing Research	9
Find the Error	10
FYI—Classroom Questioning	8
Gaming	6

Strategy	Chapter
Get in Line	4
Getting Carded	12
Google Docs Unfolding Cases	14
Grand Rounds	7
Group Concept Mapping	8
Group Research Critique	9
Group Tests	6
Group Thought	5
Guided Discussion Groups	8
Homeward Bound SBAR	14
How Do You Pick Your Shampoo?	9
Imagine [and] Remember When	6
Incident Report Exercise	10
In-Basket Exercise	6
In-Class Debate	8
In-Class Test Questions	6
Informatics	10
In the Know	9
Introduce Each Other	4
Invented Dialogues	8
Issues in Measurement	9
It Starts With the Syllabus	11
Jigsaw	6
Keep 'em Awake Quizzes	5
Learning Carts	8
Learning Contracts	6
Learning from Each Other:	7
Peer Teaching	
Peer Team Leadership	
Legal Cheat Sheets	8
Let's Be Real in Clinical	7
Let's Discuss	4
Market Research—Cookies, Candy, and the	
Research Process	9
Mock Studies	9
Mock Trials	8
Muddiest Part	6
My Biggest Challenge	4

Strategy	Chapter
NCLEX® Integrated Processes	10
Nurse Interviews	10
Nurse Practice Act Write to Learn	10
Nuts and Bolts	8
One-Minute Care Plan	7
One-Minute Class	7
Online Discussion Groups	6
Online or e-Group Concept Mapping	14
Out of the Hat	8
Pain Continuing Case Study	10
Paper Towel Ideas	9
Pass the Problem	7
Pass the Problem via Tablets	14
Pass the Stick	8
Past Experiences With	4
Patient/Family-Centered Care	10
Patient Safety Goals Clinical Assignment	12
Perioperative Care Case Study	10
Pharmacology Compare and Contrast	12
Pharmacology Critical Thinking Exercises	10
Pharmacology Field Trips	10
Poster Sessions	9
Preclinical Case Studies	11
Progressive Quizzes	10
Psychosocial Case Studies	10
Put It All Together	8
Quality Improvement	10
Quick Write via Tablet/Device	14
Quickie Quizzes	5
Quiz About Me	4
Quizzes That Count	5
Quotation Pauses	5
Read a Story	5
Reality Check	6
Reflective Journaling	11
Reliability and Validity Darts	9
Research Concept Maps	9
Research Corners—Electronic or Bulletin Board	9

Strategy	Chapter
Research Moments in Every Class	9
Rhyming Puzzlers	6
The Right Thing to Do	6
Safety	10
Same Information	8
Scavenger Hunts	7
Self-Learning Mini-Modules	6
Self-test: How Creative Are You?	4
Set the Stage	4
Setting Priorities	4
Shapes Define Your Personality	4
Short Clips	5
Six Hats Exercise	6
Skits (see Dress-up)	4
Speak UP	5
Starting With Games, Puzzles, and Brain Teasers	4
Student-Led Seminars	6
Student Puzzle Creation	14
Take-Home Quiz on NCSBN Web site	10
Teamwork and Collaboration	10
Teaching Tools	8
Teaching Trios	8
Telehealth SBAR	14
Tell 'Em Once, Tell 'Em Twice, Tell 'Em Again!	4
The Right Thing To Do	6
Think-Pair-Share	8
Think-Pair-Share via a Tablet/Device	14
Titanic 2.0	10
Twosies	6
Two Truths and a Lie	10
Use the Book	5
Use the Book in Clinical	7
Use the Star	5
Using Greeting Cards, Cartoons, and Pictures	4
Using Mnemonics	5
Using Toys, Prizes, and Props	4
V-8 Conference	7
War Stories and Clinical Anecdotes	8

Strategy	Chapter
Web Assignments	6
WebQuests	14
What Not To Do or Find the Error	10
What's the Big Deal and How Is It Treated?	10
What's the Point? or What's the Big Deal?	6
When You Think of This, Think of That	5
Why Are You Here?	4
"Why Are You in Nursing?" and Other Mysteries	4
Worksheets	5
Write to Learn	8
Write Your Own Test Questions	10
YouTube Projects	14

INDEX

Note: Illustrations are indicated by *(f)*; tables by *(t)*; boxes by *(b)*.

A

Active learning strategies, overview of, 1, 7, 357–358, 379
Active Reading Conference, 190, 193–194, 264, 329, 335
Activity Carousel, 377*(b)*
Actors, in clinical education, 189
Admit Ticket, 235–237, 359–360
   "Call Bell" Examination Questions, 313
   Current Events, 91
   delegation exercise, 311
   Feedback Lecture, 110
   flipped classroom, 377*(b)*, 379, 382, 384, 387
   FYI—Classroom Questioning, 271
   Games, Puzzles, and Brain Teasers, 46
   Guided Discussion Groups, 257
   In-Class Test Questions, 147, 236
   Invented Dialogues, 254
   It Starts With a Syllabus, 344
   In the Know, 294
   Muddiest Part, 144, 237
   online or distance education strategies, 394
   Pharmacology Field Trip, 326
   Preclass Case Studies, 74, 319
   quality improvement topics, 336
   Self-Learning Mini-Module, 162
   Web Assignments, 158
   writing own test questions, 301
Ah-Ha Journals, 29, 185–188, 187*(b)*
   on basic care and comfort, 329
   on caring, 333
   on Clinical Decision-Making Exercises, 141
   concept-based curriculum strategies, 365–366
   on Condensed Portfolios, 167
   on Day in the Life of a Client with . . ., 250, 252
   on e-Journaling, 338
   on Field Trips, 209, 326, 335
   on Film Clips in Clinical, 214
   on Film Clips in Nursing Research, 287
   flipped classroom, 383, 386
   on Grand Rounds, 196
   group-experienced (V-8 Conference), 197
   on In-Basket Exercises, 116
   on Let's Be Real in Clinical, 220
   on Mock Studies, 280
   on Muddiest Part, 144
   on One-Minute Care Plan, 184–185
   on Online Discussion Groups, 164
   on Out of the Hat, 258
   on patient/family-centered care, 334
   on quality improvement, 336
   on reflective journaling, 352
   technology and e-learning, 405, 406
   on War Stories and Clinical Anecdotes, 245
All Things Being Equal, 86–88, 87*(b)*, 325–326, 360, 381
Alternate-item practice, 302–303
Analytical learning, 249, 301
Anecdotes, clinical, 182, 243–245, 349–350
Applications of Findings, 337
Apps in the classroom, 396
Armchair Shopper, 143
As Good as It Gets (film), 215*(t)*
Assessment, 341–354
   assigning and grading written work, 348
   classroom, 343–346
   clinical, 172, 346–350
   end of program, 350–351
   of instruction, 416–417
   learning style and, 352
   newer trends in, 352–353
   student self-assessment, 351–352
   summative, 342
Assisted suicide, 222–223, 223*(b)*
Attention-grabbing, in large classrooms, 66–67
Auditory learning, 24–25, 249, 301
Author Guidelines, 296–297
Awakenings (film), 68, 215*(t)*

B

Baby boomers (1946-1964), 16
A Bag of Knees (film), 215*(t)*
Basic care and comfort, 328–329
Basics of Maternity Case Study, 317–318
A Beautiful Mind (film), 67, 68, 215*(t)*
Bedside Reports, 334
Bells and whistles, as teaching tool, 45
Be Prepared, 60–62, 320–321
Blended classroom. *See* Flipped classrooms
Blender, as teaching tool, 44
Blueprinting exams, 345
Board games, 121
Bob and Jack: A Boy and His Yak (Moss), 69
Brain
    hemisphere dominance, 25, 249, 301
    learning and memory, 23–25
Brainstorming, 249, 249*(b)*
Brain Teasers, 44, 45–46, 45*(b)*, 46*(b)*, 129
Briefings
    flipped classroom, 385, 385*(b)*
Bring in the Reinforcements, 91–95, 92*(b)*
Bring on the Evidence, 264, 294–295, 337
A Brush With Fame, 35–36
Bubbles, as teaching tool, 44–45
Build a Patient, 80–81
Bulletin boards, 285–286, 287

C

Calibration, 29
"Call Bell" Examination Questions, 312–314
Campus or Unit Research, 291–293, 296, 337
Candy research, 274–275
Capstones, clinical, 350–351
Care and comfort, basic, 328–329
Care Plan, One-Minute, 182–185, 183*(b)*, 370
    flipped classroom, 383, 389
    Grand Rounds with, 196
    Guided Discussion Groups with, 257
    NCLEX® preparation with, 332
    Pass the Problem with, 177
    Preclinical case studies with, 347
    Put It All Together with, 267
    QSEN principles with, 334
Caring, 333
Cartoons, as icebreaker, 48–49

Case studies, 29
    Basics of Maternity Case Study, 317–318
    Case Management Case Studies, 308–310
    Clinical Applications of Findings, 282–284
    Clinical Decision-Making Exercises, 134–141
    Continuing Case Studies, 75–78, 322, 329, 361
    Documentation Case Study, 198–202, 262, 332, 338, 407
    EHR Case Study, 407
    Email Exercises, 73, 74, 78, 79, 319
    End of Life Case Studies, 318–321
    exemplar, 360–363
    flipped classroom, 380, 382, 387
    Interspersed Case Studies, 74–75, 365
    Jigsaw with, 134
    large classroom strategies for, 73–81
    Learning Carts with, 264
    mini-cases, 92–93
    for NCLEX®, 308–310
    online or distance education strategies, 73, 74, 78, 79, 395
    Pain Continuing Case Study, 329
    Pass the Stick with, 265
    perioperative care, 324–326
    Preclass Case Studies, 73–74, 319, 370, 380
    Preclinical Case Studies, 185, 347, 370, 395
    psychosocial, 321–324
    Quickie Case Studies, 71–73. 382
    Reverse Case Studies, 79–81, 185, 363, 368–369, 387, 407
    safety, 336
    Same Information, 228–231
    technology and e-learning, 400, 407
    Unfolding Case Studies, 78–79, 322–323, 324, 326, 328, 344, 361–362, 387, 403–404
    "What's the Big Deal?" with, 131
    worksheet use with, 84
Centennials, 18–19
Charting, 198–202
Cheat sheets, legal, 161, 259–260, 328
Check Back, flipped classroom, 384, 384*(b)*

Cherry Ames (book series), 69
Children's books, as large-classroom strategy, 68, 69
Civility in classroom, strategies for, 19–21
Classroom
  civility in, strategies for, 19–21
  as a component of clinical, 3
  rules, policies, and guidelines for, 20
Classroom assessment, 343–346
  See also Assessment
Clean and Sober (film), 215(*t*)
Clicker, 338, 344
Clinical Ah-Ha, technology and e-learning, 405
Clinical anecdotes, 182, 243–245, 349–350
Clinical application
  defined, 368
  strategies for, 368–370
Clinical Application of Findings, 282–284, 337
Clinical Area Questioning: Research at Work, 206, 264, 287–288, 337
Clinical assessment, 172, 346–350
Clinical capstones, 350–351
Clinical Decision-Making Exercises, 134–141, 235, 380
Clinical Didactic Connect, 361
Clinical education
  challenges in, 171–172
  student evaluation in, 172
Clinical-education strategies, 171–220
  Active Reading Conference, 193–194
  Ah-Ha Journals, 185–188, 187(*b*), 406
  Clinical Puzzle, 211–212
  Clinical Questioning, 202–204
  Clinical Quick Writes, 180–182
  Cloud-Journaling, 406
  Computer Scavenger Hunts, 406–407
  Cooperative Strategies, 177–180
  Create a Client in the EHR, 407
  Creative Lab Skills, 187–191
  Documentation Case Study, 198–202
  EHR Case Study, 407
  Equipment Conference, 191–193
  Evidence-Based Practice Search/ Smartphones, 407–408
  Field Trips, 206–209
  Film Clips in Clinical, 214(*b*), 215–218, 215(*t*)–217(*t*)
  Grand Rounds, 195–196
  Group Concept Mapping, Online, 405–406
  Homeward Bound SBAR, 406
  Learning From Each Other, 209–211
  Let's Be Real in Clinical, 218–220
  One-Minute Care Plan, 182–185, 183(*b*), 405
  One-Minute Class, 212–213
  Pass the Problem, 175–177, 176(*b*), 405
  Peer Teaching and Peer Team Leadership, 209–211
  Reverse Case Study, 407
  Scavenger Hunts, 172–175, 173(*b*)
  Social Media Posting, 406
  technology and e-learning in, 404–408
  Twosies, 130
  Use the Book in Clinical, 204–206
  V-8 Conference, 196–198
  WebQuests, 408
Clinical evaluation tools (CETs), 348–350
Clinical Huddle, 368
Clinical judgment, focus on, 2–3, 2(*f*)
Clinical Judgment Exercise, 365
Clinical preceptorships, 350–351
Clinical Puzzle, 211–212, 333, 335, 347, 370
Clinical Questioning, 202–204, 213, 270, 347, 349, 369
Clinical Quick Writes, 179, 180–182
  in class debates, 224
  concept-based curricula, 360
  in flipped classroom, 387
  on FYI—Classroom Questioning, 270
  on In-Class Debate, 224
  on Invented Dialogues, 254
  on Mock Trials, 262
  on Nuts and Bolts, 247
  on Out of the Hat, 259
  on patient/family-centered care, 334
  on Preclinical case studies, 347
  reflection and, 366–367
  on Think-Pair-Share, 235
  on War Stories and Clinical Anecdotes, 245
  on Write to Learn, 239
Clinical reasoning, Worksheets and, 364
Cloud-Journaling, 406
Collaborative testing, 345

Common and Different, 46–48, 47(b), 307, 397, 404
Communication, 332
Community-Based Concepts, 366
Compare and contrast
  definition, 363
  exercises, 28
  strategies for, 364–365
Computer Scavenger Hunt, 338, 406–407
Concept-based curricula
  challenges of, 355–356
  clinical application, 368–370
  compare and contrast, 363–365
  concepts, 358–360
  exemplars, 360–363
  overview of, 356–358
  reflection, 365–367
Concept maps
  Concept map quiz, 108
  flipped classroom, 382
  group, 178, 240–242, 241(f), 334
  research and, 242, 290–291, 337
  technology and e-learning, 405–406
Concepts, definition and strategies, 358–360
Condensed Portfolios, 166–167, 338
Conflict management
  Clinical Decision-Making Exercises, 134–141
  Cooperative Strategies, 177–180
  In-Basket exercises, 114–117
  Six Hats Exercise, 112–114, 113(b), 113(f), 114(b)
  Think-Pair-Share, 233
Confusion, in Muddiest Part, 143–144
Continuing Case Studies, 75–78, 322, 329, 361, 382
Contracts, learning, 164–166, 239
Cookies research, 274–275, 275(b)
Cooperative Strategies, 177–180, 334
Coordinator of Care (PN), 308–310
Copyrighted materials, as icebreakers, 48
"Counting off," for groups, 98
Create a Client in the EHR, 407
Creative Lab Skills, 187–191, 335, 385
Creative strategies
  advantages and disadvantages, 413–414
Creativity fatigue, 9–10
Creativity quiz (Self-test), 39–41
Critical Thinking Exercises (CTE), 51–53, 52(b)

in Clinical Quick Write, 181
in flipped classroom, 380
in Guided Discussion Groups, 257
in pharmacology, 327–328
in safety field trip, 335
in Think-Pair-Share, 235
Critique, group research, 281–282, 337
Culture, institutional, 6–7
Current Events, 89–91, 237, 293–294, 316, 336, 383–384
CUS, flipped classroom and, 384, 384(b)

D

Day in the Life of a Client With . . ., 179, 250–252, 324, 367, 386
Dead Poets Society (film), 215(t)
Debate, 364
Debates, In-Class, 222–224, 223(b)
  Bring on the Evidence with, 295
  NCLEX® preparation with, 335, 336
  Out of the Hat with, 259
  Pass the Stick with, 265
  team building with, 178, 335
  Write to Learn with, 239
Decision-making
  Clinical Decision-Making Exercises, 134–141, 235
  The Right Thing to Do, 117–121, 334, 336
  Same Information, 228–231, 257, 322, 334
Deck, Michele, 31, 35–36, 187
Deck of Events (game), 125
Deep learning, 357
Delegation
  exercise on, 311–312
  Nurse Practice Act Write to Learn on, 312
Developmental Jeopardy (game show), 121–123, 122(t)
Dialogues, invented, 92, 252–254, 314, 332
Digital immigrants and natives, 393
Digital teaching. *See* Distance education; Technology
Discussion
  Clinical Huddle, 368
  current events as springboard for, 89–91
  flipped classroom, 380–383, 387, 389

Group Concept Mapping, 369
icebreaker strategies for, 37–39, 63–64
Let's Be Real in Clinical, 218–220
Online Discussion Groups, 162–164
Student-Led Seminars, 159–161, 160(t)
technology and e-learning, 400–402
Discussion groups
challenges in, 221–222
participation in, 221
Discussion-group strategies, 221–272
Admit Ticket, 235–237
Day in the Life of a Client With . . .,
250–252
FYI—Classroom Questioning,
267–270, 267(b)
Group Concept Mapping, 240–242,
241(f)
Guided Discussion Groups, 255–258, 337
In-Class Debate, 222–224, 223(b)
Invented Dialogues, 252–254
Learning Charts, 262–264
Legal Cheat Sheets, 259–260
Mock Trials, 260–262
Nuts and Bolts, 245–248, 245(b),
246(b), 247(b)
Out of the Hat, 258–259
Pass the Stick, 264–265
Put It All Together, 265–267
Same Information, 228–231
Teaching Tools, 248–250, 249(b)
Teaching Trios, 224–228
Think-Pair-Share, 231–235, 232(b), 367
War Stories and Clinical Anecdotes,
243–245
Write to Learn, 237–240
Discussion Starters, 37–39, 63–64, 326,
380–381
Disruptive innovation, 6–7
Distance education
challenges of, 391–394
class preparation strategies, 394–395
technology and e-learning for,
400–404, 401(t)
See also Technology
Doctor Dan the Bandage Man
(Gaspard), 69
Documentation, 332
Documentation Case Study, 198–202,
262, 332, 338
Domains of Nursing Practice, 299, 308(b)
Dress-up or Skits, 53–55, 54(f), 267

E

EHR Case Study, 407
Eight Slides in Eight Minutes, 403
Einstein, Albert, 341
E-Journaling, 338, 400
Elaboration, 28–29
E-Learning. *See* Online education
Electronic Admit Ticket, 394
Electronic boards, 285–286, 287
Electronic health record (EHR),
404–405, 407
Electronic In-Basket Exercise, 398–399
Electronic One-Minute Care Plan, 405
Electronic Quizzing, 394–395
Email Exercises, 148–152, 338
in Clinical Decision-making
Exercises, 141
on Condensed Portfolios, 166
on Continuing Case Studies, 78
on Critical Thinking Exercises, 52
on Current Events, 91
on End of Life Case Studies, 319
on Feedback Lecture, 110
on Film Clips in Nursing Research, 287
flipped classroom, 382, 386–387
on FYI—Classroom Questioning, 270
on Guided Discussion Groups, 257
on Imagine/Remember When, 128
on In-Class Debate, 224
on Invented Dialogues, 253, 254
on Legal Cheat Sheets, 260
on Mock Studies, 280
on Mock Trials, 262
on Muddiest Part, 144
on Nuts and Bolts, 247
on Online Discussion Groups, 164
online or distance education
strategies, 395
on Pharmacology Field Trip, 326
on Preclass Case Studies, 74
on Quickie Case Studies, 73
on Remember When, 128
on Take Home Quiz, 303–305
on Think-Pair-Share, 235
on Unfolding Case Studies, 79
on Web Assignments, 157
Emotional connection to content, 28–29
Empathy
in classroom, 20
Day in the Life of a Client With . . .,
179, 250, 324, 367, 386

Empathy (*continued*)
Imagine, 125–128, 126*(b)*, 265, 320, 329, 333, 334
Remember When, 125–128, 127*(b)*, 333, 334
Same Information, 228–231
End of Life Case Studies, 318–321
End of program assessment, 350–351
E-portfolios, 338, 351
Equipment Conference, 191–193, 329, 335
Errors, safety and infection control, 314–317
Ethical issues
Clinical Application of Findings, 283–284
Clinical Quick Write, 181
End of Life Case Studies, 318
Guided Discussion Groups, 257
In-Class Debate, 222–224, 223*(b)*
Mock Trials, 260–262
The Right Thing to Do, 117–121
Six Hats Exercise, 112–114, 113*(b)*, 113*(f)*, 114*(b)*
Think-Pair-Share, 235
Evaluation, 341–354
assigning and grading written work, 348
challenges in, 341–342
classroom, 343–346
clinical, 172, 346–350
end of program, 350–351
formative, 342
of instruction, 416–417
learning style and, 352
newer trends in, 352–353
student self-assessment, 351–352
summative, 342
Evidence-based practice (EBP), 273–274, 294–295, 337, 402
Evidence-based practice (EBP) Search, 407–408
Exemplars
defined, 360–361
strategies for, 361–363
Exit Ticket, 236, 271
assessments and, 344
concept-based curriculum strategies, 359–360
electronic, 408
flipped classroom, 377*(b)*, 379, 382, 384, 387
Muddiest Part and, 144
See also Admit Ticket
Experiential learning, 171

F

Faculty Research Sharing, 289, 337
The Fall of Freddy the Leaf (Buscaglia), 69
Family-centered care, 334
Feedback
content of, 30
learning and, 27
Feedback Lecture, 108–110, 324
Fiction, as large-classroom strategy, 68–69
Field Trips, 206–209, 319–320, 326–327, 335
Films
Cooperative Strategies, 178
Film Clips in Clinical, 213–218, 214*(b)*, 215*(t)*–217*(t)*
Film Clips in Nursing Research, 286–287
NCLEX® preparation with, 320
Short Clips (large-classroom strategy), 66–68, 178, 320, 324, 359, 361
Final Simulation Experience, 351
Find the Error, 120, 315–317, 335
Fixed mindset, 29
Flashlight, as teaching tool, 43
Fleming, Alexander, 69
Flipped classrooms
After class strategies, 386–389, 388*(b)*
challenges of, 373–374
In class strategies, 381–385, 384*(t)*, 385*(t)*
concept-based curricula and, 358
implementation of, 374–376
outcomes of, 376–379
Preclass, In Class, and After Class phases, 376, 377*b*, 378*(b)*
Preclass strategies, 379–381
Formative evaluation, 342
Freaky Friday (film), 215*(t)*
Free, Kathleen Walsh, 124
Frustration, in Muddiest Part, 144
Funnel, as teaching tool, 43
FYI—Classroom Questioning, 267–270, 267*(b)*, 344, 383

G

Games, Puzzles, and Brain Teasers, 44, 45–46, 45*(b)*, 46*(b)*, 129, 335
Game shows, 121–123, 122*(t)*, 125, 271
Gaming
flipped classroom, 385
FYI—Classroom Questioning, 270–271

Legal Cheat Sheets, 260
small-class strategies, 121–125,
122(t), 124(b)
Generational differences, 16–19, 27, 393
Get in Line, 33–34
Getting Carded, 359
flipped classroom, 381
Global learning, 249, 301
Google Docs, 403–404
Goose Chase, 407
Grand Concept Rounds, 370
Grand Rounds, 179, 195–196
Day in the Life of a Client
with . . ., 251
NCLEX® preparation with, 333
Pass the Stick with, 266
patient/family-centered care with, 334
Put it All Together with, 266
Great Confession, 402
Greeting Cards, Cartoons, and Pictures,
48–49
Group Concept Mapping, 240–242,
241(f), 369
assigning and grading written work
with, 348
Cooperative strategies with, 178
flipped classroom, 382
Preclinical case studies with, 347
Put It All Together with, 267
teamwork with, 334
technology and e-learning, 405–406
Group Research Critique, 281–282, 337
Group Tests, 153–157
flipped classroom, 385
General Nursing Review, 153–154
It Starts With a Syllabus with, 344
Management of Care and Delegation,
154–157
NCLEX® preparation with, 157, 307,
316, 329
teamwork with, 334
Group Thought (group work),
97–103, 412
assigning and grading written work
for, 348
assigning groups for, 97–98
case study strategies with, 73
delegation exercise in, 311
End of Life Case Studies with, 319
Feedback Lecture with, 110
flipped classroom, 385

grouping ideas for, 98
Legal Cheat Sheets with, 260
perioperative care case study with, 324
psychosocial case studies with, 322
team building in, 178, 334
worksheet use with, 84
Growth mindset, 29–30
Guided Discussion Groups, 254,
255–258, 337, 338–339
flipped classroom, 380–381, 382–383
technology and e-learning, 400–402

H

Harry Potter (book), 128
Healthcare Associated Infections-
Partnering to Heal-interactive, online
simulation, 316
Healthcare equipment, as teaching tool, 44
Health promotion and maintenance,
317–321
Hemisphere dominance, 249, 300
Henry, Brad, 299
Higher-level questions
Clinical Questioning, 369
examples of, 388(b)
flipped classroom, 387, 388(b)
Homeward Bound SBAR, 406
"Hot Potato," as teaching tool, 45
"How is it treated?," 330–331
How the Grinch Stole Christmas (film), 67
Huddles
Clinical Huddle, 368
flipped classroom, 385, 385(b)

I

I Am Sam (film), 215(t)
Icebreakers, 31–64, 56(b), 335
Be Prepared, 60–62
A Brush With Fame, 35–36
Campus or Unit Research, 292
challenges in, 31
Common and Different, 46–48, 47(b)
Critical Thinking Exercises, 51–53, 52(b)
Discussion Starters, 63–64
Dress-Up or Skits, 53–55, 54(f)
Email Exercises, 52
Games, Puzzles, and Brain Teasers, 44,
45–46, 45(b), 46(b)
Get in Line, 33–34

Icebreakers (*continued*)
  Greeting Cards, Cartoons, and Pictures,
    48–49
  Introduce Each Other, 34–36
  Let's Discuss, 37–39
  My Biggest Challenge, 62–63
  Past Experiences, 60
  Quiz About Me, 57–58
  Self-test (creativity quiz), 39–41
  Set the Stage, 56–58
  Setting Priorities, 58–59, 313
  Shapes Define Your Personality, 32–33,
    33(f), 314
  Teaching Tools, 248
  team building in, 335
  Tell 'Em Once, Tell 'Em Twice, Tell
    'Em Again!, 55–56, 55(b), 56(b)
  Think-Pair-Share, 235
  Toys, Prizes, and Props, 41–45
  "Why Are You Here?," 49–51, 50(b)
  "Why Are You in Nursing?," 36–37, 37(b)
iGen, 18–19
Imagine (small-class strategy), 125–128,
    126(b), 265, 320, 329, 333, 334
  flipped classroom, 384, 386
  technology and e-learning, 397, 402, 404
I Might Be a Nurse (coloring book), 69
Immunization, 208
In-Basket Exercise, 114–117, 313, 331,
    385, 398–399
Incident report exercise, 310–311
In-Class Applications, 91–95, 306–307,
    324, 384
In-Class Debate, 222–224, 223(b)
  Bring on the Evidence with, 295
  flipped classroom, 385
  NCLEX® preparation with, 335, 336
  Out of the Hat with, 259
  Pass the Stick with, 265
  team building with, 178, 335
  Write to Learn with, 239
In-Class Simulation, 189–190
In-Class Test Questions, 144–148, 145(b)
  Admit Ticket with, 236
  End-of-Life Case Studies with, 320–321
  flipped classroom, 381, 382
  informatics with, 338
  It Starts With a Syllabus with, 344
  NCLEX® preparation in, 302, 313,
    316–317

  technology and e-learning, 396–397
  writing own test questions for, 301
Infection control, 314–317
Informatics, 348–349
Information, organizing and managing
  All Things Being Equal, 86–88, 87(b),
    325–326
  Bring in the Reinforcements,
    91–95, 92(b)
  FYI—Classroom Questioning,
    267–270, 267(b)
  In-Basket Exercise, 114–117
  In-Class Applications, 91–95
  In the Know, 293–294, 337
  Legal Cheat Sheets, 161, 259–260, 328
  Mnemonics, 103–104
  Muddiest Part, 143–144
  One-Minute Care Plan, 182–185,
    183(b)
  Put It All Together, 265–267, 333
  Self-Learning Mini-Modules, 161–162,
    162(b)
  Tell 'Em Once, Tell 'Em Twice, Tell
    'Em Again!, 55–56, 55(b), 56(b)
  Use the Star, 70–71, 70(f), 269, 314
  V-8 Conference, 196–198, 211
Injection Field Trips, 208
Innovation, definition of, 1–2
Innovative strategies
  barriers to, 5–7
  enjoyment and inspiration from, 3–4
  lectures, prioritizing information in, 4–5
  use of text for, 9–10
Institutional culture, 6–7
Instructors
  care and empathy for students, 20–21
  concept-based curricula, challenges
    with, 355–356
  evaluation of, 341, 416–417
  flipped classroom, response to,
    373–374
  flipped classroom, workload of,
    377, 378
  fuel for teaching, 414
  implementing ideas into classroom,
    411–413
  motivations for teaching, 3–4, 417,
    418(f)
  online and distance education,
    challenges of, 391–394

Quiz About Me, 57–58
self-assessment of strengths, 7–8
self-confidence of, 6
student expectations of, 8–9
teaching style, 7, 412–413
Integrated processes, 331–333
Interleaving, 28
Internet etiquette, 164
Interprofessional simulation, 189
Interspersed Case Studies, 74–75,
    365, 382
Interviews, nurse, 291–293, 336
In the Know, 293–294, 337
Intro Case Studies, 382
Introduce Each Other, 34–36
Introduction, to class session, 55–56,
    55(b)
Invented Dialogues, 92, 252–254, 314,
    332, 384
Inverted classroom. *See* Flipped classrooms
Iris (film), 216
Issues in Measurement, 277–278, 277(t)
It Starts With a Syllabus, 343–344

J

Jeopardy (game show), 121–123,
    122(t), 271
Jigsaw puzzle, 132–134, 133(f), 333,
    335, 385
John Q (film), 67, 216(t)
Johnson, C., 171, 182, 209, 373
Johnson, S., 171, 182, 209, 373
Journaling, reflective, 351–352
Journals
    flipped classroom, 383, 386
    technology and e-learning, 400,
        405, 406
    use of, 29
Journals (Ah-Ha Journals), 185–188,
    187(b)
    on basic care and comfort, 329
    on caring, 333
    on Clinical Decision-Making
        Exercises, 141
    on Condensed Portfolios, 167
    on Day in the Life of a Client
        with . . ., 250, 252
    on e-Journaling, 338
    on Field Trips, 209, 326, 335

on Film Clips in Clinical, 214
on Film Clips in Nursing Research, 287
on Grand Rounds, 196
group-experienced (V-8 Conference), 197
on In-Basket Exercises, 116
on Let's Be Real in Clinical, 220
on Mock Studies, 280
on Muddiest Part, 144
on One-Minute Care Plan, 184–185
on Online Discussion Groups, 164
on Out of the Hat, 258
on patient/family-centered care, 334
on quality improvement, 336
on reflective journaling, 352
reflective practice and, 365–366
on War Stories and Clinical
    Anecdotes, 245

K

Keep 'Em Awake Quizzes, 104–108,
    381–382
Keller, Helen, 273
Kinesthetic learning, 24–25, 249, 301
Knowledge, layering of, 28–29
Koosh Ball, 43

L

Lab skills, creative, 187–191, 335
Lab supplies, 189
Large-classroom strategies, 65–110
    All Things Being Equal, 86–88, 87(b)
    Bring in the Reinforcements,
        91–95, 92(b)
    Continuing Case Studies, 75–78
    Current Events, 89–91
    Feedback Lecture, 108–110
    Group Thought, 97–103
    In-Class Applications, 91–95
    Interspersed Case Studies, 74–75
    Keep 'Em Awake Quizzes, Quickie
        Quizzes, Quizzes That Count,
        104–108
    Mnemonics, 103–104
    Preclass Case Studies, 73–74
    Quickie Case Studies, 71–73
    Quotation Pauses, 96–97
    Read a Story, 68–69, 68(b)
    Reverse Case Studies, 79–81

Large-classroom strategies (*continued*)
  Short Clips, 66–68
  Speak UP, 95–96
  Unfolding Case Studies, 78–79
  Use the Book, 81–82
  Use the Star, 70–71, 70(*f*)
  When You Think of This, Think of
    That, 88–89, 89(*b*)
  Worksheets, 82–86, 83(*t*)–84(*t*)
Layering of knowledge, 28–29
Leadership styles, 93–94, 234
Learners. *See* Student(s)
Learning
  brain and neural processes, 23–24
  digital immigrants and natives, 393
  left- and right-brain learners, 25
  sensory learning, 24–25
  time required for, 26, 28
Learning activities, 249
Learning bins, 189
Learning Carts, 193
Learning Charts, 262–264
Learning Contracts, 164–166, 239
"Learning favors," 43
Learning From Each Other, 209–211,
  266, 267
Learning management system (LMS), 394
  See also Online education
Learning Modalities, 249, 301
Learning styles, 248–249, 300–301
  sensory learning, 24–25
  today's students, changes in, 3–4
Lectures
  feedback, 108, 324
  prioritizing information in, 4–5
Left-brain learners, 25, 249, 301
Legal Cheat Sheets, 161, 259–260, 328, 387
Legal issues
  Clinical Application of Findings, 294
  Clinical Quick Write, 181
  End of Life Case Studies, 318
  In-Class Debate, 222–224, 223(*b*)
  Mock Trials, 260–262
  The Right Thing to Do, 117–121
  Six Hats Exercise, 112–114, 113(*b*),
    113(*f*), 114(*b*)
  Think-Pair-Share, 235
Let's Be Real in Clinical, 218–220,
  317, 337
Let's Discuss, 37–39, 329, 332, 333

Letter, to client, 190
Literature, as large-classroom strategy,
  68–69
Longtime Companion (film), 216

M

Make It Stick (Brown, Roediger, and
  McDaniel), 25–30, 26(*b*)
Management of Care (RN), 308–310
Mannequins, simulation, 190
Market Research (cookies and candy),
  274–275, 275(*b*)
Massed practice, 26
Matching
  match game, 124, 124(*b*)
  When You Think of This, Think of
    That, 88–89, 89(*b*)
Matching exercise, 88–89, 89(*b*)
Maternity case study, 317–318
Measurement, issues in, 277–278, 277(*t*)
Medicine cabinet assessment, 207, 327
Meet the Parents (film), 216(*t*)
Memory aids
  Legal Cheat Sheets, 161, 259–260, 328
  match game, 124, 124(*b*)
  rhyming puzzlers, 123
  strategies for remembering, 26–30, 26(*b*)
  Tell 'Em Once, Tell 'Em Twice, Tell
    'Em Again!, 55–56, 55(*b*), 56(*b*)
  Use Mnemonics, 103–104
  When You Think of This, Think of
    That, 88–89, 89(*b*), 323–324
Mental models, 28–29
Mentoring, 353
Millennials, 17–18
Mnemonics, 103–104
Mock Studies, 280–281
  Author Guidelines with, 296
  Campus or Unit Research with, 292
  evidence-based practices with, 337
  Film Clips in Nursing Research
    with, 287
  Poster Sessions with, 290
Mock Trials, 260–262, 265, 295, 332
Motivation
  for instructors, 3–4, 417, 418(*f*)
  for learning, 27, 357
Movies
  Cooperative Strategies, 178

Film Clips in Clinical, 213–218, 214*(b)*, 215*(t)*–217*(t)*
Film Clips in Nursing Research, 286–287
NCLEX® preparation with, 320
Short Clips (large-classroom strategy), 66–68, 213–214, 320, 324, 359, 361
Muddiest Part, 143–144, 360
  Admit Ticket on, 144, 237
  classroom assessment in, 343
  flipped classroom, 386, 387
  FYI—Classroom Questioning, 269
  Games, Puzzles, and Brain Teasers, 46
  Let's Discuss on, 38
  online or distance education strategies, 394
  Progressive Quizzes on, 306
  Put it All Together on, 267
  technology and e-learning, 397, 404
  textbook on, 82
  Twosies on, 130
  Write to Learn on, 239
Music, as icebreakers, 57
My Biggest Challenge, 62–63
My Flesh and Blood (film), 216, 216*(t)*

N

National Council of State Boards of Nursing (NCSBN), 2–3, 2*(f)*, 345
NCLEX®, 299–339
  basic care and comfort, 328–329
  "Call bell" Examination Questions for, 312–314
  Case Management Case Studies for, 308–310
  challenges on, 299–300
  delegation exercise for, 311–312
  Domains of Nursing Practice in, 308*(b)*
  health promotion and maintenance on, 317–321
  incident report exercise for, 310–311
  integrated processes on, 331–333
  Management of Care (RN)/Coordinate Care (PN) in, 308–310
  Nurse Practice Act Write to Learn for, 312
  pharmacology and parenterals on, 326–328
  physiological integrity on, 329–333
  psychosocial integrity on, 321–324
  QSEN principle reinforcement of, 333–335
  reduction of risk potential on, 324–326
  safety and infection control on, 314–317
  strategies for, 307–339, 308*(b)*
  test policies on, 344
"Need to know" *versus* "nice to know," 159, 212–213
Netiquette, 164
Next Generation NCLEX®, 300
The Notebook (film), 67
Nurse interviews, 291–293, 336
Nurse Nancy (Jackson), 69
Nurse Practice Act Right to Learn, 312
Nursing Competency Scale (NCS), 353
Nursing process, 332–333
Nuts and Bolts, 245–248, 245*(b)*, 246*(b)*, 247*(b)*, 333, 360

O

Objective Structured Clinical Experiences (OSCE), 353
October Sky (film), 216*(t)*
The One and Only Ivan (Applegate), 69
One-Minute Care Plan, 182–185, 183*(b)*, 370
  flipped classroom, 383, 389
  Grand Rounds with, 196
  Guided Discussion Groups with, 257
  NCLEX® preparation with, 332
  Pass the Problem with, 177
  Preclinical case studies with, 347
  Put It All Together with, 267
  QSEN principles with, 334
  technology and e-learning, 405
One-Minute Class
  clinical instruction and, 211, 212–213
  on Day in the Life of a Client with . . ., 251
  flipped classroom, 383
  NCLEX® preparation with, 332
  Out of the Hat in, 258
  Preclinical case studies with, 347
  reflection and, 366
  technology and e-learning, 405
The One Minute Teacher (Johnson and Johnson), 182

Online Discussion
  on Clinical Decision-making
    Exercises, 141
  on Continuing Case Studies, 78
  on Film Clips in Clinical, 214
  on In-Class Debate, 224
  on In-Class Test Questions, 147
  on mnemonics, 104
  on Muddiest Part, 144
  on Preclass Case Studies, 74
  on Quickie Case Studies, 73
  on Unfolding Case Studies, 79
Online Discussion Groups, 162–164,
    338–339
  Email Exercise posting in, 147
  on Field Trips, 209
  on FYI—Classroom Questioning, 270
  Group Test posting in, 153
  Guided Discussion Groups, 400–401
  on Invented Dialogues, 254
  on Legal Cheat Sheets, 260
  on Let's Be Real in Clinical, 220
  on Research Corners, 286
  Web Assignment posting in, 147
Online education
  challenges of, 391–394
  class preparation strategies, 394–395
  technology and e-learning for,
    400–404, 401(t)
  See also Technology
Oral Exams, 352
Orientation, clinical
  Active Reading Conference, 193–194
  Cooperative Strategies, 177–180
  Equipment Conference, 191–193
  Pass the Problem, 175–177
  Scavenger Hunts, 172–175
Out of the Hat
  end of program assessment with, 351
  In-Class Debates with, 223, 258–259
  Learning Carts with, 264

P

Pain continuing case study, 329
Paper Towel Ideas, 288
Parenterals, 326–328
Participation
  in discussion groups, 221
  in small classes, 111

Passion Fish (film), 216(t)
Pass the Problem, 175–177, 176(b)
  concept-based curricula, 359
  Learning From Each Other with, 211
  NCLEX® preparation with, 314,
    332–333
  Preclinical case studies with, 347
  technology and e-learning, 405
  Write to Learn with, 240
Pass the Stick, 264–265, 270
Past Experiences, 60, 333, 334
Patch Adams (film), 67, 68, 196, 216(t)
Patient education, 316
Patient/family-centered care, 334
Patient safety, 171, 172, 299, 314–317,
    335–336
Patient Safety Goals Clinical
    Assignment, 369
Pause and Do, 377(b)
Pause for Priority Setting, 362–363, 384
"Pause for thought," 96
Pearl Harbor (film), 67, 216(t)
Peer Teaching, 189, 209–211
Peer Team Leadership, 209–211
Perioperative care case study, 324–326
Perseverance, importance of, 27
Perspective
  Day in the Life of a Client
    with . . ., 179, 250–252
  Same Information, 228–231, 257,
    322, 334
  Six Hats Exercise, 112–114, 113(b),
    113(f), 114(b)
Pharmacology
  brain teasers for calculations in, 45(b),
    46, 46(b)
  Field Trips in, 206–207, 326–327
  NCLEX® testing on, 326–328
  nurses' need to learn, 36, 37(b)
  Reality Check on, 142, 142(f)
Pharmacology Compare and Contrast, 364
Pharmacology Critical Thinking Exercises,
    327–328
Pharmacology Jeopardy (game show), 123
Pharmacy visit, 207, 326–327
Phone polling websites, 396–397
Physical distance, in large classrooms, 65
Physiological Integrity, 329–333
Pictures, as icebreaker, 48–49
Polls, phone polling websites, 396–397

Portfolios, 351
  condensed, 166–167
  e-portfolios, 338, 351
Poster Sessions, 289–290, 295, 337, 351
PowerPoint, 396–397, 398, 414–416
Practice, 27
Preceptor evaluation, 353
Preceptorships, clinical, 350–351
Preclass Case Studies, 73–74, 319,
    370, 380
  online or distance education
      strategies, 395
Preclinical Case Studies, 185, 347
  online or distance education strategies,
      370, 395
Prensky, Marc, 391
Preparation, strategy for, 60–62
Presentations
  Grand Rounds, 195–196
  Mock Trials, 260–262
  Poster Sessions, 289–290, 295,
      337, 351
  PowerPoint, 396–397, 414–416
  Put It All Together, 265–267
Priority-setting
  All Things Being Equal, 86–88, 87(b),
      325–326
  In-Basket Exercise, 114–117
  Management of Care (RN)/Coordinate
      of Care (PN), 308–310
  One-Minute Care Plan, 185
  Setting Priorities (icebreaker),
      58–59, 313
  Use the Star, 70–71, 70(f), 269, 314
  "What's the Big Deal?," 130–132, 266,
      313, 325, 330–331, 336
  "What's the Point?," 130–132, 337
Prizes, 41–45, 271
Problem-solving
  Clinical Decision-Making Exercises,
      134–141
  In-Basket Exercise, 114–117
  Jigsaw, 132–134, 133(f)
  Pass the Problem, 175–177, 176(b)
  The Right Thing to Do, 117–121,
      334, 336
  Six Hats Exercise, 112–114, 113(b),
      113(f), 114(b)
Procedure, resources on, 190
Progressive Quizzes, 306–307, 326, 382

Props, as icebreaker, 41–45
Psychogeometric theory, 32
Psychomotor competency, 258
Psychosocial case studies, 321–324
Psychosocial integrity, 321–324
Put It All Together, 265–267, 333
Puzzles
  Clinical, 211–212, 333, 335, 347
  icebreakers, 44, 45–46
  Jigsaw, 132–134, 133(f), 333, 335, 385
  online or distance education
      strategies, 395
  research, 291
  small-group strategies, 123, 132–134

Q

Quality improvement (QI), 336–339
Quality Safety Education for Nurses
    (QSEN), 299, 333–335
Quickie Case Studies, 71–73, 382
Quickie Quizzes, 104–108, 301, 313,
    328, 344
  flipped classroom, 379, 380, 381–382
Quick Write, 29
  Clinical Quick Write, 360
  on Current Events, 91
  on Email exercises, 148
  in Film Clips in Clinical, 214
  on Imagine/Remember When, 127
  on In-Basket Exercises, 116
  on Let's Be Real in Clinical, 220
  technology and e-learning, 397, 400, 404
Quiz About Me, 57–58
Quizzes
  flipped classroom, 381–382
  legal cheat sheets, 260
  online or distance education strategies,
      394–395
  progressive, 306–307
  use of, 27–28
Quizzes That Count, 104–108, 301, 303,
    316, 328, 381–382
Quotation Pauses, 96–97

R

Raging Bull (film), 217(t)
Rain Man (film), 217(t)
Read a Story, 68–69, 68(b)

Reading conference, active, 190, 193–194, 264, 305, 329
Reality Check, 141–143, 142*(f)*, 265
Reflection, 28–29
  defined, 365
  strategies for, 365–367
Reflective Journaling, 351–352, 386
Reliability, 277–279, 279*(f)*, 350
Reliability and Validity Darts, 278–279, 279*(f)*
Remember the Titans (film), 67, 217*(t)*
Remember When, 125–128, 127*(b)*
  flipped classroom, 384, 386
  NCLEX®, Caring and, 333
  Pass the Stick and, 265
  QSEN principles, patient- and
    family-centered care, 334
  technology and e-learning, 397, 402, 404
Repetition
  flipped classroom and, 373
  as teaching tool, 55–56, 257
Research, 273–297
  Author Guidelines, 296–297
  Bring on the Evidence, 264, 294–295, 337
  Campus or Unit Research, 291–293
  challenges in teaching, 273–274
  Clinical Applications of Findings, 282–284, 337
  Clinical Area Questioning: Research at
    Work, 206, 264, 287–288, 337
  evidence-based practice (EBP), 273–274, 294–295, 337
  Faculty Research Sharing, 289, 337
  Film Clips in Nursing Research, 286–287
  Group Research Critique, 281–282, 337
  Issues in Measurement, 277–278, 277*(t)*
  In the Know, 293–294
  Market Research (cookies and candy), 274–275, 275*(b)*
  Mock Studies, 280–281
  Nurse Interviews, 291–293
  Paper Towel Ideas, 288
  Poster Sessions, 289–290
  Reliability and Validity Darts, 278–279, 279*(f)*
  Research Concept Maps, 242, 290–291, 337

Research Corners, 285–286
Research Moments, 206, 284–285, 285*(b)*, 337, 384
shampoo research, 275–277, 276*(b)*
Research Concept Maps, 242, 290–291, 337
Research Corners, 285–286
Research Moments, 206, 284–285, 285*(b)*, 337, 384
Resources, Active Reading Conference, 193–194
Retrieval practice, 27–28
Reverse Bingo (game), 125
Reverse Case Studies, 79–81, 185, 363, 368–369
  flipped classroom, 387
  technology and e-learning, 407
Rhyming Puzzlers, 123
Richards, Ann, 411
Right-brain learners, 25, 249, 301
The Right Thing to Do, 117–121, 334, 336
Risk potential, reduction of, 324–326
Role-play, 254, 261
Rubrics (grading scales), 348

S

Safety, patient, 171, 172, 299, 314–317, 335–336, 369
Safety topics
  clinical evaluation tools (CETs)
    and, 349
  Clinical Questioning, 202, 204
  for discussions, 109, 198
  flipped classroom, 384, 384*(b)*
  NCLEX® and, 299, 307, 314–317
  QSEN principles and, 333, 335–336
Same Information, 228–231, 257, 322, 334, 384, 399
Save the Last Dance (film), 67, 217*(t)*
SBAR (situation, background, assessment,
  recommendation)
  flipped classroom, 384, 384*(b)*, 387, 389
  Homeward Bound SBAR, 406
  One-Minute Care Plans, 185
  Speak Up, 332
  technology and e-learning, 398, 406
  Telehealth SBAR, 403

Write to Learn, 332

Scavenger Hunts, 172–175, 173(b), 208, 282, 316, 338
    technology and e-learning, 406–407

Self-assessment
    instructors, 7–8, 416–417
    students, 27–28, 29, 351–352

Self-Assessment Write to Learn, 352

Self-confidence, teachers and, 6

Self-discipline, 27

Self-Learning Mini-Modules, 161–162, 162(b), 317, 332

Self-test (creativity quiz), 39–41

Seminars, student-led, 159–161, 160(t)
    In-Class Questions with, 147
    Legal Cheat Sheets with, 260
    Out of the Hat with, 258
    Teaching Tools with, 250
    teamwork with, 335
    test preparation in, 307, 313

Seneca, 411

Sensory learning, 24–25

Set the Stage, 56–58, 380

Setting Priorities, 58–59, 313

Shampoo research, 275–277, 276(b)

Shapes Define Your Personality, 32–33, 33(f), 314, 335

Sharing, Pass the Stick for, 264–265

Shark toys, as teaching tool, 44

Shoe-tying icebreaker, 42

Short Clips (film clips), 66–68, 178, 213–214, 320, 324, 359, 361
    flipped classroom, 383
    technology and e-learning, 397, 404

Silent generation, 15–16

Simplicio, Joseph S. C., 111, 221

Simulation mannequins, 190

Simulations, technology and e-learning, 398

Six Hats Exercise, 112–114, 113(b), 113(f), 114(b)
    for faculty members, 113–114, 114(b)
    flipped classroom, 385
    for In-Class Debate, 224
    for nursing students, 112–113, 113(b)
    teamwork in, 334, 335
    test preparation with, 333

The Sixth Sense (film), 217(t)

Skits, 53–55, 267

Small-class strategies, 111–169

Clinical Decision-Making Exercises, 134–141

Condensed Portfolios, 166–167

Email Exercises, 148–152

Gaming, 121–125, 122(t), 124(b)

Group Tests, 153–157

Imagine, 125–128, 126(b)

In-Basket Exercise, 114–117

In-Class Test Questions, 144–148, 145(b)

Jigsaw, 132–134, 133(f)

Learning Contracts, 164–166

Muddiest Part, 143–144

Online Discussion Groups, 162–164

Reality Check, 141–143, 142(f)

Remember When, 125–128, 127(b)

The Right Thing to Do, 117–121

Self-Learning Mini-Modules, 161–162, 162(b)

Six Hats Exercise, 112–114, 113(b), 113(f), 114(b)

Student-Led Seminars, 159–161, 160(t)

Twosies, 128–130

Web Assignments, 157–159

What's the Big Deal?, 130–132

What's the Point?, 130–132

Smartphones, 407–408
    See also Online education

Social determinants, 395
    Community-Based Concepts/Teaching About Poverty, 366

Social Media Posting, 406

Socrates, 97

Songs, as icebreakers, 57

Spaced-out retrieval practice, 27–28

Speak UP, 95–96, 332

Staff development, use of text for, 10

Steel Magnolias (film), 217(t)

Steve's Scale, 279

Stories, as large-classroom strategy, 68–69, 68(b)

Stress management, 255–257

Student-Led Seminars, 159–161, 160(t)
    flipped classroom, 383
    In-Class Questions with, 147
    Legal Cheat Sheets with, 260
    Out of the Hat with, 258
    Teaching Tools with, 250
    teamwork with, 335
    test preparation in, 307, 313

Student presentations
  Grand Rounds, 195–196
  Mock Trials, 260–262, 265
  Poster Sessions, 289–290, 295, 337
  Put It All Together, 265–267
Student Puzzle Creation
  online or distance education
    strategies, 395
Student(s)
  assessment of, 343, 352–353
  changes in learning styles, 3–4
  characteristics of, overview, 14–15
  civility in classroom, strategies for,
    19–21
  diversity of, 13–14
  expectations of instructors, 8–9
  flipped classroom, response to, 373
  generational differences, 15–19, 393
  growth and fixed mindsets, 29–30
  individual responsibility of, 25–30, 26(b)
  learning styles of, 3–4, 24–25,
    248–249, 300–301
  Peer Teaching and Peer Team Leader-
    ship, 189, 209–211
  resistance to new methods, 7
  student self-assessment, 351–352
Student teaching assistants, 189
Suicide, assisted, 222–223, 223(b)
Summary, of class session, 55–56, 56(b)
Summative evaluation, 342
Syllabus, 343–344

T

Take Home Quiz, 303–305, 311
Teachers. *See* Instructors
Teaching About Poverty, 366
Teaching assistants, 189
Teaching Tools, 248–250, 249(b), 331
Teaching Trios, 96, 224–228, 259, 324,
  331, 334, 385
Team Leadership, peer, 209–211
Teamwork, 334–335
  Cooperative Strategies, 177–180
  Group Concept Mapping, 242
  Pass the Problem, 175–177, 176(b)
  Titanic 2.0, 334
Technology

  challenges of, 391–394
  flipped classrooms and, 374
  increasing use of, 392
  PowerPoint, guidelines for, 414–416
  use in classrooms, 396–400
  use in clinical area, 404–408
  use in online and distance education,
    400–404, 401(t)
  See also Distance education; Online
    education
Telehealth SBAR, 403
Tell 'Em Once, Tell 'Em Twice, Tell 'Em
  Again!, 55–56, 55(b), 56(b)
Test, academic
  assessment through, 344–346
  blueprinting, 345
  collaborative testing, 345
  Group Tests, 153–157
  In-Class Test Questions, 144–148,
    145(b)
  Keep 'Em Awake Quizzes, 104–108
  oral exams, 352
  Out of the Hat, 258–259
  Quickie Quizzes, 104–108, 301, 313,
    328, 344, 379, 380, 381–382
  Quizzes That Count, 104–108, 301,
    303, 316, 328, 381–382
Test, NCLEX®, 299–339
  basic care and comfort, 328–329
  "Call bell" Examination Questions
    for, 312–314
  Case Management Case Studies for,
    308–310
  challenges on, 299–300
  delegation exercise for, 311–312
  Domains of Nursing Practice in, 308(b)
  health promotion and maintenance on,
    317–321
  incident report exercise for, 310–311
  integrated processes on, 331–333
  Management of Care (RN)/Coordinate
    Care (PN) in, 308–310
  Nurse Practice Act Write to Learn
    for, 312
  pharmacology and parenterals on,
    326–328
  physiological integrity on, 329–333
  psychosocial integrity on, 321–324
  QSEN principle reinforcement of,
    333–335

reduction of risk potential on, 324–326
safety and infection control on,
    314–317
strategies for, 307–339, 308(b)
test policies on, 344
Test banks, 345
Test-taking skills, 300–307
    alternate-item practice, 302–303
    assessing learning styles, 300–301
    Progressive Quizzes, 306–307
    Take-Home Quiz, 303–305
    What's the Point?/What's the
        Big Deal?, 130
    writing own test questions, 301–302
Textbooks
    clinical use of, 204–206
    laboratory, 189
    large-classroom use of, 81–82
    Self-Learning Mini-Modules,
        161–162, 162(b)
    as Teaching Tools, 249
Text Polling, 338, 344
Think Aloud Evaluation, 352
Think-Pair-Share, 231–235, 232(b), 367
    on basic care and comfort, 329
    on End of Life Case Studies, 319
    flipped classroom, 383, 385
    Guided Discussion Groups with, 257
    on Invented Dialogues, 253
    on learning styles, 300
    on Nuts and Bolts, 248
    on Out of the Hat, 259
    on perioperative care case study, 324
    on psychosocial case studies, 322
    on Quickie Case Studies, 73
    on risk potential reduction, 324
    on safety and infection control, 316
    teamwork with, 334
    technology and e-learning, 397–398,
        400, 404
    on Two Truths and a Lie, 330
    on Unfolding Case Studies, 79
    Web Assignments with, 158
    Write to Learn with, 240
Time constraints, 5–6
Titanic 2.0, 334
Toolbox, as a teaching tool, 42–43
Total Care Test, 258
Toys, Prizes, and Props, 41–45
Traditional students, 15–16

Trainspotting (film), 217(t)
Transitions
    to concept-based curricula, 355
    signaling of, 412
Trials, mock, 260–262, 265, 295, 332
The True Story of the Three Little Pigs
    (Scieszka), 69
20 Questions, 270–271
Twosies, 128–130, 147
Two Truths and a Lie, 330

U

Unfolding Case Studies, 78–79, 322–323,
    324, 326, 328, 344, 361–362
    flipped classroom, 387
    Google Docs, e-learning and, 403–404
Uniforms, 189
Unit Research, 291–293
Use Mnemonics, 103–104
Use the Book, 81–82, 381
Use the Book in Clinical, 204–206
Use the Star, 70–71, 70(f), 269, 314

V

V-8 Conference, 196–198, 211, 336,
    347, 366
Validity, 277–278, 278–279, 279(f)
Van Doran, Mark, 1
Variance reports, 310–311
Veteran learners, 15–16
Video. *See* Films; Movies; Short Clips
    (film clips)
Visual learning, 24–25, 249, 301
Viva, 352

W

Ward, W. A., 65
War Stories and Clinical Anecdotes,
    243–245
Web Assignments, 157–159, 167, 338
WebQuests, 408
"What If? What Else? What Then?"
    (game), 124
"What Next?" (game), 124–125
What's My Line? (game show), 125
"What's the Big Deal?," 130–132, 266,
    313, 325, 330–331, 336, 362–363, 384

"What's the Point?," 130–132, 337
"What Would You Do?," 362–363, 384
When You Think of This, Think of That, 88–89, 89(b), 323–324, 359, 381
Whistles, as teaching tool, 45
"Why Are You Here?," 49–51, 50(b), 323
"Why Are You in Nursing?," 36–37, 37(b)
Wit (film), 217
Wonky Donkey (Smith and Cowley), 69
Worksheets, 82–86, 83(t)–84(t), 123, 125, 133, 328, 364
    flipped classroom, 379–380, 385
    online or distance education strategies, 394
    technology and e-learning, 398
Write a Letter to Your Client, 180
Write Their Own Test Questions, 382
Write to Learn, 29, 237–240, 360, 366–367
    on communication and documentation, 332
    compare and contrast, 364–365
    on Day in the Life of a Client with . . ., 251
    on delegation exercise, 311
    on Email Exercises, 148
    on End of Life Case Studies, 319
    on Field Trips, 320, 335
    flipped classroom, 387
    on Imagine/Remember When, 127
    on In-Basket Exercises, 116
    on In-Class Debate, 224
    on It Starts With a Syllabus with, 344
    on Muddiest Part, 239
    on Nurse Practice Act, 312
    on pharmacology, 328
    on physiological concepts, 331
    on Progressive Quizzes, 306
    on quality improvement, 336
    on risk potential reduction, 326
    on safety, 335
    on Self-Assessment Write to Learn, 352
    on Take Home Quiz, 303
    on test-taking skills, 307
    on War Stories and Clinical Anecdotes, 245
    on What's the Big Deal, 331
Write Your Own Test Questions, 386–387
Writing exercises, flipped classroom, 387
Written work, assigning and grading, 348

Y

Yeats, William Butler, 273
Young Frankenstein (film), 67, 217(t)
YouTube, 66–67, 214, 218, 286, 383, 397